MW01250522

PUBLIC HEALTH IN THE 21ST CENTURY

PERIODONTITIS

SYMPTOMS, TREATMENT AND PREVENTION

PUBLIC HEALTH IN THE 21ST CENTURY

Additional books in this series can be found on Nova's website at:

https://www.novapublishers.com/catalog/index.php?cPath=23_29&seriesp
=Public+Health+in+the+21st+Century

Additional E-books in this series can be found on Nova's website at:

https://www.novapublishers.com/catalog/index.php?cPath=23_29&seriespe
=Public+Health+in+the+21st+Century

PUBLIC HEALTH IN THE 21ST CENTURY

PERIODONTITIS

SYMPTOMS, TREATMENT AND PREVENTION

ROSEMARIE E. WALCHUCK

EDITOR

Nova Science Publishers, Inc.

New York

For permission to use material from this book please contact us:
Telephone 631-231-7269; Fax 631-231-8175
Web Site: http://www.novapublishers.com

NOTICE TO THE READER

The Publisher has taken reasonable care in the preparation of this book, but makes no expressed or implied warranty of any kind and assumes no responsibility for any errors or omissions. No liability is assumed for incidental or consequential damages in connection with or arising out of information contained in this book. The Publisher shall not be liable for any special, consequential, or exemplary damages resulting, in whole or in part, from the readers' use of, or reliance upon, this material.

Independent verification should be sought for any data, advice or recommendations contained in this book. In addition, no responsibility is assumed by the publisher for any injury and/or damage to persons or property arising from any methods, products, instructions, ideas or otherwise contained in this publication.

This publication is designed to provide accurate and authoritative information with regard to the subject matter covered herein. It is sold with the clear understanding that the Publisher is not engaged in rendering legal or any other professional services. If legal or any other expert assistance is required, the services of a competent person should be sought. FROM A DECLARATION OF PARTICIPANTS JOINTLY ADOPTED BY A COMMITTEE OF THE AMERICAN BAR ASSOCIATION AND A COMMITTEE OF PUBLISHERS.

LIBRARY OF CONGRESS CATALOGING-IN-PUBLICATION DATA

Periodontitis : symptoms, treatment, and prevention / editor, Rosemarie E.
Walchuck.
p. ; cm.
Includes bibliographical references and index.
ISBN 978-1-61668-836-3 (hardcover)
 1.Periodontitis. 2. Periodontitis--Treatment. 3.
Periodontitis--Prevention. I. Walchuck, Rosemarie E.
 [DNLM: 1. Periodontitis. WU 242 P4895 2010]
 RK450.P4P47 2010
 617.6'32--dc22
                                                        2010014101

Published by Nova Science Publishers, Inc. ✦ New York

CONTENTS

PREFACE

Periodontitis refers to a number of inflammatory diseases affecting the periodontium, that is, the tissues that surround and support the teeth. Periodontitis involves progressive loss of the alveolar bone around the teeth, and if left untreated, can lead to the loosening and subsequent loss of teeth. Periodontitis is caused by microorganisms that adhere to and grow on the tooth's surfaces, along with an overly aggressive immune response against these microorganisms. This book reviews research on periodontitis including the role of the TH17 pathway in the progression of periodontal disease; an outline of the risk factors relating to the most prevalent chronic periodontal diseases and others.

Chapter 1 - Chronic periodontal diseases include a group of inflammatory diseases that affect periodontal supporting tissues of the teeth and encompass destructive and nondestructive conditions. Periodontal diseases are multifactorial and the role of dental biofilm in their initiation is primary. However, whether dental biofilm affects a particular subject, what form the disease takes and how it progresses, are all dependent of a wide variety of factors. Therefore, the objective of this chapter is to outline the risk factors described for the most prevalent chronic periodontal diseases (plaque induced gingivitis and chronic periodontitis) and to explain some basic concepts related to the current understanding of the role of these risk factors based on *in vitro*, animal and human studies. The review will focus on the factors that may be associated with a direct increase in the likelihood of occurrence of disease or an increase in its severity. The following factors will be discussed: 1) host characteristics, such as age, gender and race; 2) social and behavioral factors (socioeconomic status, cigarette smoking and emotional stress); 3) systemic factors, e.g. diabetes mellitus and osteoporosis; 4) genetic factors; 5) tooth-level factors (root grooves, tooth position, caries, occlusal discrepancies, iatrogenic restorations, root abnormalities and periodontal parameters); and 6) the microbial composition of dental biofilm. Finally, this chapter will also present literature-based evidence on predictive factors associated with patients and tooth susceptibility for recurrence of periodontitis after the end of the active periodontal therapy and will examine the use of some prognostic models which may be useful for clinicians in the identification high-risk groups of patients.

Chapter 2 - The goals of periodontal therapy according to the American Academy of Periodontology are to alter or get rid of the microbial etiology and causative risk factors for periodontitis, thus arresting the progression of disease and preserving the dentition in a state of health, comfort, and function with appropriate esthetics; and to prevent the recurrence of periodontitis. In addition, regeneration of the periodontal attachment apparatus, where indicated, may be attempted. Mechanical debridement of the pocket has shown to significantly reduce the risk of tooth loss, slow down the rate of periodontal disease progression and improve gingival health.

Chapter 3 - The oral cavity is a warm, moist environment, in which a number of microorganisms colonize and live in harmony as a community, a so-called biofilm. In this environment, antimicrobial peptides may play a critical role in maintaining normal oral health and controlling innate and acquired immune systems in response to continuous microbial challenges in periodontal disease. Two major families of antimicrobial peptides, found in the oral cavity, are defensin and cathelicidin. Members of the defensin family are cysteine-rich peptides, synthesized by plants, insects, and mammals. These peptides vary in length and in the number of disulfide bonds, and have a beta-sheet structure. In the oral cavity, four alpha-defensins are synthesized and stored in neutrophil granules, which are converted into active peptides by proteolytic processing, while three human beta-defensins (hBDs), hBD-1, hBD-2, and hBD-3, are predominantly produced by oral epithelial cells. The only member of the cathelicidin family found in humans is LL-37, an alpha-helical peptide that contains 37 amino acids and begins with two leucines at its NH_3-terminus. LL-37 is derived from enzymatic cleavage of a precursor peptide, namely, human cationic antimicrobial peptide-18. Clinically, differential expression of antimicrobial peptides has been reported in specific types of periodontal disease, and their presence has been shown in saliva and gingival crevicular fluid. Current evidence suggests that alpha-defensins, beta-defensins, and LL-37 have distinct, but overlapping, roles in antimicrobial and pro-inflammatory activities. Several studies have shown antimicrobial activities of hBD-2, hBD-3, and LL-37 against several periodontal pathogens, suggesting their potential role as antimicrobial agents for periodontal disease. The clinical significance of antimicrobial peptides in periodontal disease has recently been demonstrated in morbus Kostmann syndrome, a severe congenital neutropenia, in which chronic periodontal infection in young patients, resulting from a deficiency of neutrophil-derived antimicrobial peptides, causes early tooth loss. Although researchers initially focused their attention on antimicrobial activities, it is now becoming evident that defensins and LL-37 are multifunctional molecules that mediate various host immune responses, and may thus represent essential molecules of innate immunity in periodontal disease. In this chapter, basic knowledge and the clinical importance of antimicrobial peptides in periodontal disease will be discussed in detail.

Chapter 4 - This comprehensive review highlights a detailed overview related to devising a periodontal prognosis. A precise predictability of the results of a disease is profound and crucial for proper treatment planning. Since the understanding of periodontal disease has progressed to include the influence of risk factors, assigning a prognosis has become more perplexing to the clinician. Various factors that influence the overall and individual tooth prognosis have been enumerated. The classification systems required to assign a prognosis has also been included. The potential adverse influences of both local and systemic factors have also been discussed. An experienced clinician should analyze all these factors, along with the patients attitude towards dental therapy, prior to arriving at a judgment for a single tooth or teeth. With newer trends in treatment modalities, patients can seek better options for treatment, thus improving the long term prognosis.

Chapter 5 - Background: Plaque-induced periodontitis is gingival inflammation at sites undergoing loss of connective tissue, apical migration of junctional epithelium and loss of alveolar bone. Non-surgical treatment of plaque-induced periodontitis typically involves removal of biofilm conducted through mechanical scaling and root planing (SRP) procedures. The antibiotic minocycline hydrochloride, delivered as a sustained-release product used for professional subgingival administration into periodontal pockets, has been shown to be beneficial as an adjunct to conventional SRP. Use of chlorhexidine rinse is also a typical adjunct therapy to SRP procedures for chemical control of supragingival plaque. Lidocaine (2.5%) and prilocaine (2.5%) provides localized anesthesia for SRP. The objective of this study is to develop and use bioluminescent recombinants of oral streptococci in determining the potential antibacterial activity of minocycline hydrochloride used either alone or in combination with the anesthetic lidocaine/prilocaine, or with the antiseptic chlorhexidine.

Methods: Recombinant plasmids containing the bioluminescence-generating *lux* gene from *Photorhabdus luminescens* were transformed into the oral bacterium *Streptococcus mutans*, strains UA159 and ATCC 25175. Transformants were verified as *S. mutans* derivatives by selection and growth on mitis salivarius agar supplemented with bacitracin, in addition to an antibody test directed specifically against *S. mutans* cell wall proteins and polymerase chain reaction experiments targeting sequences in the *S. mutans* glucosyltransferase (*gtf*) gene. *S. mutans* transformants were then subjected to growth analysis for comparison of absorbance and bioluminescence activity. Minocycline hydrochloride and lidocaine/prilocaine, or minocycline hydrochloride and chlorhexidine, were used in combination to determine the potential interactive effects of these agents on the antibacterial activity of minocycline hydrochloride.

Results: Using two distinct *S. mutans* transformants representing both strains UA159 and ATCC 25175, showed rapid and pronounced bacteriostatic activity when using high doses of minocycline hydrochloride (≥ 1 µg/ml), which were statistically distinct from untreated cultures (p=0.000058) when measured at the peak of metabolic activity. Reduced bacteriostatic activity was seen using lower doses. When lidocaine/prilocaine at doses >100 µg/ml is used in conjunction with minocycline hydrochloride, also shown was an additive antibacterial effect. The *S. mutans* transformant strain UA159, when treated with chlorhexidine (0.01%) in conjunction with either high (1 µg/ml) or low (0.1 µg/ml) doses of minocycline hydrochloride, displayed reduced levels of cell mass accumulation, as measured by absorbance, that were additive when both antimicrobial agents were deployed. Bioluminescence determinations, which are a direct measure of metabolic activity and an indirect measure of cell number when cells are in logarithmic stage of growth, displayed similar reductions when cultures were treated with minocycline hydrochloride and chlorhexidine used singularly or in combination.

Conclusions: The *S. mutans* lux transformants serve as sensitive biosensors in the determination of antimicrobial activity, and can rapidly monitor inhibition of bacterial metabolism. It was concluded that the anesthetic lidocaine/prilocaine does not interfere with the potent bacteriostatic activity of minocycline hydrochloride, and actually has an additive antibacterial effect. The potent bacteriostatic activity of minocycline hydrochloride can also be complemented with the addition of chlorhexidine. The application of the *lux* biosensor system in the assessment of minocycline hydrochloride and lidocaine/prilocaine, or minocycline hydrochloride and chlorhexidine, represents its first use in examining antimicrobial drug interactions in periodontology.

Chapter 6 - Periodontitis is a chronic inflammatory disease which destroys the tooth-supporting tissues. This disease is initiated by bacteria; in particular, facultative anaerobic

Gram-negative microorganisms. Several types of these pathogens initiate periodontal disease, and the host response determines the disease progression and ultimate tissue damage. The early periodontal lesion (gingivitis) is characterized by the presence of large numbers of T cells and macrophages within the gingiva, while the presence of beta (B) and plasma cells characterize the advanced lesion. These phenomena suggest that a shift in the type of host response occurs during the progression of periodontal disease. However, there is little specific information available concerning the characteristics of this shift.

Chapter 7 - Oral epithelia represent the first physical and chemical barrier against bacterial invasion and colonization of the underlying tissues. This protection results from the production of epithelial innate immune responses, including the secretion of cationic antimicrobial peptides with a large spectrum of activity against pathogenic microorganisms. Among these antimicrobial cationic peptides, ß-defensin 2 (hBD-2) is expressed in the gingival epithelia upon stimulation by microorganisms or inflammatory mediators such as interleukin-1β or tumour necrosis factor-α. The aim of the present study was to investigate the effect of AV119, a patented blend of two sugars from avocado, on the induction of hBD-2 in two epithelial cell lines and a primo-culture of gingival epithelial cells. Culture supernatant from epithelial cells treated with AV119 was also evaluated for its antimicrobial activity against the periodontopathogen *Porphyromonas gingivalis*. Cell ELISA assays revealed that AV119 induces the production of hBD-2 by all the epithelial cells tested. Minimal Inhibition Concentration assay also showed that the culture supernatant of epithelial cells treated with AV119 possesses antibacterial activity. In conclusion, our data revealed that AV119 component, through hBD2 induction and antibacterial activity, could be considered for potential use in the control of oral mucosal infections and reduction of microbial tissue invasion during periodontitis.

Chapter 8 - Cheilitis granulomatosa is characterized by the non-inflammatory swelling of the lips, and is considered as the incomplete expression of the Melkersson-Rosenthal syndrome, which consists of the triad of recurrent orofacial swelling, relapsing facial paralysis, and fissuring of the tongue. Rapid improvement after the treatment of periodontitis was first reported in 1961 by Kawamura et al in Japan, and 46 such cases have been reported since then in the Japanese literature. A typical case of cheilitis granulomatosa can be excperienced. The swollen lip showed marked improvement following the treatment of apical periodontitis. A 57-year-old woman presented with a swelling of the lower lip for the period of two months. Skin biopsy of the lip disclosed non-caseous giant cell granuloma. Neither facial nerve palsy nor fissuring of the tongue was present, excluding the diagnosis of Melkersson-Rosenthal syndrome. Patch testing for metal allergy was negative for all dental metallic ions, except for only mild irritation reaction for Zinc ion. The patient was first treated with topical corticosteroid ointment and oral tranilast, which inhibits the release of chemical mediators from leukocytes, for 4 months. Although the treatment was ineffective, rapid and remarkable improvement of the swelling was noted soon after the treatment of apical periodontitis. Thus, it is highly likely that the periodontitis was the cause of cheilitis granulomatosa in this case. In this article, such 46 cases are reviewed in the Japanese literature.

Chapter 9 - Periodontitis is a complex disease which is associated with multiple factors, including host immune responses, and genetic, behavioral and environmental factors. It is generally accepted that genetic polymorphisms can modulate host immune responses to bacterial challenge, hence influencing subjects' susceptibility to periodontitis. Genetic association with periodontal disease experience has been a subject of interest for more than a decade. With the completion of Human Genome Project, genetic association studies emerged in many fields of research including research into periodontitis, one of the most common human diseases. This chapter summarizes past and current research approaches with respect to periodontal disease experience and genetic polymorphisms, and suggests anticipated directions of future studies.

Chapter 10 - Coronary heart disease (CHD) shares a number of features with chronic periodontitis (CP) including risk factors such as smoking and diabetes; an aetiopathogenesis implicating a number of microbial species, as well as chronic inflammation. However, the link between these two conditions remains unclear. The prevalence of CHD increases with age and is higher in males than females. CP is a chronic inflammatory condition which destroys the supporting tissues of teeth and also increases in prevalence with age. Immune responses against heat shock proteins (HSP) can be cross-reactive among bacterial and human antigens. There is evidence that microbial HSP65 and human HSP60 is involved in periodontal disease and CHD and may therefore provide a mechanistic link between CP and CHD. The aim of this study is to investigate immune responses to the human HSP60 and microbial HSP65 in patients with CP and CHD and relate these to the level of inflammation. Serum samples was collected from 100 male subjects divided into 4 groups, each matched for age: (a) Healthy control group with minimal gingivitis, (b) CP, (c) CHD with gingivitis (d) CHD with CP. ELISA was used to determine the levels of serum anti-HSP and C-reactive protein (CRP) in the 4 groups. Peripheral blood mononuclear cells were also isolated from these 4 groups and stimulated with HSPs. Significant lymphoproliferation was seen in CHD with or without CP when stimulated with human HSP60. CRP and serum anti-human HSP60 IgG were elevated in the patients groups compared to the healthy control group, but not serum anti-microbial HSP 65 IgG,. In view of the potential confounding effects of smoking in CP and CHD, a group of current smokers (n=24) were also recruited to investigate whether smoking affects HSP immune responses.There was no significant difference in HSP-induced lymphoproliferation between smokers and non-smokers in any of the four groups. There was a significant correlation between CRP and lymphoproliferative responses to Human HSP60.

This study shows that serum anti-human HSP60 IgG and serum CRP are raised in CHD with or without CP. In CHD with or without CP, serum CRP levels correlated significantly with human HSP60-induced lymphoproliferation, but not with anti-HSP antibody levels.

Chapter 11 - Morbidity and mortality from oral cancer are high and this has not improved in decades in spite of extensive research. A significant portion of research is concentrated on chemoprevention. However, advances in this field have not translated into a visible change in mortality and morbidity. In addition, existing chemoprevention strategies have two important obstacles: toxicity and reversal of the effects after cessation of treatment. Chronic infection and inflammation have been linked to carcinogenesis in a few organs. For oral cancer, substantial evidence has accumulated for the role of *human papillomavirus* (HPV). However, the development of an effective preventive vaccine strategy for oral cancer is still years away and the target population is largely unexplored. Therefore, safe and practical additional approaches are necessary to change the status quo of oral cancer. Periodontitis is a chronic oral infection caused by inflammatory reactions in response to gram negative anaerobic bacteria in the endogenous dental plaque. It leads to irreversible destruction of tissues around teeth clinically detectable as periodontal pockets and alveolar bone loss. Periodontal pockets have been suggested as reservoirs of HPV. Chronic proliferation and ulceration of the pocket epithelium may help HPV's initial infection and persistence. Our preliminary results from existing data at Roswell Park Cancer Institute suggest a robust independent association between the history of periodontitis and incident oral cancer. Our next step is to test the synergy between periodontitis and HPV for the risk of oral cancer. If this is true, it will translate to practical and safe prevention and treatment strategies. This chapter will review the evidence supporting the association between chronic periodontitis and oral cancer as well as HPV-periodontitis synergy.

In: Periodontitis Symptoms, Treatment and Prevention ISBN: 978-1-61668-836-3
Editor: Rosemarie E. Walchuck, pp. 1-33 ©2010 Nova Science Publishers, Inc.

Chapter 1

RISK FACTORS FOR CHRONIC PERIODONTAL DISEASES

Daniela da Silva Feitosa[1], Mauro Pedrine Santamaria[1], Márcio Zaffalon Casati[2], Enilson Antonio Sallum[3], Francisco Humberto Nociti Júnior[3] and Sérgio de Toledo[3]

DDS, MS, PhD - Department of Prosthodontics and Periodontics – Division
of Periodontics, Piracicaba Dental School, University of Campinas.[1]
Associate Professor - Department of Prosthodontics and Periodontics - Division
of Periodontics, Piracicaba Dental School, University of Campinas.[2]
Professor - Department of Prosthodontics and Periodontics - Division of Periodontics,
Piracicaba Dental School, University of Campinas, Brazil[3]

ABSTRACT

Chronic periodontal diseases include a group of inflammatory diseases that affect periodontal supporting tissues of the teeth and encompass destructive and nondestructive conditions. Periodontal diseases are multifactorial and the role of dental biofilm in their initiation is primary. However, whether dental biofilm affects a particular subject, what form the disease takes and how it progresses, are all dependent of a wide variety of factors. Therefore, the objective of this chapter is to outline the risk factors described for the most prevalent chronic periodontal diseases (plaque induced gingivitis and chronic periodontitis) and to explain some basic concepts related to the current understanding of the role of these risk factors based on *in vitro*, animal and human studies. The review will focus on the factors that may be associated with a direct increase in the likelihood of occurrence of disease or an increase in its severity. The following factors will be discussed: 1) host characteristics, such as age, gender and race; 2) social and behavioral factors (socioeconomic status, cigarette smoking and emotional stress); 3) systemic factors, e.g. diabetes mellitus and osteoporosis; 4) genetic factors; 5) tooth-level factors (root grooves, tooth position, caries, occlusal discrepancies, iatrogenic restorations, root abnormalities and periodontal parameters); and 6) the microbial composition of dental biofilm. Finally, this chapter will also present literature-based evidence on predictive factors associated with patients and tooth susceptibility for recurrence of periodontitis after the end of the active periodontal therapy and will examine the use of some prognostic models which may be useful for clinicians in the identification high-risk groups of patients.

INTRODUCTION

Chronic periodontal diseases include a group of inflammatory diseases that affect the periodontal supporting tissues of teeth and encompass destructive and nondestructive conditions [12]. The term chronic periodontal diseases will refer, in this chapter, to both plaque-induced gingivitis and chronic periodontitis. Plaque induced gingivitis is the inflammation of the soft tissues without apical migration of the junctional epithelium [32]. In addition, chronic periodontitis, the most frequent form of periodontitis, results in inflammation of the supporting tissues of the teeth, progressive attachment and bone loss at a slow rate, characterized by pocket formation and/or gingival recession [34]. Cross-sectional epidemiologic studies from many countries have shown that gingivitis is highly prevalent in the primary and permanent dentitions of children [7] and affects many adults [5]. Further, chronic periodontitis is also a common entity worldwide [6]. Therefore, a knowledge of the factors that may influence the transition from health to disease and of the progression of the disease through various stages of severity are important in the development of effective strategies of prevention and treatment.

Gingivitis has already been established as a consequence of dental biofilm accumulation. It is produced as the result of a general increase in the number of microorganisms and a change in the composition of the flora associated with the increasing age of the dental biofilm [99]. Several studies show that periodontitis is preceded by gingivitis and, although the accumulation and duration of microbial dental plaque biofilm will predictably lead to the development of inflammation in the nearby gingival tissues, the duration of onset and the intensity of the inflammatory process vary considerably from person to person, as well as between teeth. Albandar et al. (1998) [4] studied a periodontally high-risk group comprising 156 young subjects that were examined twice during a period of six years to study the relationship between the presence of gingival inflammation (gingival bleeding) and the occurrence of attachment loss. They found that 9.3% of sites that had gingival bleeding and 0-2 mm of attachment loss at baseline showed a longitudinal attachment loss of ≥ 3 mm over 6 years, whereas only 4.8% of sites with no gingival bleeding at baseline showed a corresponding attachment loss. Hence, 90.7% of sites with gingival bleeding at baseline did not show any clinical attachment loss during the study period. This study showed that not all sites with gingival inflammation developed periodontitis during the study period. Thus, predisposition to periodontitis development varies significantly and may possibly be influenced by other factors. However, defining the factors involved in initiation and progression of chronic periodontitis is a more complex issue.

Chronic periodontitis is a multi-factorial disease. While the role of bacteria is primary, a number of host-related factors have been hypothesized as influencing its diverse clinical presentation and rate of progression [72]. Loe et al. (1986) [100], in a longitudinal study, evaluated a Sri Lanka population never exposed to any programs or incidents related to the prevention and treatment of dental diseases. This population did not practice any conventional oral hygiene measures. Three subpopulations were identified: 1) individuals with rapid progression of periodontal disease (8%); 2) individuals with moderate progression (81%); and 3) a group who exhibited no progression (11%). When another longitudinal study was made comprising a sample of middle-class Norwegian men who had the benefit of a comprehensive health care program, a group that represented an extreme condition of periodontal maintenance when compared to the Sri Lanka population, two subpopulations (moderate disease and no disease) were found, despite the severity of attachment loss [164]. These studies illustrate significant differences in the pattern and rates of attachment loss among individuals, even when they receive regular and adequate professional and personal health care. Based on the evidence above, the identification of factors involved in the initiation and progression rate of chronic periodontal diseases has been the focus of considerable research in recent times.

Chronic inflammatory periodontal diseases have several etiological factors for which a plausible biological model of effect exists. The term risk factors is commonly used and it refers to an aspect of personal behaviors or lifestyle, an environmental exposure, or an inborn or inherited characteristic, which on the basis of epidemiological evidence is known to be associated with a health-related condition [99]. The presence of a risk factor implies a direct increase in the likelihood of a disease occurring [95]. Prospective longitudinal studies, and in particular clinical trials, provide the most powerful evidence for the existence, and the amount, of risk. However, in most cases these types of studies are not easily conducted. For this reason, most evidence for the existence of possible risk factors for periodontal diseases comes from cross-sectional studies. Although the identification of risk factors for disease is unfeasible using cross-sectional studies, when a proper study design is employed, these studies can provide valuable information on the presence or absence of an association between the variables under study and the occurrence of periodontal diseases. In order to make a distinction between the results of the different types of studies, it is customary to refer to significant effects assessed in cross-sectional studies as associations, whereas effects disclosed using case-control studies and prospective studies have been referred to as risk determinants, risk indicators, or risk markers [8].

Usually, the overview of factors associated with chronic periodontal diseases is systematically presented as host characteristics, social and behavioral factors, systemic factors, genetic factors, tooth-level factors and microbial factors [126]. In addition to the investigation of these factors at the onset of chronic periodontal diseases, longitudinal studies of patients treated for periodontitis try to determine the patient's susceptibility to disease recurrence [64, 96]. As a result, the prognostic factors (disease predictors), defined as characteristics related to the progression of preexisting disease [133], have been the subject of much discussion. The identification of groups and individuals at risk for disease progression during maintenance therapy still represents one of the greatest challenges in the management of periodontal patients. Thus, prognostic models aimed at identifying high-risk individuals or teeth in a clinical setting have been described [56, 91]. A question remains about the safety of these models routinely used to help clinicians in decision-making.

HOST CHARACTERISTICS

Age

Several epidemiological studies have clearly demonstrated an increase in the prevalence (percentage of persons), extent (percentage of teeth per person) and severity of periodontal attachment loss with increasing age [6, 9]. Papapanou et al. (1988) [132] examined full-mouth radiographs from 531 dentate individuals aged 25-75 years and found that bone loss increased with age. Moreover, two large epidemiological studies estimated the prevalence and extent of periodontal diseases in the United States using data from the National Health and Nutrition Examination Survey (NHANES) in the years 1985 to 1986 and 1988 to 1994 [6, 23]. It was demonstrated that 48.6% of persons 35 to 44 years old and 77.3% of those 55 to 64 years old had ≥ 3 mm attachment loss in the first survey. The same trend was observed in the second study, in which 48.5% for the 40 to 49 year old cohort and 74.8% for the 60 to 69 year old group had ≥ 3 mm attachment loss. Regarding the healing of periodontal tissues following periodontal therapy, Lindhe et al. (1985) [97] evaluated 62 patients and reported that, although age did not seem to have a significant effect on the results of periodontal treatment, there was a tendency for younger patients to have a shallower probing depth and gain more periodontal attachment than older patients.

With increasing age, people have to cope with a lifelong antigenic burden encompassing several decades of evolutionary unpredicted antigenic exposure, with a major impact on survival and frailty. In fact, there is a peculiar chronic inflammatory status characterizing aging, which has been denominated by Franceschi et al. (2000) [57] as inflamm-aging, and which is considered a random process detrimental for longevity, leading to long-term tissue damage, and related to a wide range of age-related diseases, including neurodegeneration, atherosclerosis, diabetes and osteoporosis among others, which share an inflammatory pathogenesis. It may therefore be speculated that this phenomenon may also affect the periodontium, in which after a lifetime's challenge by oral periodontopathogenic bacteria and their virulence factors, periodontal tissues may develop an intense subclinical inflammatory process, but also lead to healing/regeneration outcomes after periodontal therapy [15]. In vitro studies have clearly demonstrated an age-related decrease in the proliferation of periodontal ligament cells [15, 166]. Further, aging is able to modulate the expression of genes reported to participate in periodontal homeostasis (e.g. cytokines, metalloproteinases and their inhibitors and bone-related genes) by periodontal ligament cells [14, 15]. It is important to remember the role of periodontal ligament cells on periodontal health and disease because of their ability to proliferate, migrate and synthesize several components of the periodontium and also participate in the protective host mechanism that prevents periodontitis or impedes its progression [60]. Little information on the influence of aging on the periodontium is provided by animal studies. It has been documented that the periodontal ligament presented decreased cell density and collagen synthesis, and also a decreased number of cells in the osteogenic layer of the alveolar bone has also been reported [135, 165].

Despite the well-documented loss of attachment with increasing age and the rationale behind the association, the question as to what extent aging affects periodontal homeostasis is still a controversial issue in the periodontal literature. A number of arguments have been used against the presumed association. First, there are no marked increases in the probing depth with age. Furthermore, the prevalence of moderate and advanced periodontitis increased in patients up to approximately 65 years of age, remaining steady until they were approximately 80 years of age, and decreasing thereafter [7]. There is also an indication that the effect of age may be reduced after adjusting for the effects of other confounders [1]. And finally, a diminished ability to perform daily oral hygiene activities has been blamed for the increased prevalence of periodontitis in older individuals [139].

Despite the questions that remain to be examined before consider aging as a risk factor for periodontal diseases, it may be reasonable to suggest that age is a good indicator of the degree of periodontal tissue loss that occurs due to periodontal diseases. However, more studies are needed to clarify the role of aging as a risk factor for the development and progression of periodontal tissue loss and in tissue regeneration following therapy [10].

Gender

Epidemiological surveys show an association between gender and attachment loss in adults, with men having a higher prevalence of and more severe periodontal destruction than women. In the NHANES I survey, a better periodontal status was reported for females than males in all age groups [9]. Subsequently, Hyman & Reid (2003) [76], in a study of risk factors for periodontal attachment loss among adults in the NHANES III survey, confirmed after adjustment for confounding variables, that males were at increased risk of attachment loss, deeper probing depths and a higher prevalence of periodontitis. Attachment loss thresholds of ≥ 3 mm, ≥ 4 mm and ≥ 5 mm were noted in 23%, 44% and 55% more males than females, respectively. This is attributed to a poorer standard of oral hygiene adopted by men and it is likely that hormonal and other physiological and behavioral differences between the two genders may also contribute to the higher risk for periodontal diseases in males than females [8]. Moreover, genetic predisposing factors have been related to the increased prevalence in males [10].

Race / Ethnicity

The level of attachment loss is influenced by race / ethnicity, although the exact role of this factor is not fully understood. Certain racial / ethnic groups, particularly subjects with an African or Latin American background have a higher risk of developing periodontal tissue loss than other groups [10]. In the United States, subjects of African and Mexican descent have a greater attachment loss than Caucasians [6]. However, the increased risk of periodontitis in certain racial/ethnic groups may be partly attributed to socioeconomic, behavioral and other disparities [143]. Moreover, there is evidence that increased risk may also be related to biologic/genetic predisposition [10]. A number of studies evaluating confounding variables have failed to find any differences in periodontitis prevalence and severity between different ethnic/racial groups [37, 76, 106, 107]. For example, Craig et al. (2001) [37] evaluated periodontitis progression rates among three ethnic / racial groups, Asian, African and Hispanic Americans, over a 2-month period. No significant differences in rate of attachment loss were observed between the three groups.

SOCIAL AND BEHAVIORAL FACTORS

Socioeconomic Status

Socioeconomic status is an important risk indicator of periodontal disease. Individuals with a low socioeconomic status have a higher occurrence of attachment loss and probing depth than those with a high socioeconomic status. Drury et al. (1999) [46] used an index comprising the individual's education attainment and family economic status and divided the United States population into four socioeconomic groups. They found that the prevalence of gingivitis and loss of attachment of $\geq$ 4 mm increased with the decrease in socioeconomic level. Furthermore, Dolan et al. (1997) [44] measured the attachment loss in 761 adult subjects and related these measurements to socioeconomic status and other potential risk indicators. They found that low income and residing in a rural area were significant risk indicators for attachment loss. Thus, it may be suggested that measurements of socioeconomic status, including income, education levels and urban status are fairly good risk indicators for periodontal diseases. Groups with a low socioeconomic status are at higher risk of having periodontal diseases than groups with a high socioeconomic status, and the higher level of risk in this group seems to be attributable to behavioral and environmental factors.

Smoking

It is now well established that tobacco use is among the most important, if not the most important, preventable risk factor in the incidence and progression of periodontal diseases. Cigarette smoking is associated with a two to eight-fold increased risk of periodontal attachment and/or bone loss, depending on the definition of disease severity and smoking dose [158]. For example, with the aim of examining the relationship between cigarette smoking and periodontitis and of estimating the proportion of periodontitis in the United States adult population that is attributable to cigarette smoking, Tomar & Asma (2000) [178] analyzed the data of 12,329 individuals from the NHANES III. In this study, current smokers were four times as likely to have periodontitis (the presence of $\geq$ 1 site with clinical periodontal attachment level $\geq$ 4 mm and probing depth $\geq$ 4 mm) compared to nonsmokers after adjusting for age, race or ethnicity, income, and educational level. Heavy smokers ($\geq$31 cigarettes per day) had a greater risk than light smokers ($\leq$9 cigarettes per day) with estimated odds ratios of 5.6 and 2.8, respectively. When a stricter definition of periodontitis was combined with heavy smoking in a Swedish population, the relative risk of disease ranged from 9.8 to 20.3 [19].

Summarizing the clinical findings in smokers, the gingival inflammatory response is dampened in smokers compared to non-smokers, as evidenced by a fibrotic appearance to the tissues and fewer sites that bleed upon probing smokers [18, 42]. Levels of supragingival calculus tend to be higher in smokers than in nonsmokers. This finding was independent of plaque levels. It is therefore possible to hypothesize that smoking may affect the mineralization rate of calculus [17]. Further, smokers have higher mean probing depths and more sites with deep probing [179, 182]. In addition, gingival recession is greater in smokers compared to nonsmokers [25]. Smokers have two to four times more teeth with furcation involvement [117] and demonstrate a greater loss of alveolar bone height [16]. Finally, smokers with periodontitis have a greater loss of teeth than patients with periodontitis and no history of smoking [52].

Smoking is also associated with periodontal attachment loss in individuals who are usually considered at lower risk because of their relatively young age. Rosa et al. (2008) [154], in a parallel-arm prospective study with eighty-one students considered not to have periodontitis, showed a greater clinical attachment loss and a lower mean alveolar bone height in the smokers compared to nonsmokers. Further data has revealed that even passive smoking, the exposure to environmental tobacco smoke in the home and/or workplace, has recently been associated with periodontitis. Persons exposed to tobacco had a 1.6 times greater chance of having periodontal disease compared to individuals not exposed to second-hand smoke [11]. Further, tobacco use has an adverse effect on the full spectrum of periodontal treatment approaches, ranging from mechanical debridement, local and systemic antimicrobial therapy to surgery and regenerative procedures [80, 90,144]. Interestingly, the deleterious effects of tobacco smoking may be suppressed by its cessation, despite the impossibility of reversing its past effects. In the study conducted by Tomar & Asma (2000) [178], the relative risk for developing periodontal disease was reported to be 3.97 for smokers and 1.68 for former smokers. In addition, among former smokers, the risk decreased with the number of years since quitting (3.22 after 2 years and 1.15 after 11 years).

Animal studies provide a basis of support for the evidence from human studies, since they permit the control of confounders such as behavioral and systemic factors that may also influence periodontal disease progression. Nociti et al. (2000) [122] showed, using a rat model, that nicotine administration associated with plaque infection increased the rate of periodontal loss. Subsequently, the authors, aiming to answer the question as to whether nicotine concentration could be critical in promoting a dose-dependent response, evaluated the effect of daily administration of high doses of nicotine on the bone loss rate in the furcation region of rats by histometric analysis [123]. Nicotine concentrations administered in this study were intended to reproduce the highest nicotine concentrations found in commercially available cigarette brands. The data suggested that nicotine was able to heighten the rate of bone loss in a dose-dependent manner in ligated and non-ligated teeth. However, nicotine is just one of the 2000-3000 potentially toxic substances in tobacco smoke, which presents a complex mixture of substances such as acrolein, acetaldehyde, carbon monoxide and hydrogen cyanide [158]. Therefore, in order to investigate the influence of cigarette smoke as a whole, the researchers used a cigarette smoke exposure chamber, an acrylic device where the animals were forced to breathe the cigarette smoke-contaminated air [26]. In this study, the authors first demonstrated that cigarette smoke inhalation significantly increased bone loss resulting from ligature-induced periodontitis. Furthermore, data analysis demonstrated that the cessation of cigarette smoke inhalation might positively affect the rate of bone loss resulting from periodontitis [27]. The results of these preclinical studies have thus reinforced previous clinical studies, minimizing possible confounding factors that may exist in human studies.

The mechanisms by which cigarette smoking influences the initiation and progression of periodontitis are not fully understood. It seems that tobacco smoke may affect both the composition of the microflora and the host response. Regarding microflora, while several investigators have reported no significant differences in the incidence and distribution of periodontal pathogens in the plaque biofilm of smokers [46], other studies have demonstrated significant differences in the recovery rates of periodontal pathogens in smokers [191]. Of particular interest are recent studies which demonstrate a high recovery rate of periodontal pathogens in shallow periodontal pockets and on oral mucous membrane [51, 69]. In addition, a smaller reduction in periodontal pathogens was reported in smokers than in nonsmokers, following scaling and root planning [181]. These studies points to the role of smoking in altering the load environment of the shallower pockets, thereby promoting the growth of these microbial species, as well as possible alterations in the host response that would allow for the growth of these specific microorganisms.

The influence of tobacco smoke on host response may occur in two areas: the periodontal pocket and the tissue. The first host response events occur in the periodontal pocket; it appears that cigarette smoking may tip the balance even further away from the protective functions of neutrophils and antibodies in the periodontal pockets and towards greater destructive activity [158]. For example, several studies have demonstrated reduced imunoglobulin G and imunoglobulin A levels in smokers versus nonsmokers [58, 146]. Furthermore, the effects of smoking on neutrophil function have demonstrated impaired phagocytosis, chemotaxis in neutrophils exposed to acute levels of tobacco smoke [35, 105] and increases in the release of potentially destructive oxidative products, such as superoxide and hydrogen peroxide [156]. The next stage of pathogenesis occurs when the bacterial plaque biofilm has overwhelmed the host defenses in the periodontal pocket and the bacterial products penetrate the underlying soft tissues. Here, the balance between protection and destruction is mediated largely by the type of cytokine pattern secreted by monocyte cell population. The preponderance of evidence has suggested that smoking will tip the balance toward a more inflammatory/destructive profile. For example, in vitro studies have demonstrated high secreted levels of interleukin-1β in isolated mononuclear blood cells when exposed to in vitro smoke [157]. In addition, nicotine, whether or not in association with lipopolysaccharide from periodontopathogenic bacteria, has been shown to increase interleukin-6 and interleukin-8 production by human gingival fibroblasts [185]. In vivo, César-Neto et al. (2005) [27] indicated that smoking modulation of bone destruction in periodontal disease may involve reduced levels of anti-inflammatory and anti-resorptive factors, such as interleukin-10 and osteoprotegerin, respectively, and may also involve high levels of pro-inflammatory cytokines, such as interleukin-6. However, in clinical studies, the results of the effects of tobacco smoke on inflammatory components have been inconclusive.

Emotional Stress

Stress is a state of physiological and psychological strain caused by adverse physical, mental, or emotional, internal or external stimuli that tend to disturb the functioning of an organism and which the organism naturally desires to avoid [45]. Whether or not a subject exhibits a stress response depends on a myriad of factors, including coping behaviors, genetic predisposition, concomitant stressors, levels of social support, and other lifestyle factors. Stress is compatible with good health, which is necessary to cope with the challenges of everyday life. Problems start when the stress response is inappropriate to the size of the challenge, producing neuroendocrine and biochemical changes that result in significant adverse effects on the proper functioning of the immune system [38, 151]. Potential effects of the stress response that may be observed, or even measured, include anxiety, depression, impaired cognition and altered self-steem. Stressful stimuli can induce a set of reactions that produce effects on virtually all body systems [20]. Exposure to stress may affect the host immune response, making the individual more susceptible to the development of unhealthy conditions that damage periodontal health [137].

The most documented association between stress and periodontal disease is the one between acute forms of necrotizing gingivitis and periodontitis. An increased incidence of these conditions has been amply documented in military personnel during stressful activities and in students during examination periods [62, 67]. The association between stress and chronic periodontitis has been investigated. Wimmer et al. (2002) [188] conducted a retrospective case-control study of 89 patients with different forms of chronic periodontitis undergoing treatment. All participants completed a stress coping questionnaire, which served as a psychodiagnostic survey aimed at collecting data on stress coping strategies. The results showed that periodontitis patients with inadequate stress behavior strategies (defensive coping) are at greater risk for severe periodontitis. Later, the researchers discovered, by means of a 24-month prospective clinical trial, that passive coping strategies were more pronounced in advanced disease, as well as in cases of poor response to nonsurgical periodontal treatment. Patients with active coping modes had a milder form of the disease and a more favorable course of treatment [189]. A systematic review of case-control, cross-sectional and prospective studies examining psychologic factors, such as stress and depression and periodontal disease indicated that 57.1% of the studies reported a positive correlation between stress or other psychologic factors and periodontal disease, and that 14.2% did not [137]. In addition, a subsequent study confirmed the association between stress and depression and periodontal destruction [155]. The weight of evidence therefore seems to suggest an association between stress and periodontal health.

The biologic plausibility of such an association is not as yet completely elucidated. Stress can result in the dysregulation of the immune system, mediated primarily through the hypothalamic-pituitary-adrenal axis. Activation of hypothalamic-pituitary-adrenal axis by stress results in the release of an increased concentration of corticotrophin-releasing hormone from the hypothalamus. Corticotrophin-releasing hormone, in turn, acts on the anterior pituitary, resulting in the release of adrenocorticotrophic hormone (corticotrophin). The adrenocorticotrophic hormone then acts on the adrenal cortex and causes the production and release of glucocorticoid hormones (predominantly cortisol) into the circulation. The glucocorticoids then produce a response, modifying cytokine profiles, elevating blood glucose levels, and altering levels of certain growth factors [116]. The second major pathway to be activated is the sympathetic nervous system. Stress activates the nerve fibers of the autonomic nervous system, which innervate the tissues of the immune system. The nerve bodies secrete their products (cathecolamines) directly into the bloodstream. The release of catecholamines results in the hormonal secretion of norepinephrine and epinephrine from the adrenal medulla, which results in a range of effects that may act to modulate immune responses [116]. Eventually, the impact of stress on periodontal disease may be modulated by health-impairing behaviors that include neglecting oral hygiene practices, increased consumption of cigarettes and alcohol, disturbed sleeping patterns and bruxing [116].

Animal studies reinforce the hypothesis of a relationship between stress and periodontal disease by means of the influence of stress on the immune system via nervous and neuroendocrine because the model makes it possible to exclude the impact of various behavioral changes, such as smoking and less effective oral hygiene. Takada et al. (2004) [171] demonstrated that stress modulated the progression of periodontal inflammation and increased alveolar bone loss. More recently, Peruzzo et al. (2008) [138] showed, on the basis of the same rat model of restraint stress, that chronic stress increased bone loss resulting from a ligature-induced periodontitis by a local increase in proinflammatory and proresorptive factors.

Based on the evidence described above, although further well-controlled prospective clinical trials are still required to definitively define stress as a risk factor for periodontitis, most studies point to the association between stress and periodontal disease. Stress management, therefore, may be a valuable component for current periodontal practice.

SYSTEMIC FACTORS

Diabetes Mellitus

Diabetes mellitus is a clinically and genetically heterogeneous group of metabolic disorders manifested by abnormally high levels of glucose in the blood [111]. It is a highly prevalent metabolic disorder; with 150 million cases estimated worldwide, which constitutes a global public health burden [142]. Diabetes is divided into two main forms: type 1 diabetes mellitus (formerly insulin-dependent diabetes mellitus) and type 2 diabetes mellitus (formerly non-insulin-dependent diabetes mellitus). Type 1 diabetes is caused by the immune-mediated destruction of the insulin-producing pancreatic β cells and accounts for 10% to 15% of all cases of diabetes. The more common form, type 2 diabetes, results from a combination of impaired insulin production and insulin resistance. Both forms of the disease are associated with a range of complications that increase the morbidity and mortality of affected individuals [142].

Periodontal disease has been called the sixth complication of diabetes, a view supported by several reviews which conclude that the bulk of evidence indicates there is a direct relationship between diabetes mellitus and periodontal diseases [101]. The presence of diabetes mellitus is often associated with increased gingival inflammation. Karjalainen & Knuuttila (1996) [83] observed that poorly controlled diabetes mellitus in children had higher levels of gingival inflammation than did well-controlled patients, regardless of plaque levels. Moreover, gingival bleeding significantly decreased after two weeks of insulin treatment of newly diagnosed type 1 diabetic children and adolescents. Recently, Dakovic & Pavlovic (2008) [40] confirmed that gingival inflammation is more evident in children and adolescents with type I diabetes mellitus than in healthy ones. An increased risk of periodontitis for individuals with diabetes has also been documented in several studies. The relation between diabetes and periodontal health status was first determined in a population of Pima Indians, where subjects with type 2 diabetes have an approximately three-fold increased risk of attachment loss [53]. Moreover, in a 2-year longitudinal study of the Pima Indian population, Taylor et al. (1998) [173] found that individuals with type 2 diabetes had an increased risk of progressive alveolar bone loss compared with non-diabetic subjects. The study also showed that the level of metabolic control had a significant effect on disease progression. Increased risk for progressive attachment and bone loss in poorly controlled diabetic patients have been confirmed in a meta-analysis of studies in various populations [134] and in more recent studies such as that conducted by Novak et al. (2008) [124].

Disease progression following periodontal treatment may also be related to metabolic control. Tervonen & Karjalainen (1997) [175] found that a group of type 1 diabetics with poor metabolic control had a significantly greater recurrence of deep probing depths 12 months after treatment than subjects with good or moderate diabetic control and non-diabetic controls. However, metabolically well-controlled diabetics responded to non-surgical and surgical periodontal therapy in a manner similar to that in which healthy controls responded [30, 186].

Many potential mechanisms have been studied by which diabetes could affect the periodontium. There are few differences in the subgingival microbiota between diabetic and nondiabetic patients with periodontitis [161, 162]. This suggests that alterations in the host immunoinflammatory response to potential pathogens may play a predominant role. Diabetes may result in impairment of neutrophil adherence, chemotaxis, and phagocytosis, which may facilitate the persistence of bacteria in the periodontal pocket and significantly increase periodontal destruction [108, 110]. While neutrophils are often hypofunctional in diabetes, these patients may have a hyper-responsive monocyte/macrophage phenotype, resulting in a significantly increased production of pro-inflammatory cytokines and mediators [159, 160]. This hyperinflammatory response results in high levels of pro-inflammatory cytokines in the gingival crevice fluid. In addition, high glucose concentrations induce non-enzymatic glycation and oxidation proteins, such as collagen and lipids, resulting in the accumulation of advanced glycation end-products (AGEs) in diabetic tissues, including periodontal tissues. The AGEs, through their receptors (RAGEs), may also induce the expression of pro-inflammatory cytokines. The elevated pro-inflammatory cytokines in the periodontal environment may play a role in the increased periodontal destruction seen in many people with diabetes [111]. For example, Duarte et al. (2007) [50] showed an overexpression of interleukin-1β and interleukin-6, potent pro-inflammatory cytokines, in gingival tissues of diabetic patients diagnosed with chronic periodontitis [111].

In conclusion, studies indicate that diabetics with poor glycaemic control have an increased risk of periodontitis and disease progression.

Osteoporosis

Osteopenia and osteoporosis are systemic skeletal diseases characterized by low bone mass and micro-architectural deterioration with a consequent increase in bone fragility and susceptibility to fracture. According to the World Health Organization, osteoporosis is considered to be present when mineral density is 2.5 standard deviation (SD) or more below the mean for normal young Caucasian women. Further, osteopenia is defined as a bone density level between 1 and 2.5 SD below normal bone density [82]. Both osteopenia and osteoporosis are grave public health concerns, particularly associated with estrogen deficiency among postmenopausal women. The risk factors for osteoporosis include many risk factors associated with advanced periodontal disease [61]. Since both osteoporosis and periodontal diseases are bone resorptive diseases, it has been hypothesized that osteoporosis could be a risk factor for the progression of periodontal disease.

The effects of osteoporosis induced by an estrogen-deficient state have been widely studied in a rat model. Bilateral ovariectomies of female rats were able to induce this condition. Tanaka et al. (2002) [172] histomorphometrically investigated the alveolar bone following estrogen deficiency and showed osteoporotic changes and thin alveolar bone proper in the interradicular septum of the first molar of ovariectomized rats. Later, Duarte et al. (2006) [49] confirmed that an estrogen-deficient state may negatively affect the tooth-supporting alveolar bone, resulting in a lower density of alveolar bone than that observed in estrogen-sufficient animals. It has also been shown that an estrogen-deficient state may significantly increase bone loss resulting from ligature-induced periodontitis and also at healthy sites [47, 48].

There have been a number of reports on the mechanisms involved in the estrogen regulation of bone metabolism. Since estrogen receptors in osteoblasts and osteoclasts were discovered [54, 128], it is believed that estrogen has a direct skeletal effect. It has also been shown that estrogen has an important role in controlling bone resorption through its action on osteoprotegerin (OPG) and the receptor activator of nuclear factor kB ligand (RANKL) mechanism [94, 189], as well as on bone-regulating factors such as interleukin-1, interleukin-6 and tumor necrosis factor [129, 63].

Animal studies have established a clear association between osteoporosis and oral bone density or osteoporosis and periodontitis-induced bone loss. In humans, the data gathered on the mostly cross-sectional studies appears to confirm a relationship between systemic and oral bone mineral density. For example, in a classic series of studies, Kribbs et al. (1983, 1989, 1990) [87, 88, 89] addressed this relationship in both normal and osteoporotic women. Although the technology used in those studies reflects the time at which the studies were carried out, they indicated an association between oral and systemic bone. More recent studies have included larger numbers of women with a wide range of bone mineral density in systemic bone. Wactawski-Wende et al. (1996) [183] showed positive correlations between alveolar bone loss and bone mineral density at the spine, trochanter, Ward's triangle or total femur. Further, cross-sectional data from 468 postmenopausal females enrolled in the oral ancillary portion of the Women's Health Initiative study revealed a significant correlation between basal bone density determined from intraoral radiographs and hip bone mineral density determined by DXA [79].

On the other hand, while some studies indicate osteoporosis as a risk indicator for periodontitis [153, 176], others have not detected a significant association [187]. Moreover, there is only a limited number of longitudinal studies evaluating the association of osteoporosis and periodontitis progression. Reinhardt et al. (1999) [147] prospectively analyzed the influence of serum estradiol levels and osteopenia / osteoporosis on common clinical measurements of periodontal disease over a 2-year period. No significant differences were found in attachment loss between osteoporotic and non-osteoporotic patients, although the authors reported a trend towards more attachment loss in non-smoking osteoporotic patients. In contrast, in a recent longitudinal study of 184 individuals aged 70 years [190], bone mineral density was associated with the number of progressive sites which had ≥ 3 mm additional attachment loss over 3 years, suggesting a significant relationship between periodontal disease and general bone mineral density.

It may therefore be concluded that the relationship between osteoporosis and periodontitis remains unclear. Confounding factors such as age, gender or smoking and the lack of precise methods for the assessment of osteoporosis in the jaws have been reported to affect the establishment of a clear interaction between osteoporosis and periodontitis. Larger prospective longitudinal studies are needed to further evaluate osteoporosis as a risk factor for progressive periodontitis.

GENETIC FACTORS

While microbial and other environmental factors are believed to initiate and modulate periodontal disease progression, there now exists strong supporting evidence that genes play a role in the predisposition to and progression of periodontal diseases [70, 73]. Support for this statement comes from studies in animals and humans which indicate that genetic factors influence the inflammatory and immune response in general, and periodontitis experience specifically. Different forms of genes (allelic variants) can produce variations in tissue structure (innate immunity), antibody responses (adaptative immunity) and inflammatory mediators (non-specific inflammation) [84]. Thus, complex diseases such as periodontitis may have multiple gene associations which individually have weak effects but which collectively combine with other influences, such as environmental factors, and result in various disease manifestations [120].

The hypothesis that genetic factors account for variation in phenotype expression of periodontal disease has been formally tested by comparing disease characteristics in monozygous and dizygous twins. It is assumed in these experiments that because a given set of adult twins grew up together in the same environment there is reason to believe that they should share most relevant habits and practices. Thus the similarity of such factors as personal habits, lifestyles and access to health care should not be different for members of twin pairs whether they are monozygous or dizygous. Michalowicz et al. (1991) [113, 114], in studies of both monozygous and dizygous twins reared together and apart, showed a significant genetic component for probing depth, attachment loss and radiographic alveolar bone height, supporting the role of genetics in periodontal disease. In a recent study, Michalowicz et al. (2000) [115] found that monozygous twins were found to be more similar than dizygous ones for clinical measurements such as probing depth, attachment loss, plaque and gingivitis. A statistically significant genetic variance was found for both severity and extent of the disease. Based on this study, chronic periodontitis was estimated to have approximately 50% heritability, which was unaltered following adjustments for behavioral variables including smoking. However, while monozygous twins were also more similar than dizygous twins for gingivitis scores, there was no evidence of heritability for gingivitis after behavioral covariates such as utilization of dental care and smoking were incorporated into the analyses. In short, these studies indicate that approximately half of the variance in chronic periodontitis in the population is attributed to genetic variation. Thus the basis of heritability of periodontitis seems to be biological and not behavioral.

Interest in identifying genetic risk factors for chronic periodontal diseases has been spurred by recent reports of associations with polymorphisms. Gene polymorphisms are locations within the genome that vary in sequence between individuals and are very prevalent, affecting at least 1% of the population. The rationale for studying single gene nucleotide polymorphisms is that they can be used to identify potential markers of susceptibility, severity and clinical outcome [84]. Various aspects of the host inflammatory response have attracted attention as potentially crucial variants influencing the host response in periodontitis.

Cytokines

Specific genotypes have been identified and linked to periodontal destruction. Polymorphisms of interleukin-1 (IL-1), IL-1β and IL-1RN genotypes have been identified as potential risk factors for periodontal destruction. In 1997, Kornman et al. [86] were the first to describe an association between polymorphisms and periodontal disease, creating a great interest in the topic. They found an association between polymorphisms in the gene encoding for IL-1α (-889) and IL-1β (+3953) and an increased severity of periodontitis. Functionally, IL-1 genotype is associated with high levels of IL-1 production [141]. A role has been suggested for IL-1 in the initiation and progression of periodontitis. IL-1 may activate the degradation of the extracellular matrix and bone of the periodontal tissues, and increased tissue or gingival fluid levels of IL-1β have been associated with periodontitis [84]. Moreover, it was found that the mean counts of specific bacteria species were higher in IL-1 genotype-positive individuals than in negative subjects [167]. Several studies have corroborated the association between IL-1 polymorphism and periodontal disease or tooth loss [39, 109, 184]. Furthermore, a recent systematic review and meta-analysis established a statistically significant association of IL-1A (-889) and IL-1B (+3953) polymorphisms with chronic periodontal disease [121]. However, Huynh-Ba et al. (2007) [75] in a previous systematic review suggested that there is insufficient evidence to establish whether a positive IL-1 genotype status contributes to the progression of periodontitis and/or treatment outcomes. The data thus remain inconclusive, and longitudinal studies are required to establish the extent to which this genetic factor plays a role in disease progression.

The polymorphism of tumor necrosis factor-α (TNF-α) has also been suggested as a possible risk factor for periodontitis. TNF-α is secreted as a response to bacterial stimulation by a variety of cell types [173]. It stimulates osteoclasts differentiation and together with IL-1 may result in bone resorption [103]. Furthermore, TNF-α promotes the release of collagenases (metalloproteinase) that destroy the extracellular matrix [21] and are produced in excessive amounts in inflamed periodontal tissues [66]. However, most studies have failed to link this polymorphism of the TNF-α gene to chronic periodontitis [36, 59, 121].

Human Leukocyte Antigens

Several investigations have studied populations of patients with different forms of periodontitis to determine the expression of polymorphisms of human leukocyte antigens (HLA). The HLA complex plays an important role in immune responsiveness and may be involved in antigen recognition of periodontal pathogens. Recognition of antigen peptides and their presentation to T cells is crucial for an effective antigen-specific immune response to periodontal pathogens and underlies genetic control. Because antigen presentation to and resultant activation of T cells is restricted by the major histocompatibility complex (MHC), the polymorphism of the human MHC molecules (human leukocyte antigens – HLA) may directly affect the binding capability of antigen peptides and thus the antigen-specific T-cell response [192]. A recent systematic review did not reveal any significant positive or negative associations [170]. However, few studies are available and those present significant limitations, such as the control group not always being healthy. On the other hand, when aggressive periodontitis was evaluated, an association with particular HLA polymorphisms was observed. Therefore, more studies are needed before definite conclusions can be drawn.

Immuno-Receptors

The association of immuno-receptors with periodontitis has been studied. Receptors for Fc domain of IgG FCγR) are categorized as a family of receptors, expressed on the cell surface of leukocytes, which bind IgG antibodies and immune complexes [102]. In humans, FCγRs are expressed on natural killer cells, macrophages, T lymphocytes, monocytes and mast cells [65]. The interaction between FCγRs and IgG triggers a variety of biological responses, including phagocytosis, endocytosis, antibody-dependent cellular cytotoxicity, release of inflammatory mediators, and enhancement of antigen presentation [84]. Polymorphisms that influence the binding affinity between FCγR and IgG of different subclasses are considered important in susceptibility to periodontal diseases. The few existing studies of chronic periodontitis have investigated associations between FCγR polymorphisms and susceptibility to and severity of periodontitis. The majority of them indicate that polymorphisms of FCγR tend to be associated with the chronic form of peridontitis [31, 85, 112].

Matrix Metalloproteinases

Matrix metalloproteinases (MMPs) are one of the most important groups of enzymes involved in periodontal connective tissue destruction [169]. Although few studies have suggested an association between MMP gene polymorphisms and chronic periodontitis [140, 169], there is strong controversial evidence for such an association. Itagaki et al. (2004) [140] reported that MMP-1 and / or MMP-3 single nucleotide polymorphisms were not associated with susceptibility to periodontitis in a Japanese population. More recently, polymorphisms in the gene for MMP-2 were studied and no definite correlation with periodontitis could be found [74]. Repeke et al. (2009) [150] observed a limited role for MMP-1 polymorphism in periodontitis. It seems that the extensive chronic antigenic challenge exposure overcomes the genetic control and plays a major role in the determination of MMP-1 expression. Therefore, due to the limited number of studies carried out to date, it is difficult to associate single nucleotide polymorphisms of MMP genes with chronic periodontitis.

Reports on the genetic polymorphisms associated with chronic periodontal diseases are increasing, encouraging the search for new specific markers by researchers, but the limitations of such studies have not been fully appreciated. For example, in nearly all the published studies, subjects have not been characterized as to behavioral risk factors such as smoking, stress or others. In addition, the heterogeneity of the diseases examined and the ethnic aspects of the distribution of the genetic markers may contribute to the disparity of the results [77]. In conclusion, some gene polymorphisms are associated with modest increases in the probability of periodontal disease developing. Further studies on the distribution and dynamics of genetic variation at many loci simultaneously might disclose the direct and epistatic (interaction among multiple alleles) genetic involvement in periodontitis.

MICROBIAL COMPOSITION

While periodontal disease is regarded as an opportunistic mixed microbial infection, specific periodontal pathogens have been proposed as predictors for further disease progression [72]. Although there are over 500 different intra-oral species and other that have not yet been identified, the majority of studies have focused on a subset of microorganisms including Agreggatibacter actinomycetencomitans (A.a.), Porphyromonas gingivalis (P.g.) and Tannerella forsythia (T.f.) [55, 126], presumably because they satisfy the criteria for Socransky's modifications of Koch's postulates:

> - the organism must occur at higher numbers in disease-active sites than disease-inactive sites;
> - elimination of the organism should arrest disease progression;
> - the organism should elicit a humoral or cellular immune response;
> - animal pathogenicity testing should infer disease potential;
> - the organism should possess virulence factors relevant to the disease process;

Regarding the virulence factors, A.a., P.g. and T.f. share three common features that support their role as risk factors for initiation and progression of periodontitis. First, all are Gram-negative, and therefore produce lipopolyssacharide, which can modulate the local inflammatory response in host cells that express pattern recognition receptors. Moreover, all appear capable of invasion of the mucosal barrier to infection and possibly of being sequestered inside epithelial cells. And finally, all produce factors that enable them to evade the antibacterial functions of the innate immune response either passively (anti-phagocytic capsule) or actively (leukotoxin, gingipains, proteases, induction of apoptosis) [55].

However, evaluation of these three pathogens as risk factors for attachment loss over time has resulted in conflicting evidence. Some studies do not support the detection of these specific bacterial species for the identification of individuals at risk for periodontitis progression [98, 104]. On the other hand, a number of longitudinal studies have shown that the presence of high levels of these species at baseline is a prognostic indicator for disease progression [68, 106, 177]. Individually, A.a. has been implicated only in some cases of chronic periodontitis [24, 152, 177]. Its association has been most clearly demonstrated with localized aggressive periodontitis [71]. On the other hand, the importance of P.g. and T.f. in the initiation of chronic periodontitis as well as in its progression to advanced periodontitis is more clearly established in longitudinal studies [106, 180]. Further evidence suggests that B.f. and presumably P.g. are also associated with disease recurrence when patients are followed up after therapy [29].

Although this review has focused on the three bacterial species considered most likely to initiate the events resulting in chronic periodontitis, there are several other microorganisms that have been described as moderately associated with the disease. These species include Campylobacter rectus, Eubacterium nodatum, Fusobacterium nucleatum, Prevotella intermedia, Peptostreptococcus micros, Streptococcus intermedius-complex and Treponema denticola [127].

The evidence for the prognostic value of A.a., P.g. and T.f. remains inconclusive, and the role of the other pathogenic bacteria has likewise yet to be fully appreciated. Such evidences, however, does lead us to believe that certain bacteria like P.g. and T.f. are indeed more important than others when it comes to considering risk indicators of chronic periodontitis.

Tooth-Level Factors

Individual variation in susceptibility to disease progression may be related to a number of a local clinical factors including tooth position [2], caries and defective restoration margins [3, 22], subgingival restoration margins [163], abutment tooth [145], presence of calculus [119], occlusal discrepancies [125], unsatisfactory root form [109] or root grooves [93].

A number of periodontal parameters have also been shown to influence periodontitis progression: gingivitis/bleeding on probing [43, 92], probing depth [13, 33], alveolar bone loss [145], tooth mobility [56], furcation involvement [41] and tooth type [118].

In particular, bleeding on probing, pocket depth and radiographic alveolar bone loss are considered to be of great importance by the clinicians for decision making [136]. But do these factors really predict future attachment loss?

Current theory holds that the gingival lesion is the precursor of periodontitis. Clearly, not all gingivitis lesions progress to periodontitis. It has been suggested that individuals are at lower risk for disease progression if the prevalence of bleeding on probing at a subject level is $\leq 25\%$ [81]. However, the proportion of gingival lesions progressing to periodontitis and the factors causing this conversion have not yet been sufficiently clarified. Periodontitis and mean attachment loss have been positively associated with bleeding on probing [43]. Recently, a longitudinal study of a patient cohort of 565 males was performed over a 26-year period. Sites with consistent bleeding had 70% more attachment loss than sites that were consistently non-inflamed. Moreover, teeth with sites that were consistently non-inflamed had a 50-year survival rate of 99.5%, while teeth with consistently inflamed gingivae yielded a 50-year survival rate of 63.4% [92].

Regarding pocket depth, on a site basis, the presence of deep residual pockets has been associated with disease progression [13, 33]. A systematic review addressing the use of residual pocket depth, bleeding on probing and furcation status following initial periodontal therapy to predict further attachment and tooth loss found that, at the individual level, residual pocket depth was predictive of further disease progression [149].

Furthermore, longitudinal studies of periodontal disease have shown that the amount of alveolar bone loss present at baseline, which represents the patient's previous history of periodontitis, may be also used to predict further progression of untreated and treated periodontitis [56, 133, 145].

Despite the importance of clinical findings on the progression of periodontal disease, treatment planning based only on the assessment of disease severity rather than other documented risk factors such as environmental and systemic factors leaves much to be desired [136].

MULTIFACTORIAL RISK ASSESSMENT MODELS

The management of periodontal disease patients is used to be based on a "repair" model of care, in which clinician's goal was to diagnose the problem and resolve it via treatment. In recent years, however, an increasing understanding of the aetiology and risk factors for chronic periodontal diseases has developed. As a result, their management is undergoing a transition from a repair model to the wellness model of patient care that guides the clinician toward a health care strategy based on risk reduction and disease prevention [130]. Rather than the mere application of the knowledge of the risk factors to maintain oral health and to prevent the onset of periodontal disease, attention has been drawn to the assessment of risk level for disease progression in individuals under supportive periodontal therapy, representing a population with a moderate to high level of tisk of periodontal breakdown has attracted attention. The assessment of risk level for disease progression in each individual patient would enable the practitioner to determine the frequency and extent of professional support necessary to maintain the attachment levels obtained following active therapy [91]. Moreover, the clinician often has to decide which teeth to retain, which treatment to prescribe, or how to maintain or restore a functional and aesthetically pleasing dentition. For decision making at a tooth level, it is of paramount importance to assess prognosis of each tooth in order to choose the treatment modality with the greatest probability of success [56].

Thus, as the study of prognostic factors has progressed, multi-factorial risk assessment models has been proposed using the combination of these factors to identify individuals and teeth at high risk for periodontitis progression [56, 91, 130, 136, 149].

Periodontal Risk Calculator (PRC) (Page et al., 2002)

Page et al. (2002) [130] developed a computer-based tool, the periodontal risk calculator (PRC), for assessing risk and predicting periodontal deterioration. The PRC is based on a mathematically derived algorithms that assign relative weights to various known risks that increase patients' susceptibility to develop periodontitis: patient age, smoking history, diabetes diagnosis, history of periodontal surgery, pocket depth, bleeding on probing, restorations below the gingival margin, root calculus, radiographic bone height, furcation involvements and vertical bone lesions. The aim of the PRC is to be user-friendly and to require only information that is gathered during a routine periodontal examination. The PRC determines the patient's level of risk on a scale from 1 (lowest) to 5 (highest). However, the details of the algorithm and weighting for the factors have not been published.

Page et al. (2003) [131] documented the extent of agreement between risk scores calculated using the PRC and information gathered during a baseline examination with the periodontal status 3, 9 and 15 years later. In a retrospective study, clinical records and radiographs of 523 men were used. Information from baseline examinations was entered into the risk calculator and a risk score on a scale of 1-5 for periodontal deterioration was calculated for each subject. Actual periodontal status in terms of alveolar bone loss determined using digital radiographs, and tooth loss determined from the clinical records, was assessed at 3, 9, and 15 years. The risk scores at baseline were found to be strong predictors of future periodontal status measured as worsening severity and extent of alveolar bone loss and tooth loss, especially loss of periodontally affected teeth. The authors concluded that risk scores calculated using the PRC and information gathered during a standard periodontal examination predict future periodontal status with a high level of accuracy and validity.

Periodontal Risk Assessment (PRA) (Lang & Tonetti, 2003)

Lang & Tonetti (2003) [91] constructed a functional diagram to assess patient's risk of recurrence of periodontitis based on a number of risk factors and risk indicators evaluated simultaneously. The PRA model consists of an assessment of the proportion of bleeding on probing, the prevalence of residual pockets greater than 4 mm ($\geq$ 5 mm), the tooth loss from a total of 28 teeth, the loss of periodontal support (proportion of sites with bleeding on probing) in relation to the patient's age, the systemic and genetic condition (e.g. diabetes mellitus and polymorphism of interleukin-1, respectively), and environmental factors, such as cigarette smoking. Each parameter has its own scale for minor, moderate and high risk profiles (Figure 1).

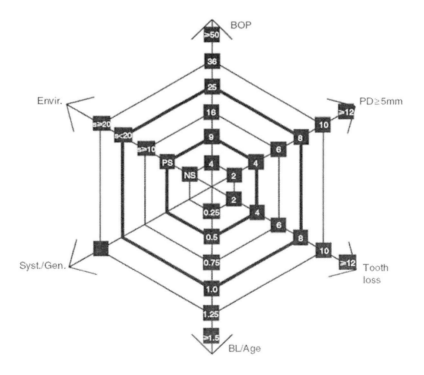

Figure 1. Schematic illustration representing a periodontal risk assessment functional diagram. Each vector represents a single risk factor or indicator. The area of low risk is found within the centre circle of the polygon, while the area of high risk lies outside the periphery of the second ring in bold. Between the two rings in bold is the area of moderate risk (Lang & Tonetti, 2003).

The authors provided evidence supporting the inclusion of each parameter within the diagram. The hexagonal risk diagram identified patients at low risk (all parameters within the low risk categories or, at the most, one parameter in the moderate) and those at moderate (at least two parameters in the moderate category, but at most one parameter in the high risk) and high risk (at least two parameters in the high risk category). Thus, a comprehensive evaluation of the functional diagram would provide an individualized total risk profile and determine the frequency and complexity of supportive periodontal therapy visits. However, this model was not validated and little evidence on its applicability is available. In a retrospective study including 100 patients who had received active treatment, Eickholz et al. (2008) [52] were the first to provide evidence that patients assigned to the high risk group according to the Lang & Tonetti risk assessment suffered from a higher rate of tooth loss after a 10-year follow-up than the other risk groups.

PRA / Multifactorial Risk Diagram (Renvert & Persson, 2004)

In this multifactorial risk diagram, a modification of the PRA model is described where the vector bone loss index (bone loss in relation to subject's age) is replaced by the proportion of sites with a distance $\geq$ 4 mm from the cementoenamel junction to the bone level [149]. The individuals were not more categorized as low, moderate or high risk. Here, the surface outlined between the various risk parameters was calculated to provide a numerical score of risk with the aid of a computer program (EXCEL XP for PC, Redmond, WA, USA). The authors suggested that in this way the risk scores can be monitored and compared over time, enabling the clinician to adjust the supportive therapy strategy as appropriate.

Prognostic Model for Tooth Survival (Faggion et al., 2007)

Faggion et al. (2007) [56] developed a prognostic model to estimate quantitatively survival rates for teeth in patients receiving treatment for periodontitis, in order to make evidence-based decisions about retaining or extracting teeth. With the aim of constructing the prognostic model, one hundred and ninety-eight patients were included in a retrospective study. At baseline, medical history (diabetes mellitus, coronary heart diseases, infectious diseases, allergies, coagulation disorders and radiation in the head and neck regions), clinical findings (teeth present, caries, dental restorations, probing depth, tooth mobility, approximal plaque index, sulcus bleeding test and tooth vitality) and full-mouth radiographs (alveolar bone level) were available. A logistic regression model revealed the following significant predictors for tooth loss during supportive periodontal therapy: a diagnosis of diabetes mellitus, the alveolar bone level, tooth mobility, root type and non-vital pulp at baseline examination. Based on these parameters, a prognostic model was constructed that provides estimates of tooth survival probability when periodontal therapy was performed (Figure 2). The authors showed that prognosis of tooth loss improved 14%, as compared with an alternative prognosis that did not consider any information provided by prognostic variables.

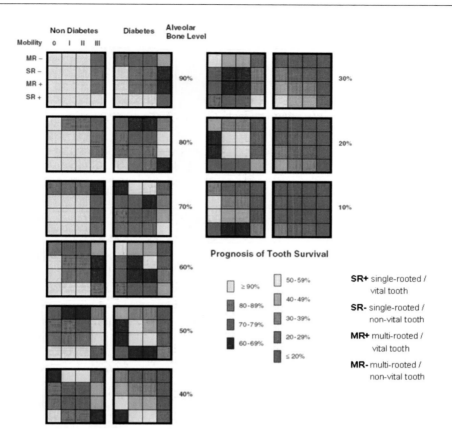

Figure 2. Schematic illustration representing a prognostic model for tooth survival. Each square represents a unique combination of predictors and the color coding on the bottom right indicates the likelihood of tooth survival probability (Faggion et al., 2007).

CONCLUSION

The above review clearly shows that chronic periodontal diseases are multifactorial disorders. Microbial dental plaque biofilm is the principal etiological factor, although several other local and systemic factors play an important modifying role in their pathogenesis. There is overwhelming evidence that both smoking and diabetes are important risk factors for periodontal tissue loss. In addition, the role of genetic factors and emotional stress has recently been highlighted. However, there is still a need for further studies to establish with great precision the contributions of other factors in the pathogenesis of these diseases.

Multifactorial risk models based on a knowledge of risk factors and risk indicators have been proposed to enhance the ability to predict risk for periodontal disease progression. However, prospective studies are virtually nonexistent to date. Moreover, few host-related factors are included in these models which may account for perhaps explain their limited improvement in predicting future disease events. Research in this field should be encouraged with the ultimate goal of helping the decision making during treatment planning and also to guide the clinician toward a strategy of risk reduction and disease prevention.

REFERENCES

[1]   Abdellatif HM, Burt BA. *An epidemiological investigation into the relative importance of age and oral hygiene status as determinants of periodontitis.* J Dent Res 1987;66:13-18.

[2]   Ainamo J. *Relationship between malalignment of the teeth and periodontal disease.* Scand J Dent Res 1972;2:104-110.

[3]   Albandar JM, Buischi YA, Axelsson P. *Caries lesions and dental restorations as predisposing factors in the progression of periodontal diseases in adolescents. A 3-year longitudinal study.* J Periodontol 1995;4:249-254.

[4]   Albandar JM, Kingman A, Brown LJ, Löe H. *Gingival inflammation and subgingival calculus as determinants of disease progression in early-onset periodontitis.* J Clin Periodontol 1998;25:231-237.

[5]   Albandar JM, Kingman A. *Gingival recession, gingival bleeding, and dental calculus in adults 30 years of age and older in the United States, 1988-1994.* J Periodontol 1999a;70(1):30-43.

[6]   Albandar JM, Brunelle JA, Kingman A. *Destructive periodontal disease in adults 30 years of age and older in the United States, 1988-1994.* J Periodontol 1999b;70:13-29.

[7]   Albandar JM, Tinoco EM. *Global epidemiology of periodontal diseases in children and young persons.* Periodntol 2000 2002a;29:153-76.

[8]   Albandar JM. *Global risk factors and risk indicators for periodontal diseases.* Periodontol 2000 2002b;29:177-206.

[9]   Albandar JM. *Periodontal diseases in North America.* Periodontol 2000 2002c;29:31-69.

[10]   Albandar JM. *Epidemiology and risk factors of periodontal diseases.* Dent Clin N Am 2005;49:517-532.

[11]   Arbes SJ Jr, Agustsdottir H, Slade GD. *Environmental tobacco smoke and periodontal disease in the United States.* Am J Public Health 2001;91:253-257.

[12]   Armitage GC. *Development of a classification system for periodontal diseases and conditions.* Ann Periodontol 1999;4:1-6.

[13]   Badersten A, Nilveus R, Egelberg J. *Scores of plaque, bleeding, suppuration and probing depth to predict probing attachment loss. 5 years of observation following non-surgical periodontal therapy.* J Clin Periodontol 1990;2:102-107.

[14]   Benatti BB, Silvério KG, Casati MZ, Sallum EA, Nociti FH Jr. *Influence of aging on biological properties of periodontal ligament cells.* Connect Tissue Res 2008;49:401-408.

[15]   Benatti BB, Silvério KG, Casati MZ, Sallum EA, Nociti FH Jr. *Inflammatory and bone-related genes are modulated by aging in human periodontal ligament cells.* Cytokine 2009;46:176-181.

[16]   Bergström J, Eliasson S, Preber H. *Cigarette smoking and periodontal bone loss.* J Periodontol 1991;62:242-246.

[17]   Bergström J. *Tobacco smoking and supragingival dental calculus.* J Clin Periodontol 1999;26:541-547.

[18]   Bergström J, Bostrom L. *Tobacco smoking and periodontal hemorrhagic responsiveness.* J Clin Periodontol 2001;28:680-685.

[19] Bergström J. *Tobacco smoking and risk for periodontal disease.* J Clin Periodontol 2003;30:107-113.

[20] Boyapati L, Wang H-L. *The role of stress in periodontal disease and wound healing.* Periodontol 2000 2007;44:195-210.

[21] Brenner DA, O'Hara M, Angel P, Chojkier M, Karin M. *Prolonged activation of jun and collagenase genes by tumour necrosis factor-alpha.* Nature 1989;337:661-663.

[22] Broadbent JM, Williams KB, Thomson WM, Williams SM. *Dental restorations: a risk factor for periodontal attachment loss?* J Clin Periodontol 2006;33:803-810.

[23] Brown LJ, Oliver RC, Löe H. *Evaluating periodontal status of U.S. employed adults.* J Am Dent Assoc 1990;121:226-232.

[24] Buchmann R, Muller RF, Heinecke A, Lange DE. *Actinobacillus actinomycetencomitans in destructive periodontal disease. Three-year follow-up results.* J Periodontol 2000;71:444-453.

[25] Calsina G, Ramon JM, Echeverria JJ. *Effects of smoking on periodontal tissues.* J Clin Periodontol 2002;29:771-776.

[26] César-Neto JB, Duarte PM, Sallum EA, Barbieri D, Moreno H Jr, Nociti FH Jr. *A comparative study on the effect of nicotine administration and cigarette smoke inhalation on bone healing around titanium implants.* J Periodontol 2003;74:1454-1459.

[27] César-Neto JB, Benatti BB, Haiter-Neto F, Sallum AW, Sallum EA, Nociti FH Jr. *Smoking cessation may present a positive impact on mandibular bone quality and periodontitis-related bone loss: a study in rats.* J Periodontol 2005;76:520-525.

[28] César-Neto JB, Duarte PM, de Oliveira MCG, Tambelli CH, Sallum EA, Nociti FH Jr. *Smoking modulates interleukin-6:interleukin-10 and RANKL:osteoprotegerin ratios in the periodontal tissues.* J Periodont Res 2007;42:184-191.

[29] Chaves ES, Jeffcoat MK, Ryerson CC, Snyder B. *Persistent bacterial colonization of Porphyromonas gingivalis, Prevotella intermedia, and Actinobacillus actinomyceten comitans in periodontitis and its association with alveolar bone loss after 6 months of therapy.* J Clin Periodontol 2000;27:897-903.

[30] Christgau M, Palitzsch KD, Schmalz G, Kreiner U, Frenzel S. *Healing response to non-surgical periodontal therapy in patients with diabetes mellitus: clinical, micro biological, and immunologic* results. J Clin Perioodntl 1998;2:112-124.

[31] Chung H-Y, Lu H-C, Chen W-L, Lu C-T, Yang Y-H, Tsai C-C. *Gm (23) allotypes and Fcγ receptor genotypes as risk factors for various forms of periodontitis.* J Clin Periodontol 2003;30:954-960.

[32] Ciancio SG. *Current status of indices of gingivitis.* J Clin Periodontol 1986;13:375-82.

[33] Claffey N, Nylund K, Kiger R, Garrett S, Egelberg J. *Diagnostic predictability of scores of plaque, bleeding, suppuration and probing depth for probing attachment loss. 3 ½ years of observation following initial periodontal therapy.* J Clin Periodontol 1990; 2:108-114.

[34] Consensus Report: chronic periodontitis. Ann Periodontol 1999;4:38.

[35] Corberand J, Laharrague P, Nguyen F, Duat G, Fontanilles M, Gleizes B, Gyrard E. *In vitro effect of tobacco smoke components on the functions of normal human poly morphonuclear leukocytes.* Infect Immun 1980;30:649-655.

[36] Craandijk J, van Krugten MV, Verweij CL, van der Velden U, Loos BG. *Tumor necrosis factor-alpha gene polymorphisms in relation to periodontitis.* J Clin Periodontol 2002;29:28-34.

[37] Craig RG, Boylan R, Yip J, Bamgboye P, Koutsoukos J, Mijares D, Ferrer J, Imam M, Socransky SS, Haffajee AD. *Prevalence and risk indicators for destructive periodontal diseases in 3 urban American minority populations.* J Clin Periodontol 2001;6:524-535.

[38] Croiset G, Heijinen C, Wied D. *Passive avoidance behavior, vasopressin and immune system: a link between avoidance latency and immune response.* Neuroendocrinology 1990;51:156-161.

[39] Cullinan MP, Westerman B, Hamlet SM, Palmer JE, Faddy MJ, Lang NP, Seymour GP. *A longitudinal study of interleukin-1 gene polymorphisms and periodontal disease in a general adult population.* J Clin Periodontol 2001;28:1137-1144.

[40] Dakovick D, Pavlovic MD. *Periodontal disease in children and adolescents with type 1 diabetes in Servia.* J Periodontol 2008;79:987-992.

[41] Dannewitz B, Krieger JK, Hüsing J, Eickholz P. *Loss of molars in periodontally treated patients: a retrospective analysis five years of more after active periodontal treatment.* J Clin Periodontol 2006;33:53-61.

[42] Dietrich T, Bernimoulin JP, Glynn RJ. *The effect of cigarette smoking on gingival bleeding.* J Periodontol 2004;75:16-22.

[43] Dietrich T, Kaye EK, Nunn ME, Van Dyke T, Garcia RI. *Gingivitis susceptibility and its relation to periodontitis in men.* J Dent Res 2006;85:1134-7.

[44] Dolan TA, Gilbert GH, Ringelberg ML, Legler DW, Antonson DE, Foerster U, Heft MW. *Behavioral risk indicators of attachment loss in adult Floridians.* J Clin Periodontol 1997;24:223-232.

[45] Dorland. *Dorland's illustrated medical dictionary.* Oxford, UK:WB Sauders, 2000.

[46] Drury TF, Garcia I, Adesanya M. *Socioeconomic disparities in adult oral health in the United States* Ann NY Acad Sci 1999;896:322-324.

[47] Duarte PM, Assis DR, Casati MZ, Sallum AW, Sallum EA, Nociti FH Jr. *Alendronate may protect against increased periodontitis-related bone loss in estrogen-deficient rats.* J Periodontol 2004a;75:1196-1202.

[48] Duarte PM, Gonçalves PF, Sallum AW, Sallum EA, Casati MZ, Nociti FH Jr *Effect of an estrogen-deficient state and its therapy on bone loss resulting from an experimental periodontitis in rats.* J Periodontol 2004b;39:107-110.

[49] Duarte PM, Gonçalves PF, Casati MZ, de Toledo S, Sallum EA, Nociti FH Jr. *Estrogen and alendronate therapies may prevent the influence of estrogen deficiency on the tooth-supporting alveolar bone: a histometric stuady in rats.* J Periodont Res 2006;41:541-546.

[50] Duarte PM, de Oliveira MCG, Tambelli CH, Parada CA, Casati MZ, Nociti FH Jr. *Overexpression of interleukin-1β and interleukin-6 may play an important role in periodontal breakdown in type 2 diabetic patients.* J Periodont Res 2007;42:377-381.

[51] Eggert FM, McLeod MH, Flowerdew G. *Effects of smoking and treatment status on periodontal bacteria: evidence that smoking influences control of periodontal bacteria at the mucosal surface of the gingival crevice.* J Periodontol 2001;72:1210-1220.

[52] Eickholz P, Kaltschmitt J, Berbig J, Reitmeir P, Pretzl B. *Tooth loss after active periodontal therapy. 1: patient-related factors for risk, prognosis, and quality outcome.* J Clin Periodontol 2008;35:165-74.

[53] Emrich LJ, Shlossman M, Genco RJ. *Periodontal disease in non-insulin-dependent diabetes mellitus.* J Periodontol 1991;2:123-131.

[54] Eriksen EF, Colvard DS, Berg NJ, Graham ML, Mann KG, Spelsberg TC, Riggs BL. *Evidence of estrogen receptors in normal human osteoblast-like cells.* Science 1988;241:84-86.

[55] Ezzo PJ, Cutler CW. *Microorganisms as risk indicators for periodontal disease.* Periodontol 2000 2003;32:24-35.

[56] Faggion CM Jr, Petersilka G, Lange DE, Gerss J, Flemmig TF. *Prognostic model for tooth survival in patients treated for periodontitis.* J Clin Periodontol. 2007;34:226-31.

[57] Franceschi C, Bonafè M, Valensin S, Olivieri F, de Luca M, Ottaviani E, De Benedictis G. *Inflamm-aging. An evolutionary perspective on immunosenescence.* Ann NY Acad Sci 2000;908:244-54.

[58] Fredriksson MI, Figueredo CM, Gustafsson A, Bergström KG, Asman BE. *Effects of periodontitis and smoking on blood leukocytes and acute-phase proteins.* J Periodontol 1999;70:1355-1360.

[59] Galbraith GM, Steed RB, Sanders JJ, Pandey JP. *Tumor necrosis factor alpha production by oral leukocytes: influence of tumor necrosis factor genotype.* J Periodontol 1998;69:428-433.

[60] Gemmell E, Seymour GJ. *Immunoregulatory control of Th1/Th2 cytokine profiles in periodontal disease.* Periodontol 2000 2004;35:21-41.

[61] Geurs NC. *Osteoporosis and periodontal disease.* Periodontol 2000 2007;44:29-43.

[62] Giddon DB, Zackin SJ, Goldhaber P. *Acute necrotizing ulcerative gingivitis in college students.* J Am Dent Assoc 1964: 68:380-386.

[63] Girasole G, Passeri G, Pedrazzoni M, Giuliani N, Passeri M. Interleukin-6: *A pathogenic role in the postmenopausal osteoporosis?* Acta Biomed Ateneo Parmense 1995;66:125-138.

[64] Goldman MJ, Ross LF, Goteiner D. *Effect of periodontal therapy on patients maintained for 15 years or longer. A retrospective study.* J Periodontol 1986;6:347-353.

[65] Gonzales JR, Kobayashi T, Michel J, Mann M, Yoshie H, Meyle J. *Interleukin-4 gene polymorphisms in Japanese and Caucasian patients with aggressive periodontitis.* J Clin Periodontol 2004;31:384-389.

[66] Graves DT, Cochran D. *The contribution of interleukin-1 and tumor necrosis factor to periodontal tissue destruction.* J Periodontol 2003;74:391-401.

[67] Grupe H, Wilder L. *Observations of necrotizing gingivitis in 870 military trainees.* J Periodontol 1956;45:255-266.

[68] Haffajee AD, Socransky SS, Smith C, Dibart S. *Relation of baseline microbial parameters to future periodontal attachment loss.* J Clin Periodontol 1991;18:744-750.

[69] Haffajee AD, Socransky SS. *Relationship of cigarette smoking to attachment level profiles.* J Clin Periodontol 2001;28:283-295.

[70] Hassell TM, Harris EL. *Genetic influences in caries and periodontal disease.* Crit Rev Oral Biol Med 1995;6:319-342.

[71] Haubek D, Ennibi OK, Poulsen K, Vaeth M, Poulsen S, Kilian M. *Risk of aggressive periodontitis in adolescent carriers of the JP2 clone of Aggregatibacter (Actinobacillus) actinomycetencomitans in Morocco: a prospective longitudinal cohort study.* Lancet 2008;371:237-242.

[72] Heitz-Mayfield LJA. *Disease progression: identification of high risk groups and individuals for periodontitis.* J Clin Periodontol 2005;32(Suppl 6):196-209.

[73] Hodge P, Michalowicz B. *Gentic predisposition to periodontitis in children and young adults.* Periodontol 2000 2001;26:113-134.

[74] Holla LI, Fassman A, Vasku A, Goldbergova M, Beranek M, Znojil V, Vanek J, Vacha J. *Genetic variations in the human gelatinase a (matrix metalloproteinase-2) promoter are not associated with susceptibility to, and severity of, chronic periodontitis.* J Periodontol 2005;76:1056-1060.

[75] Huynh-Ba G, Lang NP, Tonetti MS, Salvi GE. *The association of the composite IL-1 genotype with periodontitis progression and/or treatment outcomes: a systematic review.* J Clin Periodontol 2007;34:305-317.

[76] Hyman JJ, Reid BC. *Epidemiologic risk factors for periodontal attachment loss among adults in the United States.* J Clin Periodontol 2003;30:230-237.

[77] Ioannidis JP, Trikalinos TA, Khoury MJ. *Implications of small effect sizes of individual genetic variants on the design and interpretation of genetic association studies of complex diseases.* Am J Epidemiol 2006;164:609-614.

[78] Itagaki M, Kubota T, Tai H, Shimada Y, Morozumi T, Yamazaki K. *Matrix metalloproteinase-1 and -3 gene promoter polymorphisms in Japanese patints with periodontitis.* J Clin Periodontol 2004;31:764-769.

[79] Jeffcoat MK, Lewis CE, Reddy MS, Wang C-Y, Redford M. *Post-menopausal bone loss and its relationship to oral bone loss.* Periodontol 2000 2000;23:94-102.

[80] Johnson GK, Guthmiller JM. *The impact of cigarette smoking on periodontal disease and treatment.* Periodontol 2000 2007;44:178-194.

[81] Joss A, Adler R, Lang NP. Bleeding on probing. *A parameter for monitoring periodontal conditions in clinical practice.* J Clin Periodontol 1994;6:402-408.

[82] Kanis JA, Melton LJ III, Christiansen C, Johnston CG, Khaltaev N. *The diagnosis of osteoporosis.* J Bone Miner Res 1994;9:1137-1141.

[83] Karjalainen K, Knuuttila M. *The onset of diabetes and poor metabolic control increases gingival bleeding in children and adolescents with insulin-dependent diabetes mellitus.* J Clin Periodontol 1996;23:1060-1067.

[84] Kinane DF, Hart TC. *Genes and gene polymorphisms associated with periodontal disease.* Crit Rev Oral Biol Med 2003;14:430-449.

[85] Kobayashi T, Yamamoto K, Sugita N, van der Pol W-L, Yasuda K, Kaneko S, van der Winkel JGJ, Yoshie H. *The Fcγ Receptor genotype as a severity factor for chronic periodontitis in Japanese patients.* J Periodontol 2001;72:1324-1331.

[86] Kornman KS, Crane A, Wang Hy, di Giovine FS, Newman MG, Pirk FW, Wilson TG Jr, Higginbottom FL, Duff GW. *The interleukin-1 genotype as a severity factor in adult periodontal disease.* J Clin Periodontol 1997;24:72-77.

[87] Kribbs PJ, Smith DE, Chesnut CH. *Oral findings in osteoporosis. Part II: Relationship between residual ridge and alveolar bone resorption and generalized skeletal osteo penia.* J Prosthetic Dent 1983;50:719-724.

[88] Kribbs PJ, Chesnut CH, Ott SM, Kilcoyne RF. *Relationships between mandibular and skeletal bone in an osteoporotic population.* J Prosthetic Dent 1989;62:703-707.

[89] Kribbs PJ. *Comparison of mandibular bone in normal and osteoporotic women.* J Prosthet Dent 1990;63:218-222.

[90] Labriola A, Needleman I, Moles DR. *Systematic review of the effect of smoking on nonsurgical periodontal therapy.* Ann Periodontol 2000;5:79-89.

[91] Lang NP, Tonetti MS. *Periodontal risk assessment (PRA) for patients in supportive periodontal therapy (SPT).* Oral Health Prev Dent 2003;1:7-16.

[92] Lang NP, Schätzle MA, Löe H. *Gingivitis as a risk factors in periodontal disease.* J Clin Periodontol 2009;36(Suppl 10):3-8.

[93] Leknes KN, Lie T, Selvig KA. *Root grooves: a risk factor in periodontal attachment loss.* J Periodontol 1994;9:859-863.

[94] Lindberg MK, Erlandsson M, Alatalo SL, Windahl S, Andersson G, Halleen JM, Carlsten H, Gustafsson JA, Ohlsson C. *Estrogen receptor alpha, but not estrogen receptor beta, is involved in the regulation of the OPG/RANKL (osteo protegerin/ receptor activator of NF-kappa B ligand) ratio and serum interleukin-6 in male mice.* Endocrinol 2001;171:425-433.

[95] Lindhe J, Haffajee AD, Socransky SS. *Progression of periodontal disease in adult subjects in the absence of periodontal therapy.* J Clin Periodontol 1983;10:433-442.

[96] Lindhe J, Nyman S. *Long-term maintenance of patients treated for advanced periodontal disease.* J Clin Periodontol 1984;8:504-514.

[97] Lindhe J, Socransky S, Nyman S, Westfelt E, Haffajee A. *Effect of age on healing following periodontal therapy.* J Clin Periodontol 1985;12:774-787

[98] Listgarten MA, Slots J, Nowotny AH, Oler J, Rosenberg J, Gregor B, Sullivan P. *Incidence of periodontitis recurrence in treated patients with and without cultivable Actinobacillus actinomycetemcomitans, Prevotella intermedia, and Porphyromonas gingivalis: a prospective study.* J Periodontol 1991;62:377-386.

[99] Loe H, Theilade E, Jensen B. *Experimental gingivitis in man.* J Periodontol 1965;36:177-187.

[100] Loe H, Anerud A, Boysen H, Morrison E. *Natural history of periodontal disease in man. Rapid, moderate and no loss of attachment in Sri Lanka laborers 14 to 46 years of age.* J Clin Periodontol 1986;13:431-445.

[101] Loe H. Periodontal disease. *The sixth complication of diabetes mellitus.* Diabetes Care 1993;16:329-334.

[102] Loos BG, Leppers-van de Straat FG, Van de Winkel JG, Van der Velden U. *Fc gamma receptor polymorphisms in relation to periodontitis.* J Clin Periodontol 2003;30:595-602.

[103] Loos BG, John RP, Laine ML. *Identification of geneticrisk factors for parioodontitis and possible mechanisms of action.* J Clin Periodontol 2005;32(Suppl.6):159-179.

[104] MacFarlane TW, Jenkins WM, Gilmour WH, McCourtie J, McKenzie D. *Longitudinal study of untreated periodontitis (II). Microbiological findings.* J Clin Periodontol 1988;15:331-337.

[105] MacFarlane GD, Herzberg MC, Wolff LF, Hardie NA. *Refractory periodontitis associated with abnormal polymorphonuclear leukocyte phagocytosis and cigarette smoking.* J Periodontol 1992;63:908-913.

[106] Machtei EE, Dunford R, Hausmann E, Grossi SG, Powell J, Cummins D, Zambon JJ, Genco RJ. *Longitudinal study of prognostic factors in established periodontitis patients.* J Clin Periodontol 1997;2:102-109.

[107] Machtei EE, Hausmann E, Dunford R, Grossi S, Ho A, Davies G, Chandler J, Zambon J, Genco RJ. *Longitudinal studies of predictive factors for periodontal disease and tooth loss.* J Clin Periodontol 1999;6:374-380.

[108] Manoucher-Pour M, Spagnuolo PJ, Rodman HM, Bissada NF. *Comparison of neutrophil chemotactic response in diabetic patients with mild and severe periodontal disease.* J Periodontol 1981;52:410-415.

[109] McGuire MK, Nunn ME. *Prognosis versus actual outcome. IV. The effectiveness of clinical parameters and IL-1 genotype in accurately predicting prognoses and tooth survival.* J Periodontol 1999;70:49-56.

[110] McMullen JA, Van Dyke TE, Horoszewicz HU, Genco RJ. *Neutrophil chemotaxis in individuals with advanced periodontal disease and a genetic predisposition to diabetes mellitus.* J Periodontol 1981;52:167-173.

[111] Mealey BL, Ocampo GL. *Diabetes mellitus and periodontal disease.* Periodontol 2000 2007;44:127-153.

[112] Meisel P, Carlsson LE, Sawaf H, Fanghaenel J, Greinacher A, Kocher T. *Polymorphisms of Fcγ-receptors RIIa, RIIIa, and RIIIb in patients with adult periodontal diseases.* Genes Immun 2001;2:258-262.

[113] Michalowicz BS, Aeppli D, Kuba RK, Bereuter JE, Conry JP, Segal NL, Bouchard TJ Jr, Pihlstrom BL. *A twin study of genetic variation in proportional radiographic alveolar bone height.* J Dent Res 1991;70:1431-1435.

[114] Michalowicz BS, Aeppli D, Virag JG, Klump DG, Hinrichs JE, Segal NL, BouchardTJ Jr, Pihlstrom BL. *Periodontal findings in adult twins.* J Periodontol 1991;62(5):293-299.

[115] Michalowicz BS, Diehl SR, Gunsolley JC, Sparks BS, Brooks CN, Koertge TE, Califano JV, Burmeister JA, Schenkein HA. *Evidence of a substantial genetic basis for risk of adult periodontitis.* J Periodontol 2000;71:1699-1707.

[116] Miller DB, O'Callaghan JP. *Neuroendocrine aspects of the response to stress.* Metabolism 2002;51:5-10.

[117] Mullally BH, Linden GJ. *Mollar furcation involvement associated with cigarette smoking in periodontal referrals.* J Clin Periodontol 1996;23:658-661.

[118] Muzzi L, Nieri M, Cattabriga M, Rotundo R, Cairo F, Pini Prato GP. *The potential prognostic value of some periodontal factors for tooth loss: a retrospective multi-level analysis on periodontal patients treated and maintained over 10 years.* J Periodontol 2006;77:2084-2089.

[119] Neely AL, Holford TR, Loe H, Anerud A, Boysen H. *The natural history of periodontal disease in man. Risk factors for progression of attachment loss in individuals receiving no oral health care.* J Periodontol 2001;8:1006-1015.

[120] Nielsen R. *Population genetic analysis of ascertained SNP data.* Hum Genomics 2004;1:218-224.

[121] Nikolopoulos GK, Dimou NL, Hamodrakas SJ, Bagos PG. *Cytokine gene polymorphisms in periodontal disease: a meta-analysis of 53 studies including 4178 cases and 4590 controls.* J Clin Periodontol 2008;34:305-317.

[122] Nociti FH Jr, Nogueira-Filho GR, Primo MT, Machado MAN, Tramontina VA, Barros SP, Sallum EA. *The influence of nicotine on the bone loss rate in ligature-induced periodontitis. A hystometric study in rats.* J Periodontol 2000;71:1460-1464.

[123] Nociti FH Jr, Nogueira-Filho GR, Tramontina VA, Machado MAN, Barros SP, Sallum EA, Sallum AW. *Histometric evaluation of the effect of nicotine administration on periodontal breakdown.* J Periodont Res 2001;36:361-366.

[124] Novak MJ, Potter RM, Blodgett J, Ebersole J. *Periodontal disease in Hispanic Americans with type 2 diabetes.* J Periodontol 2008;79:629-636.

[125] Nunn ME, Harrel SK. *The effect of occlusal discrepancies on periodontitis. I. Relationship of initial occlusal discrepancies to initial clinical parameters.* J Periodontol 2001;4:485-494.

[126] Nunn ME. *Understanding the etiology of peridontitis: an overview of periodontal risk factors.* Periodontol 2000 2003;32:11-23.

[127] Offenbacher S, Zambon JJ. *Consensus report for periodontal diseases: pathogenesis and microbial factors.* Ann Periodontol 1996;1:926-932.

[128] Oursler MJ. *Estrogen regulation of gene expression in osteoblasts and osteoclasts.* Crit Rev Eukariot Gene Expr 1998;8:125-140.

[129] Pacifici R. *Is there a causal role for IL-1 in postmenopausal bone loss?* Calcif Tissue Int 1992;50:295-299.

[130] Page RC, Krall EA, Martin J, Mancl L, Garcia RI. *Validity and accuracy of a risk calculator in predicting periodontal disease.* J Am Dent Assoc 2002;133:569-576.

[131] Page RC, Martin J, Krall EA, Mancl L, Garcia R. *Longitudinal validation of a risk calculator for periodontal disease.* J Clin Periodontol 2003; 9:819-827.

[132] Papapanou PN, Wennström JL, Gröndahl K. *Periodontal status in relation to age and tooth type. A cross-sectional radiographic study.* J Clin Periodontol 1988;15:469-478.

[133] Papapanou EN, Wennstrom JL, Grondahl K. *A 10-year retrospective study of periodontal disease progression.* J Clin Periodontol 1989;16:403-411.

[134] Papapanou PN. World *Workshop in Clinical Periodontics. Periodontal diseases: epidemiology.* Ann Periodontol 1996;1:1-36.

[135] Paunio K. *Periodontal connective tissue. Biochemical studies of disease in man.* Suom Hammaslaak Toim 1969;65:249-290.

[136] Persson GR, Attstrom R, Lang NP, Page RC. *Perceived risk of deteriorating periodontal conditions.* J Clin Periodontol 2003;11:982-989.

[137] Peruzzo DC, Benatti BB, Ambrosano GMB, Nogueira-Filho GR, Sallum EA, Casati MZ, Nociti FH Jr. *A systematic review of stress and psychological factors as possible risk factors for periodontal disease.* J Periodontol 2007;78:1491-1504.

[138] Peruzzo DC, Benatti BB, Antunes IB, Andersen ML, Sallum EA, Casati MZ, Nociti FH Jr, Nogueira-Filho GR. *Chronic stress may modulate periodontal disease: a study in rats.* J Periodontol 2008;79:697-704.

[139] Phipps KR, Chan BKS, Jennings-Holt M, Geurs NC, Reddy MS, Lewis CE, Orwoll ES. *Periodontal health of older men: the MrOS dental study.* Gerodontology 2009;26:122-129.

[140] Pirhan D, Atilla G, Emingil G, Sorsa T, Tervahartiala T, Berdeli A. *Effect of MMP-1 promoter polymorphisms on GCF MMP-1 levels and outcome of periodontal therapy in patients with severe chronic periodontitis.* J Clin Periodontol 2008;35:862-870.

[141] Pociot F, Molvig J, Wogensen L, Worsaae H, Nerup J. *A TaqI polymorphism in the human interleukin-1 beta (IL-1 beta) gene correlates with IL-1 beta secretion in vivo.* Eur J Clin Invest 1992;22:396-402.

[142] Pontes-Andersen CC, Flyvbjerg A, Buschard K, Holmstrup P. *Relationship between periodontitis and diabetes: lessons from rodent studies.* J Periodontol 2007;78:1264-1275.

[143] Poulton R, Caspi A, Milne BJ, Thomson WM, Taylor A, Sears MR, Moffitt TE. *Association between children's experience of socioeconomic disadvantage and adult health: a life-course study.* Lancet 2002;360:1640-5.

[144] Preber H, Bergström J. *Effect of cigarette smoking on periodontal healing following surgical therapy.* J Clin Periodontol 1990;17:324-328.

[145] Pretzl B, Kaltschmitt J, kim T-S, Reitmeir P, Eickholz P. *Tooth loss after active periodontal therapy.2: tooth-related factors.* J Clin Periodontol 2008;35:175-182.

[146] Quinn SM, Zhang JB, Gunsolley JC, Schenkein HA, Tew Jg. *The influence of smoking and race on adult periodontitis and serum IgG2 levels.* J Periodontol 1998;69:171-177.

[147] Reinhardt RA, Payne JB, Maze CA, Patil KD, Gallagher SJ, Mattson JS. *Influence of estrogen and osteopenia/osteoporosis on clinical periodontitis in postmenopausal women.* J Periodontol 1999;70:823-828.

[148] Renvert S, Persson GR. *A systematic review on the use of residual probing depth, bleeding on probing and furcation status following initial periodontal therapy to predict further attachment and tooth loss.* J Clin Periodontol 2002;3:82-89.

[149] Renvert S, Persson GR. *Supportive periodontal therapy.* Periodontol 2000 2004;36:179-195.

[150] Repeke CE, Trombone APF, Ferreira SB Jr, Cardoso CR, Silveira EM, Martins W Jr, Trevilatto PC, Silva JS, Campanelli AP, Garlet GP. *Strong and persistent microbial and inflammatory stimuli overcome the genetic predisposition to higher matrix matalloproteinase -1 (MMP-1) expression: a mechanistic explanation for the lack of association of MMP1-1607 single-nucleotide polymorphism genotypes with MMP-1 expression in chronic periodontitis lesions.* J Clin Periodontol 2009;36:726-738.

[151] Riley V. *Psychoneuroendocrine influences on immunocompetence and neoplasia.* Science 1981;212:1100-1109.

[152] Rodenburg JP, van Winkelhof AJ, Winkel EG, Goené RJ, Abbas F, de Graff J. *Occurrence of Bacteroides gingivalis, Bacteroides intermedius and Actinobacillus actinomycetencomitans in severe periodontitis in relation to age and treatment history.* J Clin Periodontol 1990;17:392-399.

[153] Ronderos M, Jacobs DR, Himes JH, Pihlstrom BL. *Associations of periodontal disease with femoral bone mineral density and estrogen replacement therapy: cross-sectional evaluation of US adults from NHANES III.* J Clin Periodontol 2000;27:778-786.

[154] Rosa GM, Lucas GQ, Lucas ON. *Cigarette smoking and alveolar bone in young adults: a study using digitized radiographs.* J Periodontol 2008;79:232-244.

[155] Rosania AE, Low KG, McCormick CM, Rosania DA. *Stress, depression, cortisol and periodontal disease.* J Periodontol 2009;80:260-266.

[156] Ryder MI, Fujitaki R, Johnson G, Hyun W. *Alterations of netrophil oxidative burst by in vitro smoke exposure: implications for oral and systemic diseases.* Ann Periodontol 1998;3:76-87.

[157] Ryder MI, Saghizadeh M, Ding Y, Nguyen N, Soskolne A. *Effects of tobacco smoking on the secretion of IL-1ββ, TNF-αα and TGF-ββ from peripheral blood mononuclear cells.* Oral Microbiol Immunol 2002;17:331-336.

[158] Ryder MI. *The influence of smoking on host responses in periodontal infections.* Periodontol 2000 2007;43:267-277.

[159] Salvi GE, Yalda B, Collins JG, Jones BH, Smith FW, Arnold RR, Offenbacher S. *Inflammatory mediator response as a potential risk marker for periodontal diseases in insulin-dependent diabetes mellitus patients.* J Periodontol 1997a;68:127-135.

[160] Salvi GE, Collins JG, Yalda B, Arnold RR, Lang NP, Offenbacher S. *Monocytic TNF-α secretion patterns in IDDM patients with periodontal diseases.* J Clin Periodontol 1997b;24:8-16.

[161] Sastrowijoto SH, Hillemans P, van Steenberghe TJ, Abraham-Inpijn L, de Graff J. *Periodontal condition and microbiology of healthy and diseased periodontal pockets in type 1 diabetes mellitus patients.* J Clin Periodontol 1989;16:316-322.

[162] Sbordone L, Ramaglia L, Barone A, Ciaglia RN, Iacono VJ. *Periodontal status and subgingival microbiota of insulin-dependent juvenile diabetics: a 3-year longitudinal study.* J Periodontol 1998;69:120-128.

[163] Schätzle M, Lang NP, Anerud A, Boysen H, Burgin W, Löe H. *The influence of margins of restorations on the periodontal tissues over 26 years.* J Clin Periodontol 2001;1:57-64.

[164] Schätzle M, Löe H, Lang NP, Heitz-Mayfield LJA, Bürgin W, Anerud A, Boysen H. *Clinical course of chronic periodontitis: III. Patterns, variations and risks of attachment loss.* J Clin Periodontol 2003;30:909-918.

[165] Severson JA, Moffett BC, Kokich V, Selipsky H. *A histologic study of age changes in the adult human joint (ligament).* J Periodontol 1978;49:189-200.

[166] Shiba H, Nakanishi K, Sakata M, Fujita T, Uchida Y, Kurihara H. *Effects of ageing on proliferative ability, and the expressions of secreted protein, acidic and rich cysteine (SPARC) and osteoprotegerin (osteoclastogenesis inhibitory factor) in cultures of human periodontal ligament cells.* Mech Ageing Dev 2000;117(1-3):69-77.

[167] Socransky SS, Haffajee AD, Smith C, Duff GW. *Microbiological parameters associated with IL-1 gene polymorphisms in periodontitis patients.* J Clin Periodontol 2000;27:810-818.

[168] Soskolne WA, Klinger A. *The relationship between periodontal diseases and diabetes: an overview.* Ann Periodontol 2001;1:91-98.

[169] de Souza AP, Trevilatto PC, Scarel-Caminaga RM, Brito Jr RB, *Line SRP. MMP-1 promoter polymorphism: association with chronic periodontitis severity in a Brazilian population.* J Clin Periodontol 2003;30:154-158.

[170] Stein JM, Machulla HKG, Smeets R, lampert F, Reichert S. *Human leukocyte antigen polymorphism in chronic and aggressive periodontitis among Caucasians: a meta-analysis.* J Clin Periodontol 2008;35:183-192.

[171] Takada T, Yoshinari N, Sugiishi S, Kawase H, Yamani T, Noguchi T. *Effect of restraint stress on the progression of experimental periodontitis in rats.* J Periodontol 2004;75:306-315.

[172] Tanaka M, Ejiri S, Toyooka E, Kohno S, Ozawa H. *Effects of ovariectomy on trabecular structures of rat alveolar bone.* J Periodont Res 2002;37:161-165.

[173] Taylor GW, Burt BA, Becker MP, Genco RJ, Shlossman M, Knowler WC, Pettitt DJ. *Non-insulin dependent diabetes mellitus and alveolar bone loss progression over 2 years.* J Periodontol 1998;1:76-83.

[174] Taylor JJ, Preshaw PM, Donaldson PT. *Cytokine gene polymorphism and immunoregulation in periodontal disease.* Periodontol 2000;35:158-182.

[175] Tervonen T, Karjalainen K. *Periodontal disease related to diabetic status. A pilot study of the response to periodontal therapy in type 1 diabetes.* J Clin Periodontol 1997;7:505-510.

[176] Tezal M, Wactawski-Wende J, Grossi SG, Ho AW, Dunford R, Genco RJ. *The relationship between bone mineral density and periodontitis in postmenopausal women.* J Periodontol 2000;71:1492-1498.

[177] Timmerman MF, Van der Weijden GA, Abbas F, Arief EM, Armand S, Winkel EG, Van Winkelhoff AJ, Van der Velden U. *Untreated periodontal disease in Indonesian adolescents. Longitudinal clinical data and prospective clinical and microbiological risk assessment.* J Clin Periodontol 2000;27:932-942.

[178] Tomar SL, Asma S. *Smoking-attributable periodontitis in the United States: findings from NHANES III.* J Periodontol 2000;71:743-751.

[179] Torrungruang K, Nisapakultorn K, Sitdhibhisal S, Tamsailom S, Rojanasomsith K, Vanichjakvong O, Prapakamol S, Premsirinirund T, Pusiri T, Jaratkulangkoon O, Kusump S, Rajatanavin R. *The effect of cigarette smoking on the severity of periodontal disease among older Thai adults.* J Periodontol 2005;76:566-572.

[180] Tran SD, Rudney JD, Sparks BS, Hodges JS. *Persistence presence of Bacteroides forsythus as a risk factor for attachment loss in a population with low prevalence and severity of adult periodontitis.* J Periodontol 2001;72:1-10.

[181] Van der Velden U, Varoufaki A, Hutter JW, Xu L, Timmerman MF, Van Winkelhoff AJ, Loos BG. *Effect of smoking and periodontal treatment on the subgingival microflora.* J Clin Periodontol 2003;30:603-610

[182] Van der Weijden GA, de Slegte C, Timmerman MF, Van der Velden U. *Periodontitis in smokers and non-smokers: intra-oral distribution of pockets.* J Clin Periodontol 2001;28:955-960.

[183] Wactawski-Wende J, Grossi SG, Trevisan M, Genco RJ, Tezal M, Dunford RG, Ho AW, Hausmann E, Hreshchyshyn MM. *The role of osteopenia in oral bone loss and periodontal disease.* J Periodontol 1996 67(Suppl 10):1076-1084.

[184] Wagner J, Kaminski WE, Aslanidis C, Moder D, Hiller K-A, Christgau M, Schmitz G, Schmalz G. *Prevalence of OPG and IL-1 gene polymorphisms in chronic periodontitis.* J Clin Periodntol 2007;34:823-827.

[185] Wendell KJ, Stein SH. *Regulation of cytokine production I human gingival fibroblasts following treatment with nicotine and lipopolysaccharide.* J Periodontol 2001;72:1038-1044.

[186] Westfelt E, Rylander H, Blohme G, Jonasson P, Lindhe J. *The effect of periodontal therapy in diabetics results after 5 years.* J Clin Periodontol 1996;23:92-100.

[187] Weyant RJ, Pearlstein ME, Churak AP, Forrest K, Famili P, Cauley JA. *The association between osteopenia and periodontal attachment loss in older women.* J Periodontol 1999;5:85-95.

[188] Wimmer G, Janda M, Wieselmann-Penkner K, Jakse N, Polansky R, Pertl C. *Coping with stress: its influence on periodontal disease.* J Periodontol 2002;73:1343-1351.

[189] Wimmer G, Köhldorfer G, Mischak I, Lorenzoni M, Kallus KW. *Coping with stress:its influence on periodontal therapy.* J Periodontol 2005;76:90-98.

[190] Yasuda H, Shima N, Nakagawa N, Mochizuki SI, Yano K, Fujise N, Sato Y, Goto M, Yamagushi K, Kuriyama M, Kanno T, Murakami A, Tsuda E, Morinaga T, Higashio K. *Identity of osteoclastogenesis inhibitory factor (OCIF) and osteoprotegerin (OPG): A mechanism by which OPG/OCIF inhibits osteoclastogenesis in vitro.* Endocrinology 1998;139:1329-1337.

[191] Yoshihara A, Seida Y, Hanada N, Miyazaki H. *A longitudinal study of the relationship between periodontal disease and bone mineral density in community-dwelling older adults.* J Clin Periodontol 2004;31:680-684.

[192] Zambom JJ, Grossi SG, Machtei EE, Ho AW, Dunford R, Genco RJ. *Cigarette smoking increases the risk for subgingival infection with periodontal pathogens.* J Periodontol 1996;67(Suppl. 10):1050-1054.

[193] Zinkernagel RM, Doherty PC. *The discovery of MHC restriction.* Immunol Today 1997;18:14-7.

In: Periodontitis Symptoms, Treatment and Prevention   ISBN: 978-1-61668-836-3
Editor: Rosemarie E. Walchuck, pp. 35-72   ©2010 Nova Science Publishers, Inc.

Chapter 2

TREATMENT OF PERIODONTITIS

S. Raja[*]

Senior Lecturer, Modern Dental College and Research Centre, Airport Road,
Gandhinagar, Indore-453112. Madhya Pradesh, India.

RATIONALE OF PERIODONTAL TREATMENT

The goals of periodontal therapy according to the American Academy of Periodontology are to alter or get rid of the microbial etiology and causative risk factors for periodontitis, thus arresting the progression of disease and preserving the dentition in a state of health, comfort, and function with appropriate esthetics; and to prevent the recurrence of periodontitis. In addition, regeneration of the periodontal attachment apparatus, where indicated, may be attempted [1]. Mechanical debridement of the pocket has shown to significantly reduce the risk of tooth loss, slow down the rate of periodontal disease progression and improve gingival health [2,3].

After establishing a definite diagnosis of Periodontitis, a treatment plan is formulated initiated by Initial therapy. Also known as cause related therapy, initial therapy is aimed at controlling the etiologic agents for gingivitis and periodontitis and arresting further progression of periodontal tissue destruction. The Objectives of Initial therapy are: [4]

- ❖ Motivating the patient to understand and control dental disease.
- ❖ Instructions to the patient regarding self performed plaque control methods.
- ❖ Scaling and root planing.
- ❖ Removal of additional retention factors for plaque such as overhanging margins of restorations, ill fitting crowns, etc.

[*] Correspondence: B-204, Staff Quarters, Modern Dental College and Research Centre, Airport Road, Gandhinagar, Indore-453112. Madhya Pradesh, India. Phone: 09329729790, 09826642993. E-mail: drrajasridhar@rediffmail.com

TREATMENT GUIDELINES

Certain treatment considerations have been laid down by American Academy of Periodontology (AAP) for treatment of chronic periodontitis with slight to moderate amount of bone loss. There are also certain factors that affect the decision of the treatment and the expected therapeutic result which includes age and systemic health of the patient, compliance, treatment preferences and patient's ability to control plaque. Other factors include the clinician's ability to remove subgingival deposits, restorative and prosthetic demands, and the presence and treatment of teeth with more advanced chronic periodontitis[1].

FLOW CHART : TREATMENT PLAN FOR PERIODONTITIS

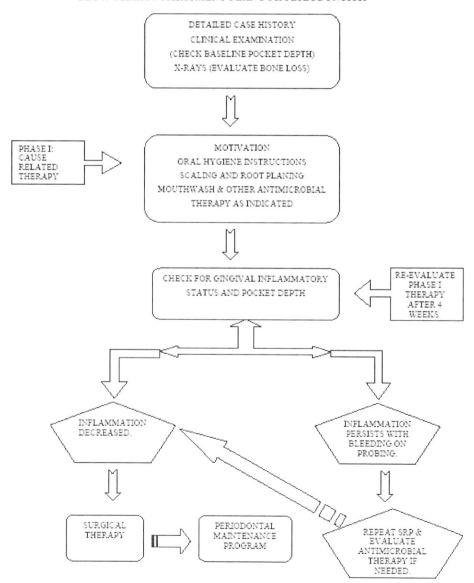

PATIENT MOTIVATION

It is the role of the dental health professional to assist patients to attain and maintain their oral health. Various effective ways are present to motivate people toward preventive dental care in general and toward preventive periodontics in particular. Each patient requires individually tailored oral health advice and information. One of the basic requirements in motivating a patient is communication between patient and the Periodontist. A well informed patient can be motivated easily and hence education and motivation goes hand in hand. Motivating patients for undergoing periodontal therapy is a task requiring considerable skills. This is because emergency care sells itself because the fear of pain and the need for self-preservation are active. The value of preventive measures is less substantial because time, effort and money must be expended to prevent possible future disease. Hence patients tend to neglect the detrimental effects caused by accumulation of plaque and calculus on the soft tissues as periodontal disease is quite painless in the initial, treatable stages and therefore, pain serves no great motivational purpose in causing people to act in a positive manner. Another factor is the lack of social pressure to have a plaque-free mouth[5]. Hence skilful communication with the patient educating him on periodontal maintenance and making him recognize the need for therapy is essential.

There are two procedures important for patient motivation [6,7]

1) Motivational interviewing
2) Stages of change model

Motivational interviewing involves a directive, patient centred counselling style that is compatible with the patient-centred clinical method. It encourages patients to speak and by doing so enables them to identify their oral health needs. The health professional acts as a medium only intervening when necessary thus allowing patients to recognise inner resistances reflected in lifestyle barriers. Although motivational interviewing was developed for use by addiction counsellors, some of its practical guidelines can be adapted for use in oral health settings. The Periodontist must take considerable time to explain to his patients regarding the importance of good periodontal health and bone support for survival of a sound tooth structure. Also the dentist should provide an atmosphere in which patients feel comfortable to speak, question and discuss the priority of their oral health needs. The dentist also has to evaluate the result of his counselling with the patient wherein the stages of change model can assist dental health professionals in their work with patients. It provides a framework by which they may evaluate their patients' progress from unawareness through motivation to compliance. The 'stages of change model' devised by Prochaska and DiClemente is divided into six different stages of behaviour change[8]. These are precontemplation, contemplation, preparation, action, maintenance and relapse. The stages reflect and hence provide a means of assessing progress from unawareness (precontemplation) through motivation (contemplation, preparation) to compliance (action, maintenance) [6]. Hence by using motivational interviewing and stages of change model, dentist can aid behavioural change in their patients and to achieve a long term goal of a stable dentition. Disclosing agents are used as motivational aids to educate patients to improve the efficiency of plaque control procedures. These agents are solutions or wafers which stain plaque on teeth and bacterial deposits on tongue and gingiva. They are applied on to teeth using cotton swabs or solution is used as rinses. Hence disclosing agents are used as plaque control instruction in the dental office.

SCALING AND ROOTPLANING

SCALING: Is defined as the instrumentation of the crown and root surfaces of the teeth to remove plaque, calculus, and stains from these surfaces [9].

ROOTPLANING: A treatment procedure designed to remove cementum or surface dentin that is rough, impregnated with calculus, or contaminated with toxins or microorganisms[9].

Instruments used for Supra and Sub Gingival Scaling and Root Planning

Treatment process in a periodontitis patient is initiated by supragingival scaling. This removal of plaque and calculus is done using either hand instruments and or ultrasonic instruments. Hand instruments used for this purpose are Supragingival Scalers (Figure 1). Sickle scalers serve as an effective instrument to remove tenacious supragingival calculus from crowns of teeth and are used in a pull motion. The working end of it has unique design characteristics like a pointed tip with a triangular cross section and two cutting edges per working end. This shape makes the tip strong so that it will not break off during use. Both anterior and posterior sickle scalers are available [10,11]

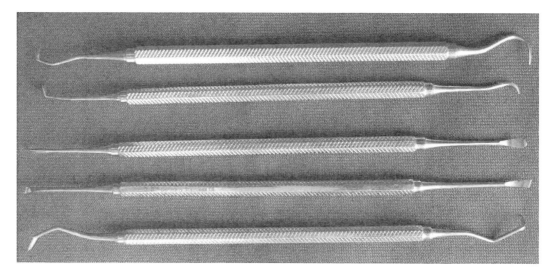

Figure 1. Set of Supragingival Scalers. L to R: Sickle,bifid,Cumine,Surface & Posterior Interdental Scalers.

Instruments with slender working ends are needed for subgingival scaling like the curettes. Curettes are finer than sickle scalers and each working end has a cutting edge on both sides of the blade and a rounded toe without any sharp points or corners. They are used to remove deep subgingival calculus, root planing altered cementum and removing the soft tissue lining the periodontal pocket. Area specific curettes were developed by Dr.Clayton gracey and are popularly known as Gracey Curettes (developed by Hu-friedy manufacturing company) (Figure 2).

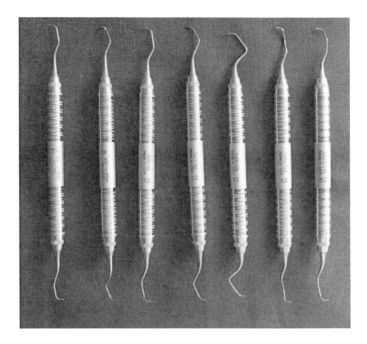

Figure 2. Set of Gracey Curettes. L to R: 1-2, 3-4, 5-6, 7-8, 9-10, 11-12 & 13-14.

Gracey Curettes are designed to adapt specific areas of dentition. Original Gracey series contains 14 single ended curettes, Gracey 1-14. Double ended Gracey curettes are paired as follows:

- Gracey 1-2 & 3-4: For Anterior teeth.
- Gracey 5-6 : For anterior teeth and Premolars.
- Gracey 7-8 & 9-10: For Posterior teeth (Facial and lingual).
- Gracey 11-12 : For Posterior teeth (Mesial).
- Gracey 13-14 : for Posterior teeth (Distal).
- Gracey 15-16 and 17-18 curettes are modifications developed to provide superior access to proximal surfaces of posterior teeth[12].

Ultrasonic and Sonic Instruments

Power driven scalers consists of Ultrasonic and sonic instruments. Sonic scalers operate at a low frequency of 3000 to 8000 cycles per second (cps) with a vibratory tip movement which is linear or elliptical in nature. Ultrasonic scalers are of two types namely Magnetostrictive and Piezoelectric working at a frequency range of 18000-45000 cps and 25000-50000 cps respectively. In magnetostrictive the vibration of the tip is elliptical, linear or circular depending on the type of unit. Here all the sides of the tip are active. In piezoelectric the vibration of the tip is linear or back and forth which allows only two sides of the tip to be active [13] (Figure 3). Removal of plaque and calculus by ultrasonic scalers is accomplished by the vibration of the tip of the instrument, acoustic streaming and cavitation effect. During operation, cooling water flows through the instrument handpiece onto the oscillating tip and the oscillating action of the tip within the water produces acoustic streaming. This causes a change in the streaming velocity to produce large hydrodynamic shear stresses which can disrupt calculus. The water droplets of the spray directed at the tip forms tiny vacuum bubbles that collapse releasing energy in a process called as cavitation which serves to dislodge the calculus and debris [14,15]. One of the disadvantages of using ultrasonic scaler is the production of aerosols. Ultrasonic and sonic scaling is considered to produce the greatest source of aerosol contamination. This occurs due to interaction between the rapidly vibrating tip and the coolant liquid that comes in contact with the tip. The aerosols may contain infectious blood borne and air borne pathogens and is considered as a potential infection threat[16].

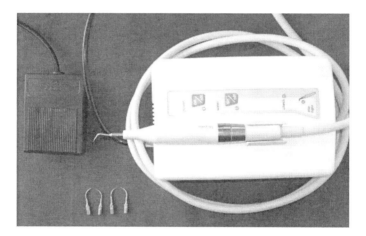

Figure 3. Ultrasonic Scaler with various tip designs.

Quadrant versus Full Mouth Scaling

Hand and power driven instruments are used for instrumentation of the root surfaces. Scaling and root planing can be performed quadrantwise or as a one stage full mouth scaling. Full mouth scaling is claimed by some researchers to be superior to standard scaling and rootplaning (SRP) quadrant wise. It was shown that a single course of SRP reduces the proportions of periodontopathic microorganisms which clearly correlates with improvement of the clinical periodontal parameters [17]. A single course of SRP unfortunately only temporarily reduces the proportions of subgingival pathogenic microorganisms [18] and hence the adjuctive use of antibiotics has been suggested [19]. However, a one stage full mouth disinfection with the use of an antimicrobial mouthrinse like chlorhexidine increases or prolongs the microbiological improvements of subgingival instrumentation without the need for antibiotics in the treatment of patients with Chronic Periodontitis [20,21,22]. Conceptually, this would reduce the microorganisms and diminish the amount of bacteria in the pockets and other intraoral habitats like the tongue, the mucosa, saliva etcs that may be responsible for reinfecting treated sites. Recent studies do not seem to prove that full mouth scaling and root planing is better than quadrantwise therapy. When short term comparison of microbiological changes following quadrantwise and full mouth SRP was done, both the treatment modalities showed similar microbiological outcomes and could not confirm that treated sites were at higher risk for bacterial reinfection in the presence of yet untreated periodontal lesions as in the case of quadrant wise root planing when compared with Full mouth root planing within 24 hours [23]. In another recent study both treatment modalities led to stabilised treatment outcomes over 6 and 12 months in pockets of 4-6mm wherein no significant difference between the groups were present with respect to clinical attachment gain, Probing depth (PD) and Bleeding on probing (BOP) reduction [24].

Greenstein in his critical commentary after reviewing various clinical trials on the topic concluded that the concept of full mouth therapy provided additional benefits compared to partial disinfection [25]. Regardless of the type of modality adapted, a thorough removal of local factors is necessary which cause an improvement in the clinical parameters like BOP, PD and Clinical attachment gain.

Hand versus Power Driven Instruments

Investigations concerning manual and power driven instrumentation of root surfaces have produced conflicting results. Certain studies have reported that hand instruments like curets produce either a smoother surface[26,27] or a rougher surface than ultrasonics[28,29]. A recent meta analysis on the topic clearly revealed that ultrasonic or sonic subgingival debridement can be completed in less time than subgingival debridement using hand instruments30. Although the time taken by power driven instruments is less, the clinical effects i.e gain in clinical attachment or decrease in pocket depth were similar for both hand or ultrasonics[30].

Healing after Scaling and Root Planing (SRP)

There is extensive evidence in support of Scaling and Root planing as an essential and effective component of therapy for inflammatory periodontal disease (Figure 4). In patients with Chronic periodontitis, subgingival debridement in conjunction with supragingival plaque control is an effective treatment in decreasing probing pocket depth and improving the clinical attachment level[31]. A review of nonsurgical mechanical pocket therapy by Cobb reveals mean probing depth reductions of 1.29mm and clinical attachment level gains of 0.55mm after mechanical therapy for initial probing depths of 4-6mm before treatment and probing depth reduction of 2.16mm and attachment level gain of 1.19mm after therapy for initial probing depths of > 6mm before treatment[32]. Lindhe et al determined the critical probing depth for scaling and root planing to be 2.9mm below which loss of attachment occurs following mechanical therapy[33].

Mechanical non surgical therapy has a profound effect on inflammatory components. The effect of scaling and rootplaning on the inflammatory cell subsets leads to a decrease in plasma cells, lymphocytes and immunoglobulin containing cells especially in periodontitis cases[34]. Marked effects are seen with the gingival tissue following mechanical therapy with distinct reduction in bleeding on probing. When collective analysis of the studies performed to evaluate the decrease in bleeding on probing and gingival inflammation was done, a 57% decrease in bleeding on probing was noted after mechanical non surgical therapy [32].

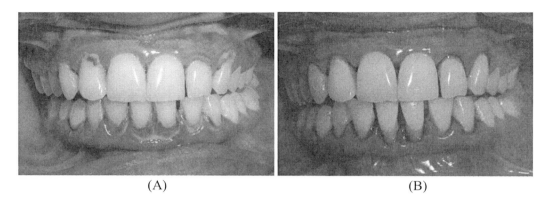

(A)   (B)

Figure 4. A – Plaque and calculus covering gingival third of the teeth. B – Immediately after scaling and root planning.

Positive results of scaling and rootplaning on alveolar bone are well noted with an increase in alveolar bone density. Longitudinal studies with regard to the same were able to demonstrate a statistically significant increase in both superficial and deep average bone densities at 6months and 1 year post treatment which was analysed using standard radiographic technique and digital substraction radiography [35,36]. At the histologic level, scaling and root planing causes a re-establishment or reepithelialization in 2 weeks[37]. Though restoration of the junctional epithelium is complete within 2 weeks, granulation tissue still remains immature and not replaced by collagen fibers. Connective tissue repair continues for 4-8 weeks with specifically oriented collagen bundle fibers [38].

MECHANICAL AND CHEMICAL PLAQUE CONTROL

The responsibility of the dentist to treat a periodontitis patient not only lies in motivating and educating the patient about periodontal procedures and performing non surgical & surgical therapy, but also includes providing instructions to the patient in adequate home care measures like proper brushing, interdental cleaning and use of mouthwashes when needed. Self performed plaque control methods include proper brushing methods, use of interdental aids and mouth washes.

Mechanical Plaque Control

Good plaque control practices are particularly important for periodontal patients. It has been proved if dentogingival plaque is allowed to accumulate freely, subclinical symptoms of gingival inflammation in the form of an exudate from the gingival sulcus appears[39]. It has been noted that plaque growth occurs within a few hours and must be completely removed at least every 48 hours to prevent inflammation in subjects with sound periodontal health[40].

Periodontal patients should completely remove plaque from the teeth at least once every 24 hours because of their demonstrated susceptibility to disease[41]. The prevention and treatment of periodontal diseases are routinely approached by inhibiting plaque formation and instituting mechanical plaque removal measures.

Brushing and flossing is the first line approach to microbial reduction. The ADA recommends brushing for 2 minutes twice a day and flossing once a day[42]. Though tooth brushing remains the bastion of oral health measures, majority of the population do not clean their teeth thoroughly enough to prevent plaque accumulation. Toothbrushes are available in myriad designs in the market. They were initially based on natural materials like hog bristles with a wooden or ivory handle. These natural materials were inherently unhygienic and hence were replaced by nylon filaments and plastic handles.

Tooth Brush Design Recommendations

Manual Toothbrushes

The European workshop on mechanical plaque control in 1998 has provided certain specifications with regard to the design of a toothbrush, the consensus of which is as follows:
43

- ❖ Inclusion of a long contoured handle and the shape of the handle should be according to a particular style of toothbrush use.
- ❖ The head size should be according to the size of the user's mouth.
- ❖ Round ended Nylon or Polyester filaments to be used not larger than 0.23mm in diameter and soft filament configurations.

Bass recommended a straight handled brush with nylon bristles (0.2mm) in diameter and 10.3mm long with rounded ends, arranged in 3 rows of tufts with 6 evenly spaced tufts per row and 80-86 bristles per tuft. Nevertheless, if a patient perceives any benefit from a particular brush design characteristics, use of that brush should be encouraged[44].

Methods of Tooth Brushing

Various tooth brushing methods have been described in the literature. Among them the Modified Bass method is the most widely recommended brushing technique by the dentist. The other techniques include, the Charter's method for cleaning healing wounds after flap surgery and the modified Stillman method for patients with progressing gingival recession and root exposure to minimize abrasive tissue destruction[44]. The modified Bass method is designed to clean the cervical one third of the crowns of teeth and the area beneath the gingival margin. It can be recommended in subjects with a sound periodontal health or even with periodontal disease or during periodontal maintenance. This technique causes removal of plaque from the gingival sulcus and the interproximal area of teeth. The method consists of placing the brush bristles at an angle of 45 degrees to the long axis of the teeth directed apically (Figure 5). Gentle force is then applied to insert the bristles into the sulcus and is moved with short vibratory back and forth strokes without removing bristle ends from the sulcus with approximately 10 strokes to be completed covering 3-4 teeth at a time. The lingual surface of the anterior teeth is brushed using the heel of the brush placed vertically along the long axis of the teeth. The Occlusal surfaces should be cleaned by pressing the bristles firmly onto the Occlusal surface and a back and forth brushing stroke is activated[44].

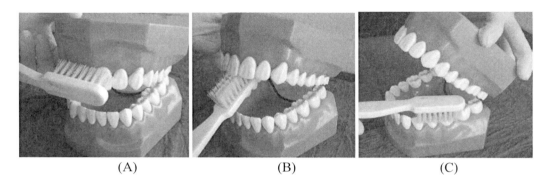

(A)   (B)   (C)

Figure 5. Modified Bass Method of Toothbrushing. Demonstration of position of toothbrush on A, B – Maxillary anterior teeth: Facial & Lingual aspect respectively. C – Occlusal surface of mandibular teeth.

Powered Toothbrushes

Electric or Powered toothbrushes enhance cleaning of the teeth especially for people with poor manual dexterity (Figure 6). Plaque removal by powered toothbrushes is faster i.e takes 1minute compared to manual toothbrushes taking 6minutes to remove the same percentage of plaque[43]. Several types of powered toothbrushes are available. The basic patterns of head motion are reciprocating back and forth movement, arcuate or up and down movement and an elliptical movement[45]. Some of the available powered toothbrushes are as follows:

- ❖ Braun Oral-B (http://www.oralb.com/en)
- ❖ Philips Sonicare (http://www.sonicare.com/)
- ❖ Colgate Motion: (http://www.colgate.com/app/colgate/US/homepage.cvsp)
- ❖ Ultreo: (http://www.ultreo.com/)
- ❖ Crest Spinbrush: (http://www.spinbrush.com/)

Ultrasonic toothbrushes use filaments that vibrate at ultrasonic frequency (>20 Khz)[43].

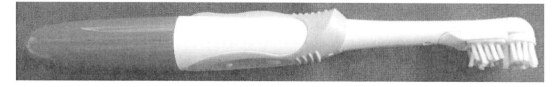

Figure 6. Powered Tooth Brush.

Ionic toothbrushes use an electric current which is applied to the filaments during brushing that alters the charge polarity of the tooth resulting in the attraction of dental plaque towards the filaments and away from the tooth. No automated action is provided[43]. The polarity of tooth surfaces is changed from negative to positive. Plaque material is actively repelled by the teeth and drawn to the negatively charged bristles. Studies have been conducted comparing the efficacy of powered versus manual toothbrushes with no consistent significant results. One study found several types of electric brushes to be as efficient as manual brushing in plaque removal from facial surfaces[46]. Literature reviews have shown that powered brushes show superior benefit with regard to plaque removal and gingival condition over manual brushes[47,48]. Nevertheless a recent systematic review on the topic has concluded the following. Limited evidence exists of the higher efficacy of powered brushes over manual in reducing dental plaque, gingival bleeding or inflammation in patients with gingivitis or periodontitis[49].

Interdental Cleaning Aids

Tough toothbrush is considered as an effective tool in plaque removal and reducing inflammation, the use of interdental aids in plaque removal is essential. It has been noted that toothbrushing is considered to be optimally capable of thoroughly cleaning the flat surfaces of the teeth while the proximal surfaces of teeth is not cleaned effectively. These areas have a high risk of developing periodontal lesions and caries. Hence interdental cleaning is crucial within the daily oral hygiene program for the treatment of periodontal diseases and the prevention of recurrence[50,51]. A wide range of interdental aids are available in the market from simple dental floss through woodensticks and brushes to mechanical or electrical devices (Figure 7). The choice of interdental cleaning aid depends on the size and shape of the interdental space. In general, embrasures with no gingival recession are adequately cleaned using dental floss while larger spaces with exposed root surfaces require the use of an interproximal brush. Interproximal spaces with no papillae covering requires single tufted brushes to remove plaque[44].

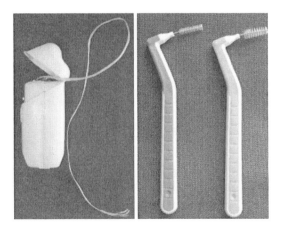

Figure 7. Interdental aids. L- R: Dental Floss and Interdental Brushes.

Chemical Plaque Control

Mechanical tooth cleaning through toothbrushing and the use of appropriate interdental aids is the most common form or oral hygiene practiced by people. Unfortunately, many individuals remove only around half of the plaque from their teeth even when brushing for 2 minutes[52]. Hence an adjunctive use of chemical plaque inhibitory mouthwash may have a major effect on improving the oral health of the individual. The most commonly used chemical plaque control agent is the Mouthwash. Other vehicles which carry the chemicals are chewing gums, varnishes, sprays, irrigators. Some of the chemicals used are Bisbigauanide antiseptics (Chlorhexidine, alexidine, Octenidine), Quaternary ammonium compounds (Cetylpyridinium chloride, banzalconium chloride), Phenols and essential oils (Thymol, ecalyptol, triclosan etc), Fluorides, Oxygenating agents (Hydrogen perioxide). The most widely used chemical agent is chlorhexidine mouthwash.

Chlorhexidine Mouthrinse

Chlorhexidine (CHX) molecule is a bisbiugnide compound, cationic agent having a desirable property of effectively inhibiting plaque and thus preventing the onset of gingivitis. Its dicationic nature makes it extremely interactive with anion which is relevant to its efficacy, safety and local side effects. Clinical efficacy of chlorhexidine as a mouthwash is achieved in two concentrations 0.2% and 0.12%. 10ml solution of 0.2% delivers 20mg and 15ml of 0.12% delivers 18mg[53].

Mechanism of Action and Unwanted Effects of Chlorhexidine

The cationic Chlorhexidine molecule binds to the negatively charged phosphate and carboxyl groups on bacterial cell surface facilitated by electrostatic forces. This alters the integrity of the bacterial cell membrane and chlorhexidine molecule is attracted towards the inner cell membrane. Further CHX binds to the phospholipids in the inner membrane leading to increased permeability of the inner membrane and leakage of low molecular weight components such as potassium ions. This occurs at low concentrations of the solution leading to bacterostatic action. At higher concentrations, coagulation and precipitation of the cytoplasm occurs by the formation of phosphated complexes leading to cell death[54,55]. Chlorhexidine's prolonged substantivity i.e ability to adsorb onto and bind to hard and soft tissues explains the long-standing bacteriostatic effect of the drug in the mouth. The main adverse effect of Chlorhexidine is extrinsic brown staining of teeth. This may be due to the precipitation of chromogenic dietary factors on to the teeth. It can alter taste sensation.

Clinical Usage

Chlorhexidine is used as an adjunct to mechanical oral hygiene and in physically and mentally challenged individuals with decreased manual dexterity to maintain an effective oral hygiene. It is also indicated in medically compromised patients predisposing to oral infections. Chlorhexidine is prescribed after periodontal surgeries as it offers the advantage of decreasing the bacterial load in the oral cavity and preventing plaque formation. There is a lack of supporting evidence that using mouthrinses on a regular basis has any therapeutic value at retarding progression of chronic periodontitis in untreated patients suffering from the disease[56]. Chlorhexidine is useful for short periods of up to 2 weeks following periodontal surgery when oral hygiene maintenance may be difficult[53]. Several studies conducted on Chlorhexidine, Listerine etc have shown that these antiseptics retard the acculumation of dental plaque and decrease the severity of gingivitis when used as a supplement. A study demonstrated that Listerine was effective in decreasing existing plaque and gingivitis scores at 1,3 and 6 months when used as an adjunct to normal oral hygiene[57.]

CHEMOTHERAPEUTIC AGENTS IN THE TREATMENT OF PERIODONTITIS

Antibiotics and other chemotherapeutic agents are a powerful group of compounds used for management of dental infections either locally or systemically administered. Microorganisms in periodontal infections are heterogeneous in nature. They vary significantly from one patient to another and is site specific even in one individual. Hence, it is difficult to recognize the need of antibiotics in periodontitis cases as an adjunctive therapy. Nevertheless local and systemic antibiotics have been used to treat periodontal diseases and earlier studies have even reported the use of these agents as a monotherapy including tetracycline hydrochloride, minocycline, metronidazole, doxycycline etc58.

Systemic Administration

There is a consensus that use of systemic antibiotics as an adjunctive therapy in the treatment of Aggressive forms of periodontitis and refractory periodontal disease along with conventional periodontal therapy and in situations that cannot be managed with mechanical therapy alone[59].

Table 1. Review of commonly used antimicrobial agents to treat periodontal diseases.

Group	Agent	Action	Suggested Dosage & duration to treat Periodontal Diseases[62,63,64].
Semisynthetic Penicillins (Extended Spectrum)	Amoxicillin	Bactericidal-inhibiting cell wall synthesis.	500 mg tid for 8-10 days
Semisynthetic Penicillins + β lactamase inhibitors.	Amoxicillin + Clavulanic acid	Clavulanic acid permeates the outer layer of cell wall of bacteria & inhibits β lactamase enzyme.	250 or 500 mg tid for 10 days.
Tetracyclines (Broad Spectrum Antibiotics)	Tetracycline Hydrochloride	Bacteriostatic- inhibits protein synthesis by binding to 30S ribosomes in susceptible organisms.	250mg QID for 14-21 days.
	Doxycycline Hyclate		100mg bid first day followed by 100mg OD for 10-14 days.
Antiamoebic agent (Nitroimidazoles)	Metronidazole	Cidal activity against protozoa & certain anaerobic bacteria by disrupting bacterial DNA synthesis in conditions with a low reduction potential.	250-500 mg tid for 10 days.
Quinolones	Ciprofloxacin	Bactericidal – inihibits enzyme bacterial DNA gyrase & digests DNA by exonucleases.	500mg bid for 8 days.
Combination therapy.	Amoxicillin + Metronidazole		250 mg of each drug tid for 8 days.
	Metronidazole + Ciprofloxacin		500 mg of each drug bd for 8 days.

Also systemic therapy has been reserved for advanced cases of periodontitis for sites that have not responded well to debridement and in progressive tissue destruction and for certain medically compromised patients[60,61]. For successful management of infections, bacterial species should be isolated, cultured and tested for antibiotic sensitivity rather than blind prescribing of drugs. When culture and sensitivity testing are not feasible, one has to choose antibiotic based on patient presentation and history. A recent review suggests the following approach to choose the appropriate antibiotic when culture and sensitivity testing is not feasible. Patients without previous history of antibiotic therapy may respond well to tetracycline group. Alternatively for patients not allergic to penicillins, amoxicillin and clavulic acid may be effective[62].

Clinical use of Systemic Antimicrobial Agents in Treatment of Periodontitis

Among the various antimicrobial agents listed, Tetracyclines are widely used in the treatment of Periodontitis. They have the ability to concentrate in the periodontal tissues and is known to inhibit the growth of microorganisms like Actinobacillus actinomy cetem comitans. These anaerobic bacteria can be cultivated from Chronic periodontitis and Aggressive Periodontitis cases. However, in mixed infections these antibiotics may not provide sufficient suppression of subgingival pathogens to arrest disease progression[65]. Tetracyclines have been investigated as adjuncts in the treatment of Aggressive periodontitis where Actinobacillus actinomycetemcomitans which is a tissue invasive bacteria is the causative microorganism. Systemic tetracycline along with mechanical removal of calculus and plaque can eliminate tissue bacteria, arrest bone loss and has even shown an increase in the post treatment bone levels[63]. A 11 month follow up study using tetracyclines in periodontitis cases revealed decreased probing depth and motile organisms[66]. Similar results were obtained in an 18 month follow up study using Doxycycline 100mg/day for 14 days in recurrent periodontal disease case[67]. Long term Tetracyclines prescription has led to infecting organism's resistance to the drug. A long term study of patients taking 250mg of tetracycline per day for 2-7 years showed persistence of deep pockets with high proportions of tetracycline resistant gram negative rods such as fusobacterium nucleatum[63]. Metronidazole has been used in a few instances as an adjunct to Scaling and Root Planing. In a 6 week follow up study, when metronidazole was administered 250mg TDS for a week, a significant reduction in probing depth and apparent gain in attachment level was found relative to patients in the positive control group. Also this was associated with a significant reduction in the need for periodontal surgery in the metronidazole treated patients[68]. Amoxicillin and Clavulanate was tested in the treatment of refractory cases with a history of periodontal surgery, tetracycline therapy and regular periodontal maintainance. 250mg of Augmentin TDS was systemically admistered for 14 days along with full mouth scaling and root planing performed under local anesthesia. Clinical evaluation after 3 months post therapy showed a gain in attachment which remained stable throughout the 1 year recall study. Probing depth decreased over 6 months with a decrease in frequency of bleeding. Hence the results proved that non surgical periodontal treatment with adjunctive use of selected antibiotic decreases the incidence of attachment loss in individuals who had been previously refractory to treatment[69]. A recent metaanalysis on the efficacy of systemically administered antimicrobial agents in the treatment of periodontal infections suggested that subjects with Aggressive periodontitis received greater benefits from these agents than Chronic Periodontitis patients but significant benefit was achieved with Chronic Periodontitis subjects. Though authors of the systematic review suggested that antimicrobial agents are useful additions in the treatment of periodontal infections, certain aspects regarding dosage, choice of drug, patient selection, duration of treatment in relation to mechanical debridement and nature of hazards such as antibiotic resistance need to be explored better in the treatment of periodontitis patients[70].

Local Delivery of Antibiotics

Antimicrobial agents must reach adequate concentration to have a therapeutic effect to kill or inhibit the growth of target microorganisms. Though systemic administration of drugs are beneficial on periodontal tissues by providing a ready exposure of all periodontal sites to the antimicrobial agent, it poses a risk of adverse reactions to non oral body sites including nausea, vomiting, headache, urticaria, GI upset, abdominal discomfort etc. Also certain drugs like penicillins may induce allergic reactions and bacterial resistance in patients. Another aspect which needs to be considered is the drug has to reach the site where the organisms exist sustaining its localized concentration at effective levels for a sufficient time and evoking minimum or no side effects. Though systemic administration of doxycycline or tetracycline was highly concentrated in the Gingival Crevicular Fluid (GCF) at levels 5-10 times more than found in serum, even this hyperconcentration of the drug in the GCF resulted in a level of antibiotic to which many organisms were notsusceptible[71,72]. Hence considering these factors local delivery of antimicrobials was developed.

Local drug delivery (LDD) agents have been classified as professional applied and home applied agents. One of the main advantages of LDD is the high concentration of the drug released in gingival crevicular fluid. For example, placement of tetracycline hydrochloride fibers subgingivally results in substantially higher dose of the drug in the pocket (1590 µg/ml in GCF & 43 µg/ml in the tissue) than in systemic dosing (2-8 µ g/ml)[61]. It has been suggested that a local concentration of 30µg/ml eliminates most pathogenic bacteria associated with periodontal disease. Though the concentration of drug in GCF is high, it's serum concentration do not exceed 0.1 µg/ml.

TABLE: LOCAL DRUG DELIVERY AGENTS.

AGENT	TRADE NAME	AVAILABLE AS
Tetracycline	Actisite	Non resorbable fibers of ethyl vinyl acetate, 25% saturated with Tetracycline Hydrochloride.
Doxycycline	Atridox	10% Doxycycline gel in a syringe.
Minocycline	Dentamycin, Periocline	2% minocycline hydrochloride gel in a syringe.
	Arestin	2% minocycline encapsulated into bioresorbable microspheres in a gel carrier.
Metronidazole	Elyzol	25% gel, a biodegradable mixture in a syringe.
Chlorhexidine	Periochip Biodegradable chip	

The other advantages being, LDD decreases potential problems with patient compliance, adverse drug reactions are eliminated, reduces the development of drug resistant microbial population at non oral body sites[73]. One of the disadvantages of LDD is difficulty in placement of the drug in deeper pockets. Placement of the drug in various sites in periodontitis patients is time consuming. Sometimes the need for a second appointment for fiber (non resorbable) removal is required. Also these agents do not markedly affect the periodontal pathogens present in the adjacent gingival connective tissue, tongue, tonsils etc which increases the risk of later reinfection[73].

Studies demonstrated that LDD agents applied with scaling and root planing improved periodontal clinical parameters. In a study comparing the efficacy of tetracycline fibers placed subgingivally in localized recurrent periodontal sites in maintainance patients with scaling and rootplaning alone revealed that at 1,3 and 6 months postoperatively, adjunctive fiber therapy was significantly better in reducing probing depth and bleeding on probing than scaling and rootplaning alone[74]. Also at 6 months, fiber therapy was significantly better in promoting clinical attachment gain. In a double blind, randomized trial, patients with pockets at least 5mm deep were selected and either minocycline 2% gel or vehicle were applied once every 2 weeks for four applications after initial scaling and root planing. Microbilogical assessment of the subgingival flora done using DNA probes at 2, 4, 6 and 12 weeks revealed statistically significant reduction of P.gingivalis, P.intermedia and Aa. Also reduction in probing depth was significantly greater with minocycline gel. Sites with 7mm pockets displayed statistically significant better results than with 5mm pockets[75]. The combination of Scaling and Root planing with metronidazole gel was proved superior to the conventional treatment of scaling and root planing alone in Chronic adult Periodontitis patients. Significantly greater reduction in pocket depths of $\geq$ 5mm at baseline was seen compared to scaling and root planing alone and the difference was maintained for a period of 9 months[76]. Studies have also shown no significant difference between groups receiving scaling and root planing alone versus scaling and root planing and LDD agent. In a study conducted to evaluate the effectiveness of a controlled release Chlorhexidine chip in the treatment of chronic periodontitis proved no statistically significant difference between the two groups for any of the clinical or microbiological parameters. Also both groups presented a significant improvement in papillary bleeding score, probing depths and relative attachment level but no significant difference was seen between the two groups. Also for both treatments, there was a significant reduction in the percentage of BANA positive sites and the improvements in the BANA test were similar for both groups after 3 and 9 months[77]. Another interesting finding in the study was the adverse reaction seen in patients treated with Chlorhexidine chip. The most common reactions were gingival pain, discomfort, local irritation and gingival edema. Gingival abscesses were found in three sites; however, this side-effect was minor and transient, with resolution usually complete within a few days and requiring no intervention or medication.

Metanalysis on local drugs like tetracycline, minocycline, metronidazole and Chlorhexidine revealed some interesting results. Adjunctive use of local antibiotics though appeared to have an impact on probing depth improvements or gain in attachment level, it was only in the range of about 0.25 – 0.5mm and 0.1 – 0.5mm respectively. According to the results obtained from the analyses of numerous studies with respect to probing depth and clinical attachment level, local minocycline might be the most promising adjunctive therapy followed by tetracycline. Side effects from these adjunctive therapies are relatively minor.

Adjunctive therapies may be used routinely as treatment alternatives when isolated sites do not respond adequately to scaling and root planing. The difference between the added effects of the adjunctive treatment and scaling and root planing alone narrows with time. Nevertheless at all time periods, Scaling and root planing with adjunctive therapy seems to be more effective than scaling and root planing alone[78].

HOST MODULATION

In periodontitis which is initiated by bacteria, the "host" harbors these pathogens. Though the presence of these pathogens especially gram negative bacteria is required, it is not sufficient to induce periodontal disease[79]. Ultimately it is the host's reaction to the presence of bacteria that mediates tissue destruction which is also influenced by certain risk factors like environmental, acquired and genetic factors[80]. Hence modulating the host in periodontal management strategies has a significant potential for improving treatment outcomes. Host modulation is a new concept introduced in dentistry and in the periodontal context host modulation means modifying or modulating destructive or damaging aspects of the inflammatory host response that develops in the periodontal tissues as a result of the chronic challenge presented by the subgingival bacterial plaque[81]. Bacterial challenge to the host leads to an upregulation of inflammatory mediators and destructive enzymes such as IL-1α, IL-1β and IL-6. In response there is an increase in the anti inflammatory mediators such as IL-1ra (receptor antagonist) and tissue inhibitors of matrix metalloproteinases (TIMPs)[82,83]. An imbalance with an excessive level of the proinflammatory or destructive mediators present in the host tissues will lead to tissue destruction. Hence host modulatory therapy is to restore balance between, on the one hand, pro-inflammatory mediators and destructive enzymes, and, on the other hand, anti-inflammatory mediators and enzyme inhibitors.

Host modulatory therapy (HMT) can be included as one of the available adjunctive treatment. This is achieved by downregulating or modifying destructive aspects and / or upregulating protective or regenerative components of the host response. HMT consists of systemically or locally delivered pharmaceutical agents that are prescribed as part of periodontal therapy and are used as adjuncts to conventional periodontal treatment such as scaling-root planing and surgery. Numerous agents have been evaluated as host response modulators, including the nonsteroidal anti-inflammatory drugs, bisphosphonates, and tetracyclines.

Non Steroidal Anti-Inflammatory Drugs (NSAID)

They inhibit the formation of inflammatory mediators like PGE$_2$ produced by variety of cells like neutrophils, macrophages, fibroblasts etc in response to bacterial lipopolysaccharides (LPS). PGE$_2$, a potent inflammatory mediator elevated in periodontitis patients is known to upregulate bone resorption by osteoclastic activity[84]. Studies have shown that NSAIDs like Flurbiprofen, indomethacin and others administered daily for 3 years significantly decreased the rate of alveolar bone loss[85,86]. NSAIDs need to be administered for an extended period of time (years) for the periodontal benefits to become apparent. However, these agents have some disadvantages like gastro intestinal problems, hemorrhage, renal and heparic impairment. Also a patient may experience a 'rebound effect' once he stops taking the drug leading to an increase in the rate of bone loss[81]. Selective clyclo-oxygenase-2 inhibitors were investigated as HMT agents. However serious adverse effects of these agents were identified and were withdrawn from the market. Hence NSAIDs due to their unwanted effects, their use as adjuncts to periodontal treatment is not justified.

Tetracyclines

Tetracyclines molecules have been modified by removing all the antibiotic properties but retaining the host modulatory, anticollagenolytic effects. Such agents are known as Chemically Modified Tetracyclines (CMT). CMT-3 and CMT-8 have shown to inhibit osteoblastic bone resorption and promote bone formation, enhance wound healing and inhibit proteinases produced by periodontal pathogens[87].

Subantimicrobial Dose Doxycycline (SDD)

Are an effective HM agent indicated in the treatment of Periodontitis. It is marketed as "Periostat" and has the ability to downregulate certain enzymes like Matrix Metallo Proteinases (MMP) which degrades a variety of extracellular matrix molecules including collagen[81]. Doxycycline has several benefits when used as an adjunctive treatment. It inhibits connective tissue breakdown by a multiple non-antimicrobial mechanisms. They may have a direct inhibition of the MMPs, promote excessive proteolysis of pro-matrix metalloproteinases into enzymatically inactive fragments, decrease cytokine levels and also may have a pro anabolic effect such as increase in collagen production and osteoblastic activity[88].

Bisphosphonates

Are bone sparing agents which have been used in the management of osteoporosis. They are absorbed by the bones and locally released during acidification with osteoclastic activity[89]. Bisphosphonates at the tissue level decrease bone turnover by decreasing bone resorption and by reducing the number of new bone multicellular units. At the cellular level they decrease osteoclast and osteoblast recruitment, decrease osteoclast adhesion and also decrease the release of cytokines by macrophages[90]. Clinical trials have been performed to examine the role of bisphosphonates in the management of periodontal bone loss. A study was conducted on type II diabetic subjects with established periodontitis. Patients treated with scaling and root planing and alendronate- 10 mg/day for 6 months induced improvement in alveolar bone crest height than control therapy. Alendronate induced a significant decrease in urine N-telopeptide which was used as a biochemical marker of bone resorption[91]. Some bisphosphonates have undesirable effects such as inhibiting bone calcification and inducing changes in white blood cell count[87].

Host response modulation has emerged as a convincing treatment concept for the management of periodontal disease. To date, only subantimicrobial dose doxycycline has been approved specifically as a host response modulator for the treatment of periodontitis[81] and the majority of clinical trials of this drug have clearly demonstrated a benefit. The prevention of bone loss associated with periodontal disease progression may be enhanced by modulating the host response which in turn may be an auxillary to the management of Periodontitis.

SURGICAL PHASE

Rationale for Periodontal Surgery

The aim of effective treatment of periodontal disease is to arrest the inflammatory diseases process and establish an environment compatible with periodontal health. The success of periodontal therapy is measured in terms of improvement in clinical attachment levels, decrease in probing pocket depths, reduction in bleeding on probing and maintenance. With regard to the ecological environment, periodontal therapy results in a microbiota more representative of health. Presumptive periodontopathogens like P.gingivalis, F.nucleatum and C.rectus are decreased and gram positive facultative organisms are increased[92]. Numerous studies have utilized probing depth measurements to assess the need for therapy and to evaluate the response to treatment. Deep sites experience greater disease progression and further when the risk/ratio of developing disease progression in deep sites as compared to shallow sites evaluated over 5-36 months was usually found around 3 times greater at deep sites[92]. Also there is a direct relationship between the type of pathogens and increased probing depths. Deep periodontal pockets are associated with increased levels of spirochetes and motile forms[92].

A thorough mechanical therapy brings about improvements in both clinical and microbiological parameters of the gingival tissue. Clinician needs to evaluate their ability to instrument deep pockets and decide if non surgical therapy can achieve the preferred outcomes of periodontal therapy i.e resolution of clinical signs of inflammation, attaining shallow probing depths, stabilization and gain of clinical attachment, radiographic resolution of osseous defects, occlusal stability and decreased plaque to a level associated with health[92]. With respect to these objectives, non surgical therapy should be used as long as it attains favourable results. However, numerous investigations have shown that the difficulty of this task increases as the pocket becomes deeper [92,93]. As the pocket deepens, the surface to be scaled increases, more irregularities appear on the root surface and accessibility is impaired especially in the furcation involved sites[94]. Hence the need for surgical access therapy is needed by displacing the soft tissue wall of the pocket which increases the visibility and accessibility of the root surface[95].Therefore surgical therapy for access and pocket reduction should be considered when non surgical treatment is unsuccessful or the desired result cannot be achieved[92]. A classic study by Lindhe et al determining the critical probing depths stated an improvement in attachment level occurs when surgery is performed in pocket depths measuring >4.2mm[33]. However, A final decision on the need for periodontal surgery should be made only after a thorough evaluation of Phase I therapy. The assessment is made not less than 1-3months and sometimes as much as 9 months after completion of phase I therapy[96]. Clinicians have to evaluate every case and determine what type of treatment will best preserve the dentition in a state of health.

Evaluation of Patients after Phase I Therapy

The purposes of re-evaluation of the tissue are to determine the need for further therapy and to determine the effectiveness of scaling and root planing and to review the proficiency of home care[97]. Re-evaluation consists of examination of the gingival tissues, bleeding on probing, probing depth and occlusal factors. A study performed on a group of teenagers with gingivitis, showed a decrease in plaque index and bleeding on probing from baseline to 15 and 30 days after being treated with ultrasonic scaling[98]. The American Academy of Periodontology world workshop agreed that a 4-6 week interval was usually adequate to assess the initial response to phase I therapy[99]. As stated earlier, reepithelialization of attachment (junctional epithelium) occurs in 1-2 weeks. Hence revaluation of the soft tissue response should not be done earlier than 2 weeks after instrumentation[100]. Repopulation of periodontal pockets by microbes after instrumentation occurs within 2 months in the absence of improved plaque control. The ideal time for reevaluation is between 4-8 weeks[101].

Objectives of Periodontal Surgery

The surgical phase consists of techniques performed for pocket therapy and for correction of certain mucogingival defects. The objectives are to improve the prognosis of teeth and improve esthetics. The purposes of periodontal surgery as proposed by Barrington 1981[102] are as follows:

❖ To eliminate pockets by removing and or recontouring soft tissues or bone.
❖ To remove diseased periodontal tissues by creating a favourable environment for new attachment and/or readaptation of soft tissues or bone.
❖ To correct mucogingival defects.
❖ To establish tissue contours to facilitate oral hygiene.
❖ To establish esthetics by reducing soft tissue in cases of gingival enlargement.
❖ To establish a favourable restorative environment.
❖ To establish drainage (periodontal abscess).
❖ To facilitate regeneration of bone and soft tissue.

Indications for Periodontal Surgery

Carranza and Takei proposed the following indications[96] :

❖ Sites with irregular bony contours, deep craters and other defects.

❖ When complete removal of root irritants is not considered clinically possible especially in pockets of posterior teeth.

❖ Grade II or grade III furcation involved teeth wherein surgery ensures the removal of irritants.

❖ Root resection or hemisection requires surgical intervention.

❖ Intrabony pockets on distal areas of last molars, frequently complicated by mucogingival problems, are usually unresponsive to nonsurgical methods.

❖ Persistant inflammation in areas with moderate to deep pockets may require surgical approach.

Surgical Methods for Periodontal Pocket Therapy

The most common method is the removal of the periodontal pocket wall which can be accomplished by non surgical and surgical methods. Scaling and root planing procedures resolve tissue inflammation thereby causing shrinkage of the gingiva and hence reduction in the pocket depth. Surgical therapy consists of tissue resection performed by gingivectomy technique or by means of flap procedure (undisplaced flap). Apically displaced flap technique leads to an apical displacement of the flap thereby reducing the pocket wall. Elimination of pocket depth is carried out by New Attachment technique. New attachment is defined as the union of connective tissue or epithelium with a root surface that has been deprived of its original attachment apparatus. This new attachment may be epithelial adhesion or connective tissue adaptation or attachment and may include new cementum[103].

Treatment Guidelines for Periodontal Pocket Problems

In sites with gingival or pseudo pockets, gingivectomy (excision of the gingiva) is the treatment of choice for pockets with a fibrotic wall[96]. In cases involving larger areas of the dentition flap technique is needed. A conservative approach and satisfactory oral hygiene is sufficient to control the disease in cases with slight periodontitis with shallow to moderate pockets. Sites with deeper pockets as in case of moderate periodontitis, surgical procedure of choice in the anterior teeth with wide interproximal spaces, the papilla preservation flap technique is considered as the first choice[96]. This technique offers less recession and reduced soft tissue crater formation interproximally[104]. In teeth very close interproximally, the sulcular incision flap is the next choice and Modified Widman flap is chosen when esthetics are not the primary consideration. Access to posterior teeth for periodontal therapy is difficult due to their root morphology, furcation involvement etc.. Accessibility can be obtained by either the undisplaced flap or the apically displaced flap. The flap of choice for regeneration of osseous defects in the posterior teeth is the papilla preservation flap and followed by sulcular flap and the modified widman flap[96].

Periodontal Surgical Procedures

Gingivectomy

Excision of the gingiva is performed to eliminate suprabony pockets which are fibrotic and to eliminate gingival enlargements. The technique is performed by means of scalpel, electrosurgery or lasers. The pockets are marked with pocket marker after careful exploration of the pockets using a periodontal probe. Periodontal knives (Kirkland and orban) are used for making the incisions other than Bard-Parker knives. Incision must be placed at a level more apical to the level of the points marked and should be beveled at approximately 45 degrees to the tooth surface[105,106]. As far as possible, the normal festooned pattern of the gingiva is created. The excised pocket wall is removed and granulation tissue is curetted. Plaque and calculus is removed and the wound areas are covered with a periodontal pack. The pack is removed after a week (Figure 8).

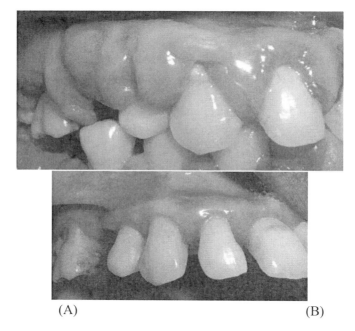

(A)   (B)

Figure 8. Gingivectomy A – Gingival enlargement in relation to the first quadrant. B – Post operative view after Gingivectomy.

Modified Widman Flap

Is defined as a scalloped, replaced, mucoperiosteal flap, accomplished with an internal bevel incision that provides access for root planning[107]. This flap procedure was described by Ramfjord and Nissle in 1974[108]. The initial incision is the internal bevel incision given 1.0 mm away from the gingival margin following the contour of the gingival margin. This may be performed using a bard parker blade (no.11) which should be parallel to the long axis of the tooth. A similar incision technique is used on the palatal aspect. The incisions should be placed as far as possible between the teeth such that sufficient amounts of tissue can be included in the palatal flap to allow for proper coverage of the interproximal bone when the flap is sutured. Next a periosteal elevator is used to reflect the flap such that a few millimetres of the alveolar crest is exposed. A second crevicular incision is made around the teeth to facilitate the separation of the collar of pocket epithelium and granulation tissue from the root surfaces. After the flap is reflected, a third incision is made in the interdental space close to the surface of the alveolar bone crest to remove the gingival collar. Granulation tissue is removed using curettes. The exposed root surfaces are scaled and planed. The flaps are then trimmed and the facial and lingual interproximal tissue is adapted such that there is complete coverage of the interproximal bone. Recontouring of bone from the outer aspect of the alveolar process may be needed if it prevents good tissue adaptation. The flaps are sutured together with interrupted direct sutures. Finally surgical dressing (periodontal pack) may be placed. The sutures and dressing is removed after 7 days. Advantages of modified widman flap are the ability to coapt the tissues to the root surfaces, access to the root surfaces, less likelihood of root sensitivity and caries and a positive environment for oral hygiene maintenance. The disadvantage being the presence of a flat or concave interproximal soft tissue contours may be seen after the surgery[107].

Modified Flap Operation

Kirkland described this technique which is an access flap for proper root debridement. It makes use of only intracrevicular incisions through the bottom of the pocket. Both buccal and lingual flaps are reflected and debrided. The flaps are then replaced to the original position and sutured interproximally (Figure 9 and Figure 10).

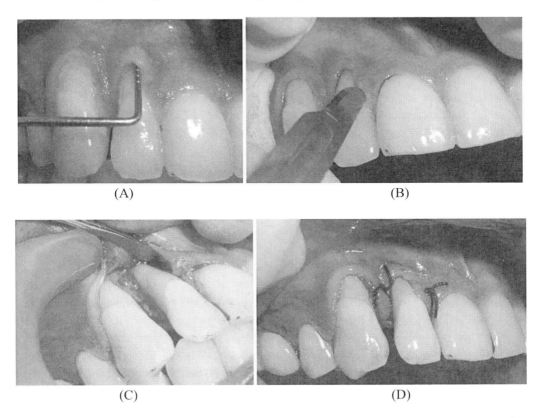

(A)

(B)

(C)

(D)

Figure 9. Flap Surgery A – Deep Pocket on facial aspect of maxillary right lateral incisor. B – Incision given, C – Flap reflected and debridement performed, D – Sutures placed

Coronally Advanced Flap

The periosteum is considered as having a regenerative potential due to the presence of osteoprogenitor cells. The barrier type effect by the repositioned periosteum and the cellular activity of the periosteum is considered as the reason for its regenerative potential[103].

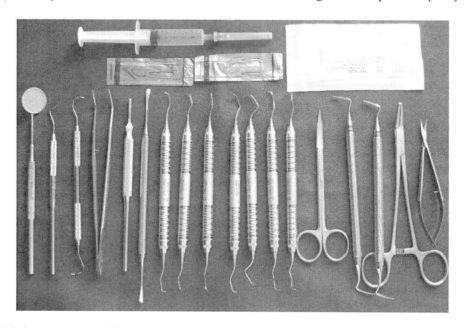

Figure 10. Instruments used for Periodontal flap Surgery.

Reconstructive Periodontal Surgery

Periodontal regeneration is defined as the restoration of lost periodontium or supporting tissues and includes formation of new alveolar bone, new cementum and new periodontal ligament[103]. New attachment is defined as 'the reunion of connective tissue with a root surface which has been deprived of its periodontal ligament. The reunion occurs by the formation of new cementum with inserting collagen fibers'[109]. Though new attachment is the ideal treatment outcome, achieving this end point requires repopulation of a detached root surface by cells from the periodontal ligament which is a prerequisite for new attachment formation. Other therapeutic results may be seen such as formation of a long junctional epithelium, root resorption and ankylosis, recession or reccurrence of periodontal pockets[110].

A study was undertaken to evaluate four periodontal regenerative procedures on the connective tissue attachment level. Tissue sections analyzed 12 months after surgery revealed that healing following the 4 different regenerative procedures resulted in the formation of a long junctional epithelium along the treated root surface with no connective tissue attachment[111]. It has been reported that granulation tissue derived from gingival connective tissue produced root resorption and granulation tissue derived from bone produced ankylosis of roots deprived of their PDL and root cementum[109]. Despite the various treatment outcomes seen, regeneration of the periodontal tissues with new attachment seems to be the ultimate goal.

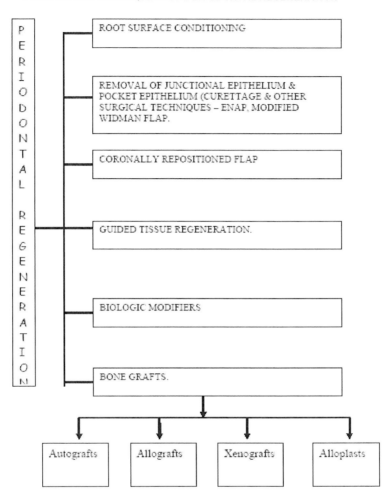

FLOW CHART: TECHNIQUES FOR PERIODONTAL REGENERATION

Root Surface Conditioning

This method is perhaps the oldest and most frequently attempted type of regeneration. Periodontal disease leads to structural and biochemical damage of the root surface including decreased insertion of collagen fibers, alterations in mineral density and surface composition and root surface contamination by bacteria and their endotoxins[112]. Use of certain chemical modifying agents on the altered root surfaces serve for cell attachment and fiber insertion. Agents which are commonly used for root conditioning are citric acid, ethylenediaminetetra acetic acid (EDTA), tetracyclines and fibronectin.

Citric acid (pH 1 for 2min) when used on denuded root surfaces in dogs led to formation of cementum pins extending into dentin tubules to facilitate regeneration[113]. Citric acid treated root surfaces produced wide zones of demineralization dominated by exposed collagen fibrils[114]. Removal of smear layer from root planed surfaces was seen with citric acid resulting in depressions corresponding to open dentinal tubules[115]. It also initiated wound healing by clot stabilization which may result in new connective tissue attachment[116]. Citric acid is also known to reduce aerobic and anaerobic bacteria[117] and endotoxins from root surfaces. Effect of tetracycline root conditioning on cell adhesion, migration and proliferation of fibroblasts was seen in a study and was concluded that tetracyclines increased attachment of fibroblastic cells[118]. Though studies on animals show the beneficial effects of root conditioning agents, human studies have shown contradictory results[119].

A recent systematic review concluded that the use of citric acid, tetracyclines or EDTA to modify the root surfaces provides no clinical benefit to the patient with respect to decrease of probing depth or gain in clinical attachment level in chronic periodontitis patients[112].

Bone Grafts

Bone replacement grafts remain among the most widely used therapeutic approaches for the correction periodontal osseous defects. Many investigators have focused upon bone regeneration as the prerequisite for new attachment formation and hypothesizede that this will also lead to induction of new cementum[109].The rationale behind the clinical use of grafting procedures is that the complete regeneration of the attachment apparatus (including new bone formation and new connective tissue attachment) would be improved by various biomaterials due to their osteogenetic (Any tissue or substance with the potential to induce growth or repair of bone is said to be osteogenic[9]) potential if the graft contained viable bone-forming cells, osteoinductive capacities (exerted by the release of boneinducing substances), or osteoconductive properties (i.e. the possibility to create a scaffold to support bone formation)[120].

Bone grafts are classified as Autogenous bone grafts, Allografts, Xenografts Alloplasts.

Autografts are tissue transferred from one position to another in the same person[9]. Iliac crest of the pelvis is the most common extraoral site for procuring graft. Common intraoral sites are healing extraction sockets, edentulous sites, tuberosity region distal to the last molar and mental symphisis below the teeth. Trephines, saws or drills are used to procure intraoral autogenous bone with profuse faline irrigation to prevent overheating and also to maintain viability of the bone cells. Techniques like osseous coagulum (a mixture of bone dust with patient's blood) and bone blend (a triturated mixture of cortical or cancellous bone with saline) have been used in periodontal regeneration with successful results of new bone, cementum and new attachment seen at the interdental osseous defect site[121]. A technique also know as bone swaging has been proposed which requires the existence of an edentulous area adjacent to the defect from which the bone is pushed into contact with the root surface without fracturing the bone [122].

The main advantage of Autogenous bone grafts is that they contain viable cells which may go on to actively form new bone. The disadvantages are creation of a second surgical site for harvesting the bone which may lead to increased risk of morbidity due to post operative complications, availability of limited quantity of bone and difficulty in procuring the same from intraoral sites and chances of root resorption when fresh ilac grafts are used[123].

Allografts are grafts between genetically dissimilar members of the same species; a processed human bone graft obtained from a tissue bank[9]. Allografts are available from commercial tissue banks. Grafts are obtained from cadaver bone, freeze dried and treated to prevent transmission of disease to get Freeze dried bone allografts (FDBA) or may be demineralised to obtain demineralised freeze dried bone allografts (DFDBA). The antigenic properties of allografts are reduced by radiation, freezing or chemical treatment[109].

FDBA is regarded as an osteoconductive material wherein it acts as a scaffold for natural bone to grow into but does not activate bone growth. Eventually the graft is resorbed and replaced by new bone. A recent academy report on periodontal regeneration revealed bone fill ranging from 1.3-2.6 mm when FDBA was used in controlled clinical trials to treat periodontal defects[124]. DFDBA stimulates bone formation due to the influence of bone inductive proteins called as Bone Morphogenetic Proteins (BMP) a group of polypeptides belonging to the transforming growth factor- β (TGF-β) family which gets exposed during the demineralization process. They stimulate bone formation through osteoinduction by inducing pleuripotential stem cells to differentiate into osteoblasts. Hence DFDBA elicits mesenchymal cell migration, attachment and osteogenesis when implanted in well vascularized bone[125]. It has been reported that DFDBA have demonstrated bone fill similar to that achieved with FDBA ranging from 1.7-2.9 mm[103]. Variability has been reported in the ability of DFDBA to induce new bone. In a study conducted to compare the ability of DFDBA, Guided tissue regeneration (GTR) membrane and growth factors, it was seen that DFDBA were least effective in promoting bone growth[126]. Variability in results could be attributed to insufficient quantity of BMPs present especially in adult cortical bone[127] or bone inductive components of the graft may be in an inactive form. Further natural variation in human donors may exist which may explain the variation in the osteoinductive capacity of DFDBA[125].

Human mineralized bone has been developed recently. It contains human mineralized component, organic matrix and collage. This mineralized bone allograft (MBA) which is solvent preserved by tutoplast process and low dose gamma irradiation is more osteoconductive material than FDBA[103]. This treatment has been claimed to preserve the bony trabecular pattern and is shown to exhibit increased porosity than FDBA[128]. MBA with or without membrane when compared with open flap debridement in the regenerative ability of class II furcation defects in molars revealed significantly improved bone fill. Hence MBA has been introduced to periodontal therapy and recently been evaluated for its use in regenerative and bone augmentation [129,130].

Alloplast is a synthetic graft or inert foreign body implanted into tissue[9]. These are synthetic, inorganic bone graft materials which are osteoconductive in nature. Various alloplasts are available namely Hydroxyapatite (HA), β-tricalcium phosphate, Polymethyl methacrylate/hydroxyethylmethacrylate (PMMA/HEMA), calcium layered polymer and bioactive glass. Alloplastic materials must possess certain properties which will make it ideal as a regenerative material. The material should be biocompatible with host tissues, non allergenic, non carcinogenic and non inflammatory. They should possess sufficient porosity to allow bone conduction and have the ability to stimulate bone induction, resorbability with replacement of bone and be radiopaque[107]. The bioactive glass showed a greater increase in bone fill and significantly greater probing depth reduction than open flap debridement procedure[120].

Xenograft is a graft taken from a donor of another species and is referred to anorganic bone[9]. There are minimal clinical data supporting the use of xenografts in periodontal defects. An anorganic bovine derived graft marketed as bio-oss has been used to treat osseous defects in periodontitis with successful new attachment and bone regeneration. They contain porous matrix containing minerals from cancellous or cortical bone which is bovine derived. Though the organic components of the bone are excluded, the bony trabecular architecture is still retained[131].

Guided Tissue Regeneration

It provides a barrier to epithelial downgrowth and excludes gingival connective tissue cells thereby allowing cells with regenerative potential i.e periodontal ligament and bone cells to enter the wound first. A biocompatible membrane is used to isolate the defect from the gingival epithelium and connective tissue. Resorbable and non resorbable membranes are available. Increase in gain of clinical attachment and probing depth reduction in the treatment of furcation defects and intrabony defects has been noted[132].

Biologic Modifiers

Certain naturally occurring molecules with matrix proteins known as growth factors regulate the biologic events necessary for regeneration namely mitogenesis, migration and metabolism[133]. Numerous growth factors have been identified and characterized. Studies in non human primate model showed Platelet derived growth factors (PDGF) has the capacity to stimulate bone formation and periodontal regeneration[133]. It has also shown to be an important stimulator of cellular chemotaxis, proliferation and matrix synthesis enhancing influx of fibroblasts into the wound site and increases extracellular matrix production[133]. Combination of recombinant PDGF and Insulin like growth factors (IGF) has shown promising results in the treatment of intrabony defects and furcation involvement[134]. Bone Morphogenetic Proteins (BMP) are natural proteins which play important roles during embryogenesis and mediate in specific aspects of skeletal growth and development. They are osteoinductive in nature. BMP-2 & BMP-7 have shown improved regenerative results when used for treatment of periodontal defects[103]. Certain proteins are secreted by hertwig's epithelial root sheath during development of tooth and induces acellular cementum formation. These proteins which are known as enamel matrix proteins are believed to favour periodontal regeneration[135]. One of the enamel matrix derivative (EMD) has been approved by the U.S Food and drug administration for use in achieving periodontal regeneration in osseous defects. They are marketed under the trade name of Emdogain. It consists of a viscous gel of enamel derived proteins from tooth buds in a polypropylene liquid and is delivered by a syringe to the defect site[110]. Amelogenin is the major protein present in the mixture[136]. Emdogain has promoted increased gain of radiographic bone and clinical attachment onto diseased root surfaces associated with intrabony defects in periodontitis subjects compared to control group who received a placebo application[137]. A recent systematic review has shown the beneficial effects of EMD in periodontal regeneration and decreasing probing depth[136] and also there is a strong evidence that EMD favours wound healing and new periodontal tissue formation[138].

Resective Osseous Surgery

Osseous Surgeries are procedures to modify bone support altered by periodontal disease, either by reshaping the alveolar process to achieve physiologic form without the removal of alveolar supporting bone, or by the removal of some alveolar bone, thus changing the position of the crestal bone relative to the tooth root[9]. The rationale of osseous resective surgery is that the discrepancies in level and shapes of the bone and gingiva may predispose patients to the recurrence of pocket depth post surgically. Thus resective osseous surgery leads to reshaping the marginal bone to resemble that of alveolar process undamaged by periodontal disease[139]. Osteoplasty (reshaping of the alveolar process to achieve a more physiologic form without removal of alveolar bone proper[9]) and Ostectomy (the excision of a bone or portion of a bone[9]) procedures are utilised in osseous surgery. Osteoplasty is used to reduce buccal and lingual bony ledges, shallow intrabony defects and incipient furcation involvements that do not necessitate removal of supporting bone[140]. Ostectomy is used to treat shallow (1-2mm) to medium (3-4mm) intrabony and hemiseptal osseous defects and to correct reverse osseous architecture. The apically displaced flap design is utilized with this technique to provide minimum probing depth and gingival tissue morphology that enhances good self performed oral hygiene and periodontal health.

Healing after Flap Surgery

Following flap surgery, the area between the flap and tooth / bone surface is established by blood clot consisting of fibrin reticulum with numerous neutrophils, erythrocytes, debris of injured cells and blood capillaries[141]. 1-3 days post surgery the epithelial cells migrate over the border of the flap and by one week and epithelial attachment to the root is established. The clot is replaced by granulation tissue derived from gingival connective tissue, bone marrow and periodontal ligament. Collagen fibers appear parallel to the tooth surface 2 weeks after surgery and a fully epithelialized gingival crevice with a well defined epithelial attachment is seen one month after surgery[141]. Full thickness flaps results in necrosis of bone which peaks at 4-6 days following surgery[141]. Repair of the osseous lesion may be seen when flap surgery is carried out in an area with a deep infrabony lesion. Various factors influence the amount of bone fill such as the anatomy of the defect, crestal bone resorption and extent of inflammation[106]. The presence of retained cementum on the root surface is beneficial during the healing process. It was seen that resorption occurred prior to new cementum formation and connective tissue attachment in those areas where cementum had been planed from the root[142].

PERIODONTAL MAINTENANCE
(SUPPORTIVE PERIODONTAL THERAPY)

Upon completion of active periodontal therapy, a routine periodontal maintainance (PM) visits should be formulated for patients which is also known as Supportive periodontal therapy. The importance of regular maintenance visits should be made aware to patients for a long term control of the disease. This will include the following:

❖ To revise medical and dental histories of the patients.
❖ To assess oral hygiene status.
❖ To Evaluate periodontal soft tissues and dental hard tissues.

❖ To perform mechanical scaling to remove plaque, stains and calculus with adjunctive chemotherapeutic agents when indicated.

❖ To identify any new risk factors and formulating an appropriate treatment for the same.

Achieving a stable attachment level with absence of clinical signs of inflammation after periodontal therapy is important. Hence prevention of the progression and recurrence of periodontal disease in patients previously treated for gingivitis and periodontitis is one of the objectives of periodontal maintenance[143]. Another objective is to decrease the incidence of tooth loss by monitoring patients' dentition. Also concurrent diseases within the oral cavity can be recognized and treated in periodic maintenance visits. It has been reported that there was decreased probing depth and tooth loss in patients who had received periodic periodontal maintenance compared to subjects who had not received the same for 10 years following completion of periodontal therapy[144]. It was also seen in a study that subjects who adhered to strict periodontal maintenance lost fewer teeth. Also patients were assessed for percentage of compliance (total number of visits the patient should have made divided by the number of visits actually made) wherein it was seen that patients whose percentage of compliance was higher maintained their teeth longer than those less compliant[145].

Bacteria present within the tissues in Chronic and Aggressive Periodontitis patients[146,147] may not be eliminated completely in certain areas[148] and these bacteria may recolonize the pocket and may be the cause for recurrent periodontal disease. Debridement of pockets in periodontitis patients suppresses the components of the subgingival microflora but may return to their baseline levels in approximately less than 3 months[144]. Hence constant monitoring and mechanical debridement is needed for good maintenance results. Healing after periodontal surgery often leads to the formation of a weak long junctional epithelium and inflammation may lead to the separation of this epithelium from the tooth leading to recurrence of disease activity. Hence treated periodontal patients may be at a risk of developing recurrent periodontal disease if regular maintenance care is not optimal which is essential for a long term preservation of the dentition. The frequency and quality of such recall visits is important and has been reported that an average periodontal maintenance visit should last for an hour and should be scheduled every 3 months[149].

REFERENCES

[1]   The American Academy of Periodontology. *Parameter on Chronic Periodontitis with Slight to Moderate Loss of Periodontal Support*. J Periodontol 2000;71:853-855.

[2]   Morrison EC, Ramfjord SP and Hill RW. *Short term effects of initial, non surgical periodontal treatment (hygiene phase)*. J Clin Periodontol 1980;7: 199-211.

[3]   Badersten A, Nilveus R and Egelberg J. *Effect of nonsurgical periodontal therapy II. Severely advanced periodontitis*. J Clin Periodontol 1984;11: 63-76.

[4]   Rylander H and Lindhe J. *Cause Related Periodontal Therapy in: Lindhe J, Karring T & Lang NP. Clinical Periodontology and Implant* Dentistry,4th edn, Blackwell Munksgaard Publishing Company, UK, pg:433-448.

[5]   Derbyshire J C. *Patient Motivation in Periodontics*. J Periodontol 1970, 70: 630-635.

[6]   Ruth Freeman. the psychology of dental patient care: *Strategies for motivating the non-compliant patient.* Br Dent J 1999; 187:307-312.

[7]   Butler C, Rollnick S, Stott N. *The practitioner, the patient and resistance to change: recent ideas on compliance.* Can Med Assoc J 1996; 154: 1357–1362.

[8]   Prochaska, James O, DiClemente, Carlo C. *J Consult Clin Psychol* 1983, 51(3), 390-395.

[9]   Cohen RE, Mariotti A, Rethman M and Zackin SJ. *Glossary of periodontal terms.* 4th edition. Chicago: The American Academy of Periodontics; 2001.

[10]   Pattison AM and Pattison GL. *Scaling and Root Planing in: Newman MG, Takei HH, Klokkevold PR and Carranza FA.* Clinical Periodontology, 10th edition, Saunders-an imprint of Elsevier, St.Louis, Missouri: Pg 749-797.

[11]   Jill S Nield Gehrig. 'Sickle Scalers' in: Jill S Nield Gehrig. *Fundamentals of periodontal instrumentation and advanced root instrumentation.* Lippincott Williams and Wilkins, Baltimore & Philadelphia, 2008. 285-306.

[12]   Jill S Nield Gehrig. 'Area Specific Curets' in: Jill S Nield Gehrig. *Fundamentals of periodontal instrumentation and advanced root instrumentation.* Lippincott Williams and Wilkins, Baltimore & Philadelphia, 2008. 335-360.

[13]   Drisko CL, Cochran DL, Blieden T et al: *Position paper, Sonic and ultrasonic scalers in periodontics. Research, Science and Therapy Committee of the American Academy of Periodontology.* J Periodontol 2000, 71:1792-1801.

[14]   Walmsley AD, Laird WRE and Williams AR. *A Model System to Demonstrate the Role of Cavitational Activity in Ultrasonic Scaling.* J Dent Res 1984; 63; 1162.

[15]   Khambay BS, Walmsley AD. *Acoustic Microstreaming: Detection and Measurement Around Ultrasonic Scalers.* J Periodontol 1999;70(6): 626-636.

[16]   Harrel SK and Molinari J. *Aerosols and splatter in dentistry: A brief review of the literature and infection control implications.* J Am Dent Assoc 2004;135;429-437

[17]   Mousquès T, Listgarten MA, Philips RW. *Effect of scaling and root planing on the composition of the human subgingival microbial flora.* J Periodontal Res 1980;15:144-151.

[18]   Curd M.L. Bollen and Marc Quirynen. *Microbiological Response to Mechanical Treatment in Combination with Adjunctive Therapy. A Review of the Literature.* J Periodontol 1996;67:1143-1158.

[19]   M. Quirynen, C.M.L. Bollen, B.N.A. Vandekerckhove, C. Dekeyser, W. Papaioannou, and H. Eyssen. *Full- vs. Partial-mouth Disinfection in the Treatment of Periodontal Infections: Short-term Clinical and Microbiological Observations.* J Dent Res 1995; 74: 1459 - 1467.

[20]   Betty N.A. Vandekerckhove, Curd M.L. Bollen, Chris Dekeyser, Paul Darius, and Marc Quirynen. Full- *Versus Partial-Mouth Disinfection in the Treatment of Periodontal Infections. Long-Term Clinical Observations of a Pilot Study.* J Periodontol 1996; 67: 1251 – 1259.

[21]   Quirynen M, Claudio Mongardini, Martine Pauwels, Curd M.L. Bollen, Johan Van Eldere, Daniel Van Steenberghe. *One Stage Full- Versus Partial-Mouth Disinfection in the Treatment of Chronic Adult or Generalized Early-Onset Periodontitis.* J Periodontol 1999;. 70: 646-656.

[22]   Claudio Mongardini, Daniel van Steenberghe, Christel Dekeyser, Marc Quirynen. *One Stage Full- Versus Partial-Mouth Disinfection in the Treatment of Chronic Adult or*

Generalized Early-Onset Periodontitis. I. Long-Term Clinical Observations. J Periodontol 1999; 70: 632-645.

[23] Jervoe-Storm PM, H. AlAhdab, E. Semaan, R. Fimmers, S. Jepsen. *Microbiological outcomes of quadrant versus full-mouth root planing as monitored by real-time PCR.* J Clin Periodontol 2007;34:156-163.

[24] Gerhild U. Kno¨fler, Regina E. Purschwitz, and Holger F.R. Jentsch. *Full-Mouth Scaling in the Treatment of Chronic Periodontitis.* J Periodontol 2007;78:2135-2142.

[25] Greenstein G. *Full-Mouth Therapy Versus Individual Quadrant Root Planing: A Critical Commentary.* J Periodontol 2002; 73: 797-812.

[26] Hunter RD, O'Leary TJ, Kafrawy AT. *The effectiveness of hand versus ultrasonic instrumentation in open flap root planing.* J Periodontol 1984;55:697–703.

[27] Jones SJ, Lozdan J, Boyde A. *Tooth surfaces treated in situ with periodontal instruments.* Br Dent J 1972;132:57–64.

[28] Moskow BS, Bressman E. *Cemental response to ultrasonic and hand instrumentation.* J Am Dent Assoc 1964;68:698–703.

[29] Ewen SJ, Scopp IW, Witkin RT, Ortiz-Junceda M. *A comparative study of ultrasonic generators and hand instruments.* J Periodontol 1976;47:82–86.

[30] Tunkel J, Heinecke A, Flemmig T.F: *A systematic review of efficacy of machine-driven and manual subgingival debridement in the treatment of chronic periodontitis.* J Clin Periodontol 2002; 29(Suppl. 3): 72–81.

[31] Van der Weijden GA, Timmerman MF. *A systematic review on the clinical efficacy of subgingival debridement in the treatment of Chronic periodontitis.* J Clin Periodontol 2002; 29 (Suppl.3): 55-71.

[32] Cobb CM. *Non surgical pocket therapy:Mechanical. Ann Periodontol 1996;1:443-490.*

[33] *Lindhe J, Socransky SS, Nyman S, Haffajee A, Westfelt E. "Critical probing depths" in periodontal therapy.* J Clin Periodontol 1982;9:323–336.

[34] Klienfelder JW, Dieter EL, Werner B. *Some effects of non surgical therapy on gingival inflammatory cell subsets in patients with adult and early onset periodontitis.* J Periodontol 2000;71: 1561-1566.

[35] Dubrez B, Graf JM, Vuagnat P, Cimasoni G. *Increase of interproximal bone density after subgingival instrumentation: A quantitative radiographical study.* J Periodontol 1990; 61: 725–731.

[36] Hwang YJ, Matthew Jonas Fien, Sam-Sun Lee, Tae-Il Kim, Yang-Jo Seol, Yong-Moo Lee, Young Ku, In-Chul Rhyu, Chong-Pyoung Chung, and Soo-Boo Han. *Effect of Scaling and Root Planing on Alveolar Bone as Measured by Subtraction Radiography.* J Periodontol 2008; 79:1663-1669.

[37] Waerhaug J. *Healing of the dento-epithelial junction following subgingival plaque control. I. As observed in human biopsy material.* J Periodontol 1978;49:1-8.

[38] Biagini G, Checchi L, Miccoli MC, Vasi V, Castaldini C. *Root curettage and gingival repair in periodontics.* J Periodontol 1988;59:124-129.

[39] Lang NP, Cumming BR, Loe H. *Toothbrushing frequency as it relates to plaque development and gingival health.* J Periodontol 1973: 44: 396–405.

[40] Straub AM, Salvi GE, Lang NP: *Supragingival plaque formation in the human dentition.* In Lang NP, Attstrom R, Loe H, editors: Proceedings of the European Workshop on Mechanical plaque control, Chicago, 1998, Quintessence.

[41] American Academy of Periodontology: *Position paper: treatment of gingivitis and periodontitis,* J Periodontol 1997;68:1246

[42] Ryan ME. *Non Surgical Approaches for the treatment of periodontal diseases.* Dent Clin North Am 2005;49:611-636.

[43] Claydon NC. *Current concepts in toothbrushing and interdental cleaning.* Periodontol 2000; 2008, 48: 10–22.

[44] Perry DA. '*Plaque control for the periodontal patient' in : Newman MG, Takei HH and Carranza FA.* Carranza's Clinical Periodontology 9th edition, Elsevier Science, Pennsylvania, 2003. pg 651-674.

[45] Cancro LP and Fischman SL. *The expected effect on oral health of dental plaque control through mechanical removal in: Ciancio SG. Mechanical and chemical supragingival plaque control.* Periodontol 2000; 1995;8:60-74.

[46] Khocht A, Spindell L, Person P. *A comparative clinical study of the safety and efficacy of three toothbrushes.* J Periodontol 1992;63:603-610.

[47] Saxer UP, Yankell SL. *Impact of improved toothbrushes on dental diseases II.* Quintessence Int. 1997: 28: 573–593.

[48] Walmsley AD. The electric toothbrush: a review. Br Dent J 1997: 182: 209–218.

[49] Sicilia A, Arregui I, Gallego M, Cabezas B, Cuesta S: *A systematic review of powered vs. manual toothbrushes in periodontal cause-related therapy.* J Clin Periodontol 2002; 29(Suppl. 3): 39–54.

[50] Kinane DF. *The role of interdental cleaning in effective plaque control. Need for interdental cleaning in primary and secondary prevention.* In: Lang NP, Attstrom R, Loe H, editors. Proceedings of the European Workshop on Mechanical Plaque Control. Berlin: Quintessenz Verlag, 1998: 156–168.

[51] Loe H. *Oral hygiene in the prevention of caries and periodontal disease.* Int Dent J 2000: 50: 129–139.

[52] de la Rosa M R, Guerra J Z, Johnson D A and Radike A W. *Plaque growth and removal with daily tooth brushing.* J Periodontol 1979, 50:661-664.

[53] Eley BM. *Antibacterial agents in the control of supragingival plaque – a review.* Br Dent J 1999;186:286-296.

[54] Greenstein S, Berman C & Jaffin R. Chlorhexidine. *An adjunct to periodontal therapy.* J Periodontol 1986;57 (6): 371-376.

[55] Heasman PA and Seymour RA. *Pharmacological control of periodontal disease.I. Antiplaque agents.Review.* J Dent 1994;22:323-335.

[56] Moran JM. *Home-use oral hygiene products: mouthrinses.* Periodontol 2000., 2008.; 48: 42–53.

[57] Lamster IB, Alfano MC, Seiger MC & Gordon JM. *The effect of Listerine antiseptic on the reduction of existing plaque and gingivitis.* Clin Prev Dent. 983;5;12-16.

[58] Novak MJ, Polson AM, Adair SM. *Tetracycline therapy in patients with early juvenile periodontitis.* J Periodontol 1988;59:366–372

[59] Slots J. *Systemic antibiotics in periodontics.* J Periodontol 2004;75(11):1553-1565.

[60] Greenstein G. *Nonsurgical periodontal therapy in 2000: a literature review.* J Am Dent Assoc 2000;131:1580-1582.

[61] Ryan ME. *Nonsurgical approaches for the treatment of periodontal diseases.* Dent Clin North Am. 2005;49:611-636.

[62] Walker C and Karpinia K. *Rationale for use of antibiotics in periodontics.* J Periodontol 2002;73:1188-1196.

[63] Jolkovsky DL & Ciancio S. *Chemotherapeutic agents in: Newman MG, Takei HH, Klokkevold PR and Carranza FA.* Clinical Periodontology, 10th edition, Saunders-an imprint of Elsevier, St.Louis, Missouri: Pg 798-812.

[64] Committee on Research, Science and Therapy and approved by the Board of Trustees of The American Academy of Periodontology. *Position Paper. Systemic Antibiotics in Periodontics.* J Periodontol 1996;67:831-838.

[65] Van Winkelhoff AJ, Rams TE, Slots J. *Systemic antibiotic therapy in periodontics.* Periodontol 2000.; 1996;10:45-78.

[66] Rams TE, Keyes PH, Wright WE, Howard SA. *Long-term effects of microbiologically modulated periodontal therapy on advanced adult periodontitis.* J Am Dent Assoc 1985; 111:429-441.

[67] Lundstrom A, Johansson LA, Hamp SE. *Effec1 of combined systemic antimicrobial therapy and mechanical plaque control in patients with recurrent periodontal disease.* J Clin Periodontol 1984; 11:321 330.

[68] Loesche WJ, Glordano JR, Hujoel P, Schwarcz J & Smith A. *Metronidazole in periodontitis: reduced need for surgery.* J Clin Periodontol 1992; 19:103-112.

[69] Magnusson I, Clark WB, Low SB, Maruniak J, Marks RG, Walker CB. *Effect of non-surgical periodontal therapy combined with adjunctive antibiotics in subjects with "refractory" periodontal disease. (I) Clinical results.* J Clin Periodontol 1989;16:647-653.

[70] Haffajee AD, Socransky SS, Gunsolley JC. Systemic *Anti-Infective Periodontal Therapy. A Systematic Review.* Ann Periodontol 2003;8:115-181.

[71] Gordon JM, Walker CB, Murphy JC et al. *Tetracycline:levels achievable in gingival crevice fluid and in vitro effect on subgingival organisms. Part I. Concentrations in crevicular fluid after repeated doses.* J Periodontol 1981;52(10):609-612.

[72] Pascale D, Gordon J, Lamster I et al. *Concentration of doxycycline in human gingival fluid.* J Clin Periodontol 1986;13(9):841-844.

[73] Rams TE & Slots J. *Local delivery of antimicrobial agents in the periodontal pocket.* Periodontol 2000.;1996;10:139-159.

[74] Newman MG, Kornman KS, Doherty FM. *Source: A 6-Month Multi-Center Evaluation of Adjunctive Tetracycline Fiber Therapy Used in Conjunction With Scaling and Root Planing in Maintenance Patients: Clinical Results.* J Periodontol 1994: 65: 685–691.

[75] Steenberghe DV, Bercy P, Kohl J, DeBoever J, Adriaens P, Vanderfaeillie A, Adriaenssen C, Rompen E, DeVree H, McCarthy EF, Vandenhoven G. *Subgingival Minocycline Hydrochloride Ointment in Moderate to Severe Chronic Adult Periodontitis: A Randomized, Double-Blind, Vehicle-Controlled, Multicenter Study.* J Periodontol 1993;64:637-644.

[76] Griffiths GS, Smart GJ, Bulman JS, Weiss G, Schrowder J, Newman HN: *Comparison of clinical outcomes following treatment of chronic adult periodontitis with subgingival scaling or subgingival scaling plus metronidazole gel.* J Clin Periodontol 2000; 27: 910–917.

[77] Grisi DC, Salvador SL, Figueiredo LC, Souza SLS, Novaes AB Jr, Grisi MFM. *Effect of a controlled-release chlorhexidine chip on clinical and microbiological parameters of periodontal syndrome.* J Clin Periodontol 2002; 29: 875–881.

[78] Bonito AJ, Lux L, and Lohr KN. *Impact of Local Adjuncts to Scaling and Root Planing in Periodontal Disease Therapy: A Systematic Review.* J Periodontol 2005;76: 1227-1236.

[79] Page RC, Kornman KS. *The pathogenesis of human periodontitis: An introduction.* Periodontol 2000.; 1997; 14:9-11.

[80] Salvi GE, Lawrence HP, Offenbacher S, Beck JD. *Influence of risk factors on the pathogenesis of periodontitis.* Periodontol 2000.;1997;14:173-201.

[81] Preshaw PM. *Host response modulation in Periodontics.* Periodontol 2000 2008;14:173-201.

[82] Ryan ME and Preshaw PM. *Host Modulation in: Newman, Takei, Klokkevold and Carranza.* Clinical Periodontology, 10th edition, Saunders-an imprint of Elsevier, St.Louis, Missouri: Pg 275-282.

[83] Offenbacher S. *Periodontal diseases:Pathogenesis.* Ann Periodontol 1996;1:821-878.

[84] Offenbacher S, Heasman PA, Collins JG: *Modulation of host PGE2 secretion as a determinant of periodontal disease expression.* J Periodontol 1993, 64: 432- 444.

[85] Williams RC, Jeffcoat MK, Howell TH et al: *Indomethacin or fluribiprofen treatment of periodontitis in beagles comparison of effect on bone loss,* J Periodontal Res 1987; 22: 403 – 407.

[86] Williams RC, Jeffcoat MK, Howell TH et al: *Altering the progression of human alveolar bone loss with the non steroidal anti-inflammatory drug flurbiprofen.* J Periodontol 1989, 60: 485-490.

[87] Preshaw PM, Ryan ME and Giannabile WV. *Host Modulation Agents in Newman MG, Takei HH, Klokkevold PR and Carranza FA.* Clinical Periodontology, 10th edition, Saunders-an imprint of Elsevier, St.Louis, Missouri: Pg 813-827.

[88] Paquette D & Williams RC. *Modulation of host inflammatory mediators as a treatment strategy for periodontal diseases.* Periodontol 2000; 2000;24: 239–252.

[89] Reddy MS, *Geurs NC and Gunsolley JC. Periodontal host modulation with antiproteinase, anti-inflammatory and bone sparing agents. A systematic review.* Ann Periodontol 2003;8:12-37.

[90] Giannobile WV. *Host-Response Therapeutics for Periodontal Diseases.* J Periodontol 2008;79:1592-1600.

[91] Rocha M, Nava LG, Vázquez de la Torre C, Sánchez-Marín F, Ma. Eugenia Garay-Sevilla, Malacara JM. *Clinical and Radiological Improvement of Periodontal Disease in Patients With Type 2 Diabetes Mellitus Treated With Alendronate: A Randomized, Placebo-Controlled Trial.* J Periodontol 2001; 72: 204-209.

[92] Greenstein G. *Contemporary Interpretation of Probing Depth Assessments: Diagnostic and Therapeutic Implications. A Literature Review.* J Periodontol 1997;68: 1194-1205.

[93] Bower RC. *Furcation morphology relative to periodontal treatment:furcation root surface anatomy.* J Periodontol 1979, 50:23-27.

[94] Rabbani GM, Ash MM, Caffesse RG. *The effectiveness of subgingival scaling and root planing in calculus removal.* J Periodontol 1981,52:119-123.

[95] Caffesse RG, Sweeney PL, Smith BA: *Scaling and root planing with and without periodontal flap surgery.* J Clin Periodontol 1986,11: 205-210.

[96] Carranza FA and Takei HH. *Phase II Periodontal Therapy in: Newman MG, Takei HH, Klokkevold PR and Carranza FA.* Clinical Periodontology, 10th edition; Saunders-an imprint of Elsevier, St.Louis, Missouri: 881-886.

[97] McGuire MK. *Mild chronic adult periodontitis: Clinical applications. In: Wilson TG, Kornman KS, Newman MG, eds.* Advances in Periodontics, 1st ed. Chicago: Quintessence Publishing; 1992:130-142.

[98] Novaes AB Jr., Souza SL, Taba M Jr., Grisi MF, Suzigan LC, Tunes RS. *Control of gingival inflammation in a teenager population using ultrasonic prophylaxis.* Braz Dent J 2004;15:41-45.

[99] Ciancio SG. *Non-surgical periodontal treatment.* In: Proceedings of the World Workshop in Clinical Periodontics.Chicago: American Academy of Periodontology 1989:II-4.

[100] Pattison GL, Pattison AM. *Principles of periodontal instrumentation.* In: Carranza FA, Newman MG, eds. Clinical Periodontology, 8th ed. Philadelphia: W.B. Saunders; 1996:451-465.

[101] Segelnick SL and Weinberg MA. *Reevaluation of Initial Therapy: When is it Appropriate Time?* J Periodontol 2006;77:1598-1601.

[102] Barrrington EP. *An overview of Periodontal Surgical Procedures.* J Periodontol 1981;52: 518-528.

[103] Wang HL, Cooke J. *Periodontal Regeneration techniques for treatment of periodontal diseases.* Dent Clin North Am. 2005;49:637-659.

[104] Takei HH, Han TJ, Carranza F.A. Jr., Kenney E.B., Lekovic V. Flap *Technique for Periodontal Bone Implants—Papilla Preservation Technique* J Periodontol 1985;56:204-209.

[105] Takei HH and Carranza FA. *Gingival Surgical Techniques in: Newman MG, Takei HH, Klokkevold PR and Carranza FA.* Clinical Periodontology, 10th edition; Saunders-an imprint of Elsevier, St.Louis, Missouri:909-917.

[106] Wennstrom JL, Heijl L and Lindhe J. *Periodontal Surgery: Access therapy in: Lindhe J, Karring T and Lang NP.* Clinical Periodontology and Implant Dentistry, 4th edition, Blackwell Munksgaard, UK, 2003, pg 519-560.

[107] Hallmon WW, Chair, Carranza FA Jr., Drisko CL, Rapley JW & Robinson P. *Surgical Therapy in: Periodontal Literature Reviews.* The American Academy of Perio dontology 1996, Chicago, Illinois.pg 145-203.

[108] Ramfjord S, Nissle RR. *The Modified Widman flap.* J Periodontol 1974;45:601-607.

[109] Gottlow J. *Periodontal regeneration in Lang NP and Karring T.* Proceedings of the 1st European Workshop on Periodontology, Quintessence Publishing Co., Ltd; 1993:172-192.

[110] Carranza FA, Takei HH and Cochran DL. *Reconstructive periodontal surgery in: Newman MG, Takei HH, Klokkevold PR and Carranza FA.* Clinical Periodontology, 10th edition, Saunders-an imprint of Elsevier, St.Louis, Missouri: Pg 968-990.

[111] Caton J, Nyman S, Zander H. *Histometric evaluation of periodontal surgery II. Connective tissue attachment levels after four regenerative procedures.* J Clin Periodontol 1980; 7:224 - 231 .

[112] Mariotti A. *Efficacy of chemical root modifiers in the treatment of periodontal disease. A systematic review.* Ann Periodontol 2003;8:205-226.

[113] Register A, Burdick F. *Accelerated reattachment with cementogenesis to dentin, demineralised in situ. I. Optimum range.* J Periodontol 1975; 46:646-655.

[114] Garrett J, Crigger M, Egelberg J. *Effects of citric acid on diseased root surfaces.* J Periodont Res 1978;3:155-163.

[115] Polson A, Frederick G, Ladenheim S, Hanes P. *The production of a root surface smear layer by instrumentation and its removal by citric acid.* J Periodontol 1984;54:443-446.

[116] Hanes P, Polson A, *Frederick G. Initial wound healing attachments to demineralised dentin.* J Periodontol 1988;59:176-183.

[117] Daly C. *Antibacterial effect of citric acid treatment of periodontally diseased root surfaces in vitro.* J Clin Periodontol 1982;9:386-392.

[118] Terranova V, Franzetti L, Hic S et al. *A biochemical approach to periodontal regeneration: tetracycline treatment of dentin promotes fibroblast adhesion and growth.* J Periodontal Res 1986;21: 330-337.

[119] Stahl SS, Froum SJ. *Human clinical and histologic repair responses following the use of citric acid in periodontal therapy.* J Periodontol 1977;48:261-266.

[120] Trombelli L. *Which reconstructive procedures are effective for treating the periodontal intraosseous defect?* Periodontol 2000.;2005;37: 88–105.

[121] Froum SJ, Thaler R, Scopp IW and Stahl SS. *Osseous autografts II. Histological responses to osseous coagulum-bone blend grafts.* J Periodontol 1975;46:656-661.

[122] Carranza FA, McClain P and Schallhorn. *Regenerative Osseous Surgery in : Newman MG, Takei HH, and Carranza FA.* Clinical Periodontology, 9th edition, Saunders-an imprint of Elsevier, St.Louis, Missouri: Pg 804-824.

[123] Dragoo MR, Sullivan HC. *A clinical and histological evaluation of autogenous iliac bone grafts in humans. I. Wound healing 2 to 8 months.* J Periodontol 1973;44(10):599-613.

[124] American Academy of Periodontology. *Position Paper:Periodontal Regeneration.* J Periodontol 2005;76:1601-1622.

[125] American Academy of Periodontology. Position Paper: *Tissue banking of bone allografts in Periodontal Regeneration.* J Periodontol 2001; 72: 834-838.

[126] Becker W, Lynch S, Lekholm U, Becker BE, Caffesse R, Donath K, Sanchez R. *A Comparison of ePTFE Membranes Alone or in Combination with Platelet-Derived Growth Factors and Insulin-Like Growth Factor-I or Demineralized Freeze-Dried Bone in Promoting Bone Formation Around Immediate Extraction Socket Implants.* J Periodontol 1992;63:929-940.

[127] Zohar R and Tenenbaum HC. *How Predictable Are Periodontal Regenerative Procedures?* J Can Dent Assoc 2005; 71(9):675–680.

[128] Gunther KP, Scharf HP, Pesch HJ, Puh W. *Osteointegration of solvent-preserved bone transplants in an animal model.* Osteologie 1996;5:4-12.

[129] Block MS, Degen M. *Horizontal ridge augmentationusing human mineralized particulate bone: Preliminary results.* J OralMaxillofac Surg 2004;62(Suppl.2)67-72.

[130] Block MS, Finger I, Lytle R. *Human mineralized bone in extraction sites before implant placement: Preliminary results.* J Am Dent Assoc 2002;133:1631-1638.

[131] Carmelo M, Nevins M, Schenk R et al. *Clinical, radiographic and histologic evaluation of human periodontal defects treated with bio-oss and bio-guide.* Int J Periodont Restor Dent 1998;18:321

[132] Murphy K, Gunsolley J. *Guided tissue regeneration for the treatment of periodontal intrabony and furcation defects. A systematic review.* Ann Periodontol 2003;8:266-302.

[133] Raja S, Byakod G, Pudakalkatti P. *Growth factors in periodontal regeneration.* Int J Dent Hygiene 7, 2009; 82–89

[134] Howell TH, Fiorellini JP, Paquette DW, Offenbacher S, Giannobile WV, and Lynch SE. *A Phase I/II Clinical Trial to Evaluate a Combination of Recombinant Human Platelet-Derived Growth Factor-BB and Recombinant Human Insulin-Like Growth Factor-I in Patients with Periodontal Disease.* J Periodontol 1997;68: 1186-1193.

[135] Hammarstrom L. *Enamel matrix, cementum development and regeneration.* J Clin Periodontol 1997;4: 658-668.

[136] Giannobile WV and Somerman MJ. *Growth and amelogenin like factors in periodontal wound healing. A systematic review.* Ann Periodontol 2003;8:193-204.

[137] Heijl L, Heden G, Svardstrom G, Ostgren A. *Enamel matrix derivative (EMDOGAIN) in the treatment of intrabony periodontal defects.* J Clin Periodontol 1997;24:705-714. 705-714.

[138] Bosshardt DD. *Biological mediators and periodontal regeneration: a review of enamel matrix proteins at the cellular and molecular levels.* Clin Periodontol 2008; 35 (Suppl. 8): 87–105

[139] Sims TN & Ammons W Jr. *Resective Osseous surgery in: Newman MG, Takei HH and Carranza FA.* Clinical Periodontology, 9th edition; Saunders-an imprint of Elsevier, St.Louis, Missouri: pg 786-803.

[140] Carnevale G & Kaldahl WB. *Osseous resective surgery.* Periodontol 2000.;2000;22: 59–87.

[141] Carranza FA & Takei HH. *The flap technique for pocket therapy in: Newman MG, Takei HH, Klokkevold PR and Carranza FA.* Clinical Periodontology, 10th edition, Saunders-an imprint of Elsevier, St.Louis, Missouri: Pg 926-936.

[142] Hiatt W H, Stallard RE, Butler ED & Badgett B. *Repair Following Mucoperiosteal Flap Surgery with Full Gingival Retention.* J Periodontol 1968; 11-16.

[143] Kerry GJ. *Supportive periodontal treatment.* Periodontol 2000.;1995;9: 176-185.

[144] American *Academy of Periodontology. Position paper-Periodontal maintenance.* J Periodontol 2003,74:1395-1401.

[145] Wilson TJ, Glover ME, Malik AK, Schoen JA, Dorsett D. *Tooth loss in maintenance patients in a private periodontal practice.* J Periodontol 1987;58:231-235.

[146] Pertuiset JH, Saglie FR, Lofthus J, Rezende M. and Sanz M. *Recurrent Periodontal Disease and Bacterial Presence in the Gingiva.* J Periodontol 1987;58:553-558.

[147] Christersson LA, Albini B, Zambon JJ, Wikesjo UME, Genco RJ. *Tissue Localization of Actinobacillus actinomycetemomitans in Human Periodontitis—I. Light, Immunofluorescence and Electron Microscopic Studies.* J Periodontol 1987;58:529-539.

[148] Cortellini P, Pini-Prato G, Tonetti M. *Periodontal regeneration of infrabony defects (V). Effect of oral hygiene on long-term stability.* J Clin Periodontol 1994;21:606-610.

[149] Wilson TG, Jr. *Maintaining periodontal treatment.* J Am Dent Assoc 1990; 121: 491-494.

In: Periodontitis Symptoms, Treatment and Prevention
Editor: Rosemarie E. Walchuck, pp. 73-103

ISBN: 978-1-61668-836-3
©2010 Nova Science Publishers, Inc.

Chapter 3

THE ROLE OF ANTIMICROBIAL PEPTIDES IN PERIODONTAL DISEASE

Suttichai Krisanaprakornkit[1] and Sakornrat Khongkhunthian[2]
Center of Excellence for Innovation in Chemistry, Department of Oral Biology
and Diagnostic Sciences[1], Department of Restorative Dentistry and Periodontology[2]
Faculty of Dentistry, Chiang Mai University, Chiang Mai, Thailand

ABSTRACT

The oral cavity is a warm, moist environment, in which a number of microorganisms colonize and live in harmony as a community, a so-called biofilm. In this environment, antimicrobial peptides may play a critical role in maintaining normal oral health and controlling innate and acquired immune systems in response to continuous microbial challenges in periodontal disease. Two major families of antimicrobial peptides, found in the oral cavity, are defensin and cathelicidin. Members of the defensin family are cysteine-rich peptides, synthesized by plants, insects, and mammals. These peptides vary in length and in the number of disulfide bonds, and have a beta-sheet structure. In the oral cavity, four alpha-defensins are synthesized and stored in neutrophil granules, which are converted into active peptides by proteolytic processing, while three human beta-defensins (hBDs), hBD-1, hBD-2, and hBD-3, are predominantly produced by oral epithelial cells. The only member of the cathelicidin family found in humans is LL-37, an alpha-helical peptide that contains 37 amino acids and begins with two leucines at its NH_3-terminus. LL-37 is derived from enzymatic cleavage of a precursor peptide, namely, human cationic antimicrobial peptide-18. Clinically, differential expression of antimicrobial peptides has been reported in specific types of periodontal disease, and their presence has been shown in saliva and gingival crevicular fluid. Current evidence suggests that alpha-defensins, beta-defensins, and LL-37 have distinct, but overlapping, roles in antimicrobial and pro-inflammatory activities. Several studies have shown antimicrobial activities of hBD-2, hBD-3, and LL-37 against several periodontal pathogens, suggesting their potential role as antimicrobial agents for periodontal disease. The clinical significance of antimicrobial peptides in periodontal disease has recently been demonstrated in morbus Kostmann syndrome, a severe congenital neutropenia, in which chronic periodontal infection in young patients, resulting from a deficiency of neutrophil-derived antimicrobial peptides, causes early tooth loss. Although researchers initially focused their attention on antimicrobial activities, it is now becoming evident that defensins and LL-37 are multifunctional molecules that mediate various host immune responses, and may thus represent essential molecules of innate immunity in periodontal disease. In this chapter, basic knowledge and the clinical importance of antimicrobial peptides in periodontal disease will be discussed in detail.

INTRODUCTION

The warm and moist environment in the oral cavity is a unique niche suitable for a number of microorganisms to colonize, proliferate, and live in harmony as a community, a so-called biofilm. Oral epithelium plays a main role as a physical barrier between the microbial biofilm in the external environment and underlying connective tissue and blood vessels. Naturally, this barrier can be disrupted, since the oral epithelium is the only site in the body normally penetrated by a hard tissue, namely, a tooth. The junction between oral epithelium and the tooth is, therefore, considered a site that is readily susceptible to infection from various microorganisms living in dental plaque. Previously, the role of oral epithelium was viewed as that of an innocent bystander. However, it is now apparent that oral epithelial cells can respond to continuous microbial challenges from the dental plaque by production of cytokines, chemokines, and antimicrobial peptides, which enhance inflammation and immune response in periodontal tissues. Uncontrolled inflammation and immune response from excessive production of these pro-inflammatory molecules is considered one of the etiological factors in the pathogenesis of periodontal disease.

In the oral cavity, antimicrobial peptides may play a critical role in maintaining balance between periodontal health and disease. Therefore, their biological and clinical significances, particularly the ones that are pertinent to periodontal disease, will be emphasized in this chapter. These include the differential expression of antimicrobial peptides in healthy and diseased periodontal tissues and in gingival crevicular fluid (GCF), their antimicrobial effects against a variety of periodontal microorganisms, and their novel functions, related to host immune responses in periodontal disease. Furthermore, some recent studies have demonstrated a connection between the deficiencies in antimicrobial peptide production or function and patients affected with some types of periodontitis, highlighting the clinical importance of these antimicrobial peptides.

Two well-characterized families of antimicrobial peptides, including defensin and cathelicidin, are present in saliva and GCF, and localized in the oral mucosa (Dale and Fredericks, 2005). These peptides include β-defensins that are expressed in the oral epithelial cells, α-defensins that are secreted from neutrophil granules, and LL-37, the only human antimicrobial peptide in the cathelicidin family, which mainly derives from neutrophil granules and to a lesser extent from oral epithelial cells (Dale et al, 2001). The synthesis of some of these antimicrobial peptides can be considerably up-regulated upon exposure to oral microorganisms; thus, these peptides are regarded as essential effector molecules in innate immunity. In this chapter, basic knowledge, regarding expression and regulation of defensins and LL-37, as well as their antimicrobial activities and other functions, will be extensively reviewed. However, a review of other antimicrobial peptides present in the oral cavity, such as calprotectin, adrenomedullin, histatins, etc., is beyond the scope of this chapter and will not be discussed.

GENERAL INFORMATION ON HUMAN CATHELICIDIN AND DEFENSIN

Cathelicidin is a family of antimicrobial peptides that contain a cathelin domain at their NH$_3$-terminus and an antimicrobial domain at their COOH-terminus (Zanetti et al, 1995). Whereas the amino acid sequence of the cathelin domain is conserved throughout animal species tested to date, the sequence of the antimicrobial domain exhibits considerable variations, accounting for various molecular structures, such as α-helix, β-sheet, etc., possibly reflecting the nature of microbial diversity. The cathelin domain, categorized as a member of the cystatin family (Ritonja et al, 1989), primarily functions as a cathepsin L inhibitor, from which the name of this domain is derived (Kopitar et al, 1989). However, it was later demonstrated that this domain also possesses an antimicrobial function against *Escherichia coli* and methicillin-resistant *Staphylococcus aureus* (Zaiou et al, 2003), yet its antimicrobial mechanism is still largely unknown. The first cathelicidin antimicrobial peptide was isolated from bovine neutrophils (Romeo et al, 1988). Subsequently, several cathelicidin peptides were identified in various mammals, particularly humans. The only cathelicidin in humans, LL-37, is derived from proteolytic processing of a precursor peptide, human cationic antimicrobial protein-18 (hCAP-18), and contains two leucines at its NH$_3$-terminus (Agerberth et al, 1995; Cowland et al, 1995).

Defensin is a family of small cationic antimicrobial peptides, containing six unique cysteine amino acids that form three disulfide bonds, functioning in stabilization of their β-sheet structure (Zasloff, 2002; Ganz, 2003). Moreover, these peptides, comprising several positively charged amino acids that favorably interact with negatively charged microbial membranes, can form a complex structure, such as a dimeric structure (Hill et al, 1991). In addition, the defensin peptides contain both hydrophobic and hydrophilic domains in their molecules, a so-called amphipathic structure. All of these properties, thus, make the defensins suitable for membrane integration that eventually leads to a pore formation in the membrane. The pore-forming mechanism of the defensins is then believed to be a crucial process in their antimicrobial function. Therefore, it has been shown by a number of studies that the defensins exert their broad spectrum of antimicrobial activities against gram-negative and gram-positive bacteria, fungi, and some enveloped viruses (Ganz, 2003).

The human defensin family can be further divided into two subfamilies, i.e., α-defensin and β-defensin subfamilies. In the α-defensin subfamily, four of the six α-defensins, human neutrophil peptide-1, -2, -3, and -4 (HNP-1, -2, -3, and -4), are synthesized and stored in neutrophil granules (Ganz et al, 1985; Wilde et al, 1989), while the other two α-defensins, human defensin-5 and -6 (HD-5 and -6), are synthesized and stored in the granules of Paneth cells, specialized epithelial cells located at the crypts of Lieberkühn of the small intestine (Jones and Bevins, 1992; 1993). Being encoded by the same gene, the pro-peptide of HNP-1, -2, and -3 comprises 94 amino acids, which is successively cleaved by putative proteolytic enzymes, yielding different sizes of the mature peptides that are stored in azurophilic granules (Valore and Ganz, 1992). The number of amino acids in the mature peptides of HNP-1 to HNP-3 varies from 29 to 30 amino acids. On the other hand, HD-5 and HD-6 are stored in Paneth cell granules as pro-peptides, and are subsequently activated by trypsin digestion upon release into the intestinal lumen (Ghosh et al, 2002). HNP-4 is encoded by another gene, and its amino acid sequence completely differs from that of HNP-1, HNP-2, and HNP-3, leaving only the identical characteristic cysteines and some arginines (Wilde et al, 1989).

In the β-defensin subfamily, four human β-defensins, human β-defensin-1, -2, -3, and -4 (hBD-1, -2, -3, and -4), are principally expressed in epithelial cells that cover several tissues and organs, particularly skin and the mucosal surfaces of gastrointestinal, respiratory, and urogenital tracts, whereas hBD-5 and hBD-6 are expressed only in epididymis (Semple et al, 2003). However, only hBD-1, -2, and -3 are found in the oral cavity (Abiko et al, 2007). HBD-1 and hBD-2 peptides are localized in differentiated epithelial cells within the suprabasal layers of normal gingival epithelium (Dale et al, 2001), whereas hBD-3 peptide is expressed in undifferentiated epithelial cells within the basal layer (Lu et al, 2005), suggesting a potential role for hBD-3 as a mediator to signal the underlying connective tissue cells. HBD-1 is constitutively expressed in several epithelial cell types studied to date, especially gingival epithelial cells (Krisanaprakornkit et al, 1998), whereas expression of hBD-2, hBD-3, and hBD-4 is inducible upon stimulation with pro-inflammatory cytokines or contact with microorganisms. The regulation of human β-defensins will be discussed below.

EXPRESSION AND REGULATION OF HUMAN CATHELICIDIN AND DEFENSINS

Human cathelicidin is mainly isolated from neutrophil granules in the amount of 0.627 micrograms per one million neutrophils (Sørensen et al, 1997). After synthesis, human cathelicidin is stored in granules distinct from those that store proteolytic enzymes, such as neutrophil elastase, proteinase-3, etc., to prevent premature activation of the cathelicidin peptide inside the neutrophils. Upon being released into neutrophil phagosomes after bacterial phagocytosis or being released into extracellular environment, the neutrophil cathelicidin is proteolytically cleaved into a mature LL-37 peptide by the proteinase-3 (Sørensen et al, 2001). In addition to regulation of cathelicidin activation by enzymatic cleavage in human neutrophils, cathelicidin expression in other cell types is controlled by exposure to microorganisms, growth factors, and differentiating agents. For instance, LL-37 expression in skin keratinocytes and gastric epithelial cells is induced by Staphylococcus aureus and Helicobacter pyroli, respectively (Midorikawa et al, 2003; Hase et al, 2003). Furthermore, LL-37 expression in skin keratinocytes is up-regulated by insulin-like growth factor-I and vitamin D, known to promote wound healing and differentiation, respectively (Sørensen et al, 2003; Weber et al, 2005). In addition, LL-37 expression in gastric and small intestinal epithelial cells is induced by short chain fatty acids, including butyrate, via mitogen activated protein (MAP) kinases (Schauber et al, 2003).

Expression of LL-37 can also be found in natural killer cells, monocytes, B- and T-lymphocytes (Agerberth et al, 2000), mast cells (Di Nardo et al, 2003), epithelial cells lining respiratory (Bals et al, 1998) and gastrointestinal tracts (Tollin et al, 2003), reproductive organs (Agerberth et al, 1995; Frohm Nilsson et al, 1999; Malm et al, 2000), salivary glands (Murakami et al, 2002a), sweat glands (Murakami et al, 2002b), and in inflammatory skin disorders (Frohm et al, 1997). In the oral cavity, LL-37 is expressed in buccal and tongue mucosa (Frohm Nilsson et al, 1999), and its expression is up-regulated in the inflamed gingival tissues (Hosokawa et al, 2006). Correspondingly, the concentrations of LL-37 in the gingival tissue, whether derived from neutrophils or from gingival epithelium, correlate positively with the depth of the gingival crevice, suggesting that the LL-37 levels may be used as one diagnostic tool in inflammatory periodontal disorders (Hosokawa et al, 2006). In addition, LL-37 peptide is detected in saliva (Murakami et al, 2002a) and GCF (Puklo et al, 2008), and LL-37 levels in GCF are significantly elevated in patients with chronic periodontitis compared to those in patients with gingivitis or to those in healthy volunteers (Türkoğlu et al, 2009). However, it is likely that LL-37 present in saliva and GCF originates mostly from neutrophil granules (Dale and Fredericks, 2005).

The neutrophil α-defensin gene (*DEFA1*) is located on chromosome 8 (8p23) (Sparkes et al, 1989), and the number of such genes in different individuals varies from two to three genes per diploid cell (Mars et al, 1995). HNP-1, HNP-2, and HNP-3 mRNAs are mainly expressed in neutrophils, and their respective proteins were first characterized from azurophilic granules (Ganz et al, 1985) that also comprise other antimicrobial peptides, such as myeloperoxidase, cathelicidin, etc. Moreover, expression of HNP-1, HNP-2, and HNP-3 can be detected in lymphocytes (Blomqvist et al, 1999; Agerberth et al, 2000) and Langerhans cells in the vicinity of epithelial dysplasia adjacent to precancerous lesions and oral squamous cell carcinoma (Mizukawa et al, 1999), but their expression is not found in normal oral mucosa. They are also present in ductal cells of submandibular salivary glands from patients with oral cancer (Mizukawa et al, 2000).

With respect to periodontal tissue, the detectable amounts of HNP-1, HNP-2, and HNP-3 in GCF can vary from 270 to 2000 nanogram per site (or approximately equivalent to mg/ml) (McKay et al, 1999), which is sufficient for their antimicrobial function in periodontium. By virtue of matrix assisted laser desorption ionization mass spectrometry (MALDI-MS), it has been demonstrated that HNP-1 is most abundant in GCF, whereas HNP-3 is least abundant (Lundy et al, 2005). Moreover, the concentrations of HNP-1 to HNP-3, as well as those of LL-37 and hBD-3, have been quantified in saliva. These concentrations (up to twelve μg/ml) are variable in the human population (Tao et al, 2005). In addition, the median levels of HNP-1 to HNP-3 in saliva are significantly higher in children without dental caries than in those with dental caries experience, whereas the median levels of LL-37 and hBD-3 do not correlate with caries experience (Tao et al, 2005), suggesting the protective role of neutrophil α-defensins against dental caries.

Enteric α-defensin genes are located on chromosome 8 in the same vicinity as *DEFA1*, suggesting the duplication of α-defensin genes during evolution (Bevins et al, 1996). Up to now, only very weak HD-5 expression has been identified in a few oral tissue samples, whereas HD-6 expression is not detectable at all, indicating that enteric α-defensins do not play any role in the innate immunity of the oral cavity (Dunsche et al, 2001).

β-defensins are somewhat larger than α-defensins. Although 28 β-defensin genes have been discovered by computer searching of the human genome (Schutte et al, 2002), expression of only six human β-defensins, hBD-1 to hBD-6, has been characterized to date in human tissues and organs. HBD-1 is the first human β-defensin, isolated from hemofiltrate passing through the kidney at the nanomolar levels (Bensch et al, 1995). The gene encoding hBD-1, *DEFB1*, is on chromosome 8, in close proximity to *DEFA1*, around 100-150 kilobases apart (Liu et al, 1997). However, both the amino acid sequence and the pairing between two cysteine amino acids that form the disulfide bond in hBD-1 greatly differ from both the sequence and pairing in HNP-1; thus, creating a new β-defensin subfamily. *DEFB1* contains two exons with one large 6962 base pair (bp) intron (Liu et al, 1997). The two exons encode a 362 bp complementary DNA (cDNA) that is translated into an hBD-1 pro-peptide

(Liu et al, 1997). The hBD-1 pro-peptide is subsequently cleaved to yield several hBD-1 mature peptides, ranging from 36 to 47 amino acids long. Widespread and low expression of hBD-1 has been detected in various epithelia lining several organs, including trachea, bronchus, prostate gland, mammary gland, placenta, thymus, testis, skin, small intestine (Zhao et al, 1996), pancreas and kidney – especially, the collecting duct, distal tubule, and loop of Henle – (Schnapp et al, 1998), vagina, endometrium, Fallopian tube (Valore et al, 1998), and salivary glands (Bonass et al, 1999; Sahasrabudhe et al, 2000).

In the oral mucosa, hBD-1 expression is found in gingival epithelium, but is not associated with the amount of IL-8 expression in the gingival tissue (Krisanaprakornkit et al, 1998). In other words, the amount of hBD-1 expression in gingival tissue does not correlate with the degree of tissue inflammation, but varies among different individuals (Krisanaprakornkit et al, 1998). Moreover, confluent cultured gingival epithelial cells constitutively express hBD-1 mRNA at baseline levels; however, its expression is up-regulated in a post-confluent culture, representing the state of cellular differentiation *in vitro* (Dale et al, 2001). In this study, the state of differentiation is shown by increased mRNA expression of profilaggrin, a late marker for differentiation. Consistent with the increased hBD-1 mRNA expression in the post-confluent culture, hBD-1 mRNA and peptide are localized in the suprabasal layers of oral epithelium *in vivo* (Dale et al, 2001). On the other hand, it has been demonstrated that increased hBD-1 expression can, in turn, induce differentiation in skin keratinocytes (Frye et al, 2001).

By using a protein chip array together with surface enhanced laser desorption/ionization (SELDI) and time-of-flight mass spectrometry, hBD-1 peptide at a molecular mass of about 4.7 kilodalton (kDa) is detected in culture medium of gingival epithelial cells (Diamond et al, 2001). Unlike known concentrations of neutrophil α-defensins in GCF, the precise levels of hBD-1 present in GCF have not yet been accurately quantified. Highly variable amounts of hBD-1 peptide have been found in saliva and GCF, collected from different normal individuals (Diamond et al, 2001). It is possible that salivary ductal cells may also contribute some hBD-1 peptide detected in saliva in addition to hBD-1 peptide synthesis by oral epithelial cells (Sahasrabudhe et al, 2000). It is noteworthy that hBD-1 and hBD-2 are neither expressed in cultured gingival fibroblasts (Krisanaprakornkit et al, 1998; 2000) nor found in the underlying connective tissue of the oral mucosa (Dale et al, 2001).

The second human β-defensin, hBD-2, was first isolated in large amounts from psoriatic skin keratinocytes (Harder et al, 1997a). The gene encoding hBD-2 is *DEFB4*, which is located on chromosome 8, region 8p22-p23.1, in close proximity to *DEFA1* and *DEFB1* (Harder et al, 1997b). *DEFB4* contains one 1639 bp intron (Liu et al, 1998), and two small exons that encode a signal peptide domain and a mature peptide, whose sizes are 23 and 41 amino acids long, respectively (Harder et al, 1997b). Expression of both hBD-1 and hBD-2 is localized in the suprabasal layers of normal epidermis (Ali et al, 2001), identical with their expression in normal oral mucosa (Dale et al, 2001). HBD-2 peptide is stored in lamellar granules in the spinous layer of epidermis, and later released into the extracellular environment with other lipids in the granular layer, suggesting that lipids covering the skin function as a natural barrier against water permeability and microbial invasion due to the presence of antimicrobial peptides (Oren et al, 2003).

As with the inducible expression of hBD-2 by microorganisms and pro-inflammatory cytokines in other cell types, hBD-2 mRNA is up-regulated in cultured gingival epithelial cells in response to stimulation with IL-1β, TNF-α, phorbol ester, a potent epithelial activator, and Gram-negative periodontal bacteria, including *Aggregatibacter actinomycetemcomitans*, *Fusobacterium nucleatum*, and *Porphyromonas gingivalis* (Mathews et al, 1999; Krisanaprakornkit et al, 2000; Noguchi et al, 2003; Chung et al, 2004; Taguchi and Imai, 2006; Laube et al, 2008). Nevertheless, unlike the critical role of CD14, a lipopolysaccharide (LPS) co-receptor, and nuclear factor-kappa B (NF-κB) in hBD-2 induction in respiratory epithelial cells and mononuclear phagocytes (Becker et al, 2000; Harder et al, 2000; Tsutsumi-Ishii and Nagaoka, 2002), CD14 and NF-κB are neither critical nor essential for hBD-2 up-regulation in gingival epithelial cells (Krisanaprakornkit et al, 2002). In fact, a purified LPS fraction of either *Fusobacterium nucleatum* or *Aggregatibacter actinomycetemcomitans* is a poor hBD-2 activator in gingival epithelial cells (Krisanaprakornkit et al, 2000; Laube et al, 2008, respectively). Furthermore, p38 MAP kinase and c-Jun N-terminal MAP kinase (JNK) control hBD-2 mRNA up-regulation in response to *Fusobacterium nucleatum* in gingival epithelial cells (Krisanaprakornkit et al, 2002). Likewise, the MAP kinase pathways, but not the NF-κB transcription factor, are critical for hBD-2 up-regulation by the outer membrane protein 100 (Omp100; named after its molecular mass) of *Aggregatibacter actinomycetemcomitans* (Ouhara et al, 2006). Taken together, these findings suggest different cellular receptors and intracellular signaling mechanisms to control hBD-2 up-regulation by different stimulants in distinct cell types.

In addition to the involvement of p38 MAP kinase and JNK in hBD-2 up-regulation by *Fusobacterium nucleatum*, it is shown that an increase in intracellular calcium ion and phosphorylated phospholipase D, two important molecules in regulating epithelial cell differentiation (Exton, 1999; Bollag et al, 2005), are involved in hBD-2 up-regulation by *Fusobacterium nucleatum* (Krisanaprakornkit et al, 2003; 2008). It is noteworthy that treatment of gingival epithelial cells with either exogenously added calcium ions or thapsigargin, an inhibitor of the sarcoendoplasmic reticulum calcium (SERCA) pump, an inhibitor that leads to continuous calcium ion release from its intracellular storage, induces hBD-2 mRNA, whereas BAPTA-AM, a cell permeable calcium chelator, blocks hBD-2 mRNA up-regulation by *Fusobacterium nucleatum* and thapsigargin in a dose-dependent manner (Krisanaprakornkit et al, 2003). In summary, the regulation of hBD-2 expression can be controlled by both inflammation from bacteria and epithelial differentiation.

Consistent with this conclusion, the strongest hBD-2 expression in gingival tissue is found at the gingival margin, adjacent to microbial plaque accumulation, and hBD-2 expression is localized in differentiated epithelial cells within the suprabasal layers of gingival epithelium (Dale et al, 2001). Moreover, the localization of hBD-2 peptide is found not only in cultured gingival epithelial cells that express involucrin, another marker for differentiation, but also in stimulated cells with infectious and pro-inflammatory stimulants (Dale et al, 2001). In contrast, neither hBD-1 nor hBD-2 is expressed in junctional epithelium (Dale et al, 2001), which consists of relatively undifferentiated epithelial cells, implying that the junctional epithelium may be more susceptible to infection than other areas of gingival epithelium because of the lack of some antimicrobial peptides. However, it is probable that other antimicrobial peptides, such as α-defensins, LL-37, etc., released from neutrophils that transmigrate from blood vessels into the junctional epithelium and gingival crevice, may perform this antimicrobial function instead (Dale and Fredericks, 2005).

Using biochemical and molecular biology techniques, the gene encoding hBD-3 (*DEFB103*) has been cloned from human skin keratinocytes and alveolar epithelial cells, and the amino acid composition of hBD-3 has been sequenced and classified as a novel peptide in the β-defensin subfamily (Harder et al, 2001). *DEFB103*, containing two small exons, is located 13 kb upstream from *DEFB4* that encodes hBD-2 on chromosome 8 (Jia et al, 2001). HBD-3 cDNA is translated into an hBD-3 pro-peptide that comprises a signal peptide domain (22 amino acids long) and a mature peptide (45 amino acids long). The amino acid sequence of hBD-3 is 43% identical to that of hBD-2 (Jia et al, 2001).

In addition to skin keratinocytes, hBD-3 is expressed in various epithelia lining several tissues, including gingiva (Jia et al, 2001; Dunsche et al, 2002), tonsils (Harder et al, 2001), esophagus, trachea, placenta, and fetal thymus glands (Jia et al, 2001). In the oral cavity, hBD-3 mRNA and peptide are localized in the basal layer of normal gingival epithelium (Lu et al, 2005), whereas hBD-1 and hBD-2 are expressed in the suprabasal layers (Dale et al, 2001). Furthermore, hBD-3 mRNA is expressed in both inflamed and non-inflamed epithelium and salivary glands (Dunsche et al, 2001), and its expression is up-regulated in leukoplakia and oral lichen planus (Nishimura et al, 2003). *In vitro*, hBD-3 mRNA expression is induced in cultured epithelial cells that are stimulated with IFN-γ, TNF-α, and IL-1β (García et al, 2001; Harder et al, 2001; Jia et al, 2001), although IFN-γ does not up-regulate hBD-2 mRNA (García et al, 2001). Consistent with the findings obtained from these studies, it was later demonstrated that IFN-γ is a primary inducer for hBD-3 expression, whereas IL-1β and TNF-α are major stimulants for hBD-2 expression (Joly et al, 2005).

With respect to up-regulation of hBD-3 by oral microorganisms, hBD-3 mRNA expression is induced by live nonperiodontopathic bacteria (Ji et al, 2007a), including *Streptococcus sanguinis* and *Streptococcus gordonii*, and some periodontopathic bacteria, including *Aggregatibacter actinomycetemcomitans* (Feucht et al, 2003), *Prevotella intermedia*, and *Fusobacterium nucleatum* (Ji et al, 2007a). In contrast, three well known causative pathogens in chronic periodontitis, including *Porphyromonas gingivalis*, *Tanerella forsythia*, and *Treponema denticola*, down-regulate hBD-3 mRNA expression, as well as IL-8 production and secretion in an oral epithelial cell line (Ji et al, 2007a). This indicates that these so-called "red-complex" periodontal pathogens may suppress innate immune responses of oral epithelial cells by an immune-evading mechanism, known as "chemokine paralysis" (Darveau et al, 1998). Furthermore, the red-complex bacteria can tolerate the host immune response by being more resistant to LL-37 and phagocytosis by neutrophils (Ji et al, 2007b), indicating their strong implication with chronic periodontal infection.

ANTIMICROBIAL ACTIVITY

Up to the present, there have been an enormous number of *in vitro* studies, showing the antimicrobial activity of LL-37 and human defensins against various pathogens associated with a variety of human diseases. All of these studies cannot be completely mentioned in this chapter due to the space limitation. Therefore, the scope of this topic will be restricted to the antimicrobial effects on oral pathogens, especially the ones associated with periodontal disease. In the oral cavity, the warm temperature and moistened mucosal and tooth surfaces are suitable for microbial colonization and then the formation of biofilm, so-called dental plaque. The dental plaque is essential for some specific oral microorganisms to survive and thrive in this complex community. It is conceivable that the exopolysaccharide-producing plaque can protect oral microorganisms from exposure to antibiotics, or antimicrobial peptides in the context of this discussion. As with antibiotics, it is, therefore, likely that plaque microorganisms are more resistant to destruction by antimicrobial peptides than are planktonic microrganisms present in the saliva. Consequently, antimicrobial peptides can be regarded as one of the selective pressures that oral microorganisms must overcome in order to establish colonies in the dental plaque.

Furthermore, it should be emphasized that the results obtained from most studies that examine the susceptibility of one or more microbial species to individual antimicrobial peptides *in vitro* may not represent the real effectiveness of antimicrobial peptides due to the complexity of interactions between host and microorganisms or between two different types of microorganisms in the dental plaque. However, it is rather difficult to evaluate the effectiveness of antimicrobial peptides in such a complicated situation *in vivo*. Fortunately, some recent *in vivo* studies have shed light into the clinical significance of antimicrobial peptides for periodontal homeostasis. In this regard, it has been shown that genetic and acquired deficiencies of some antimicrobial peptides are associated with the pathogenesis of some types of periodontitis (Pütsep et al, 2002; Puklo et al, 2008), and this will be discussed under the next heading.

Other factors that influence the antimicrobial effects of some antimicrobial peptides are high salt concentrations that are shown to inhibit antimicrobial functions in other parts of the body (Goldman et al, 1997; Midorikawa et al, 2003) and the presence of inhibitors in serum (Tanaka et al, 2000). However, in the oral cavity, antimicrobial peptides may not be affected by these factors, since the peptides function at the mucosal surface, where the concentrations of salt or inhibitors, diluted with saliva, are too low to exert any significant inhibitory action.

At the outset of the study of the antimicrobial effects on oral bacteria, the bactericidal activity of LL-37 was tested against different strains of *Aggregatibacter actinomycetemcomitans* and *Capnocytophaga* spp., which are implicated in the pathogenesis of juvenile periodontitis and gingivitis, respectively (Tanaka et al, 2000). It was found that the concentrations of LL-37 (below 12 μg/ml) already killed all strains of these two bacteria by 99%. Subsequently, under a more detailed investigation into the antimicrobial effects of LL-37 against different kinds of periodontal bacteria, involved with various stages of dental plaque formation, it was demonstrated that the early colonizing yellow-complex bacteria, such as oral *Streptococci*, *Actinomyces*, etc., and the bridging orange-complex bacterium, i.e., *Fusobacterium nucleatum*, are susceptible to the bactericidal activity of LL-37 with low minimum inhibitory concentrations (MICs) in μg/ml (Ji et al, 2007b). Similar results have also been obtained from another study (Ouhara et al, 2005), which shows the antimicrobial effects of LL-37 against various gram-positive oral *Streptococci*. In contrast, the red-complex periodontopathic bacteria, including *Porphyromonas gingivalis*, *Tannerella forsythensis*, and *Treponema denticola*, are more resistant to LL-37 than are other bacteria (Ji et al, 2007b), suggesting their strong involvement with periodontitis.

Furthermore, LL-37 exerts its candidacidal activity by disrupting the yeast cell membrane, leading to membrane fragmentation and a release of intracellular contents, such as adenosine triphosphate (den Hertog et al, 2005). With respect to the antimicrobial activity of neutrophil α-defensins, oral microorganisms are usually resistant to HNP-1 to HNP-3, even though a synergistic antimicrobial effect is revealed between HNP-1 and LL-37 against *Escherichia coli* and *Staphylococcus aureus* (Nagaoka et al, 2000).

The antimicrobial activities of hBD-1, hBD-2, and hBD-3 peptides have been tested against different strains of gram-negative and gram-positive oral bacteria and fungi in several *in vitro* studies. In brief, it is found that, among these three human β-defensins, hBD-3 has the strongest antibacterial activity against oral *Streptococci* and some periodontal bacteria, especially all strains of *Fusobacterium nucleatum*, while hBD-1 and hBD-2 are less effective against both oral gram-positive and gram-negative bacteria (Ouhara et al, 2005). This may be owing to the strong basic property of hBD-3 due to several positively charged amino acids in its molecule (Schibli et al, 2002). However, hBD-2 exerts its antimicrobial activity well with cariogenic bacteria, including *Streptococcus mutans* and *Streptococcus sobrinus* (Nishimura et al, 2004). Generally, aerobic bacteria are more susceptible to hBD-2 and hBD-3 peptides than are anaerobic bacteria (Joly et al, 2004). Although the antimicrobial activity of β-defensins is normally inhibited by high salt concentrations, as shown in other studies (Goldman et al, 1997; Midorikawa et al, 2003), the antimicrobial activity of hBD-3 against periodontal and cariogenic bacteria is not much influenced by high salt concentrations (Ouhara et al, 2005). It can be concluded that, among the antimicrobial peptides of the defensin and cathelicidin families, hBD-3 and LL-37 exhibit the greatest degrees of antimicrobial effects against various oral bacteria, especially most aerobic bacteria and some periodontal bacteria. Although the red-complex periodontopathic bacteria are more resistant to hBD-3 and LL-37, it is likely that hBD-3 and LL-37 may still play a role in the pathogenesis of periodontal disease by reducing the number of early colonizing and bridging bacteria so that the late colonizers, including the red-complex periodontopathic bacteria, cannot colonize and thrive in dental plaque.

Interestingly, some pathogenic bacteria have evolved other virulence mechanisms that enable them to resist the activity of antimicrobial peptides. For example, antimicrobial peptides can be degraded by distinct enzymes secreted from bacterial pathogens, including SufA, a novel subtilisin-like serine protease of *Finegoldia magna* (Karlsson et al, 2007), streptopain of *Streptococcus pyogenes*, elastase of *Pseudomonas aeruginosa*, gelatinase of *Enterococcus faecalis* (Schmidtchen et al, 2002), and the 50 kDa metalloprotease (ZapA) of *Proteus mirabilis* (Belas et al, 2004). By analogy, *Porphyromonas gingivalis*, one of the red-complex bacterial triad, can also be resistant to the bactericidal activity of antimicrobial peptides due to its ability to synthesize a group of enzymes, called gingipains. In fact, it has been recently demonstrated that the gingipains efficiently degrade several different antimicrobial peptides, including HNP-1, hBD-1, hBD-2, and hBD-3 (Carlisle et al, 2009). However, it was formerly shown that the degradation of antimicrobial peptides by gingipains does not appear to contribute to the resistance of *Porphyromonas gingivalis* to the antimicrobial action (Bachrach et al, 2008).

The possible alternative mechanisms for the resistance of *Porphyromonas gingivalis* may be due to the possibility that gingipains secreted from *Porphyromonas gingivalis* may prevent destruction of its commensal bacteria, i.e., *Fusobacterium nucleatum*, which is easily destroyed by antimicrobial peptides. Otherwise, gingipains and proteases released from *Porphyromonas gingivalis* and *Prevotella intermedia*, respectively, may inactivate cystatins, inhibitors that function against endogenously-derived proteases, such as host cathepsins, etc.

This ultimately releases cathepsins from their tight control by cystatins. The active cathepsins, including cathepsin B, L, and S in the cysteine protease family, may then proteolytically degrade antimicrobial peptides, resulting in depletion of antimicrobial activity (Taggart et al, 2003). The gingipains and other virulence factors make *Porphyromonas gingivalis* one of the critical periodontal pathogens, and antimicrobial peptides may then be regarded as an important determinant for the "normal" and "diseased" states of periodontium.

As with *Porphyromonas gingivalis*, *Treponema denticola*, another red-complex periodontal pathogen, is resistant to the antimicrobial activity of human β-defensins, but by other distinct mechanisms, since *Treponema denticola* does not produce degrading enzymes. These mechanisms include an efflux pump of defensin peptides that enter the cytoplasm (Brissette and Lukehart, 2007) and reduction of defensin binding to the microbial surface due to the lack of LPS (Brissette and Lukehart, 2002). Furthermore, *Treponema denticola* cannot induce the host innate immune response, i.e., expression of hBD-2 and IL-8, in gingival epithelial cells (Brissette et al, 2008). The immune tolerant mechanisms of *Treponema denticola*, including resistance to the antimicrobial effect of antimicrobial peptides and silencing host innate immunity, may, therefore, partly explain the strong association of *Treponema denticola* with chronic periodontitis.

IMMUNOREGULATORY EFFECTS

In addition to its antimicrobial activities, LL-37 can elicit host innate and acquired immune responses. For example, LL-37 inhibits the binding of endotoxin LPS to its receptor complex, comprising Toll-like receptors (TLRs) and CD14, which results in prevention of sepsis (Fukumoto et al, 2005; Mookherjee et al, 2006) and suppression of the synthesis of nitric oxide (Ciornei et al, 2003), TNF-α, prostaglandin E$_2$ (PGE$_2$), monocyte chemoattractant protein-1 (MCP-1), and macrophage inflammatory protein-2 (MIP-2) (Ohgami et al, 2003). Moreover, LL-37 can block macrophage stimulation with lipoteichoic acid and lipoarabinomannan, indicating that LL-37 can bind to various molecules on bacterial cell membranes (Scott et al, 2002).

LL-37 chemoattracts monocytes, neutrophils, CD4 T lymphocytes, and eosinophils along its concentration gradient via a G-protein coupled receptor, namely, formyl peptide receptor-like 1 (FPRL1), on these cells (De Yang et al, 2000; Tjabringa et al, 2006). However, the appropriate LL-37 concentrations fall within the range between 10^{-7} and 10^{-5} molar, which are far greater than those of chemokines used in chemotaxis. In this regard, it is possible that LL-37 can play a role as a chemoattractant at inflamed periodontal sites only when elevated concentrations of LL-37 derived from inflamed gingival epithelial cells and granules of neutrophils, which are abundant in diseased tissues, are sufficient to exert the chemotactic effect. Moreover, LL-37 attracts migration of mast cells in rats (Niyonsaba et al, 2002a) and induces histamine release from mast cell granules via intracellular calcium mobilization (Niyonsaba et al, 2001), leading to enhanced phagocytosis of opsonized microorganisms. LL-37 can also induce dendritic cell differentiation, which then activates cell-mediated acquired immunity through a Th1 profile (Davidson et al, 2004).

Several studies have also shown the inducible effect of LL-37 on the expression of several immune-related genes. For instance, LL-37 can induce expression of chemokines and chemokine receptors (Scott et al, 2002) via MAP kinase pathways (Bowdish et al, 2004). It can also induce expression of intercellular adhesion molecule-1 (Edfeldt et al, 2006), implying an indirect role for LL-37 in chemotaxis in addition to its direct role, as indicated above. LL-37 transactivates an epidermal growth factor receptor (EGFR) through induction of matrix metalloproteinase activity, resulting in interleukin-8 (IL-8) up-regulation and increased cell proliferation in human bronchial epithelial cells (Tjabringa et al, 2003). Similarly, LL-37 enhances IL-8 expression and release by human airway smooth muscle cells, albeit through purinergic receptors (Zuyderduyn et al, 2006). In addition, in the presence of IL-1β, lower LL-37 concentrations can synergistically induce IL-8 synthesis in both human keratinocytes and bronchial epithelial cells (Filewod et al, 2009), and up-regulate expression of IL-6, IL-10, MCP-1, and MCP-3 in peripheral blood mononuclear cells (Yu et al, 2007).

With respect to periodontal cells, we have recently found similar IL-8 mRNA up-regulation by LL-37 in both gingival epithelial cells and gingival fibroblasts in dose- and time-dependent manners (Figure 1). Interestingly, the kinetics of IL-8 up-regulation between these two cell types shows distinct profiles, indicating different signaling pathways controlling IL-8 expression (Figure 1). Therefore, it is possible that LL-37 may be responsible for controlling neutrophil transmigration from blood vessels into diseased periodontal tissue in chronic periodontitis.

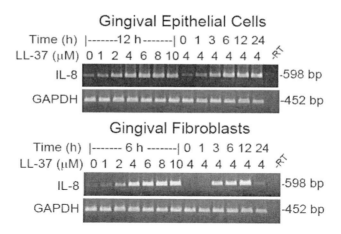

Figure 1. Up-regulation of IL-8 mRNA expression by treatment with various doses (0-10 μM) of LL-37 for indicated times (0-24 hours) in gingival epithelial cells and gingival fibroblasts. Note a dose-dependent increase in IL-8 expression. While IL-8 mRNA was transiently induced by LL-37 in gingival fibroblasts, up-regulation of IL-8 mRNA in gingival epithelial cells accumulated from 0 to 24 hours. Expression of glyceraldehyde phosphate dehydrogenase (GAPDH) was equivalent among all samples, indicating the equal mRNA loadings in this experiment. –RT represents a negative control sample where a reverse transcriptase enzyme was omitted from the reaction.

As with LL-37, neutrophil α-defensins also exert their immunomodulating effects on various types of immune cells. For example, HNP-1 and HNP-2 can induce chemotaxis of T-lymphocytes (Chertov et al, 1996), dendritic cells (Yang et al, 2000), macrophages, and mast cells (Grigat et al, 2007). Neutrophil α-defensins enhance cytokine expression in T-lymphocytes and immunoglobulin G production in B-lymphocytes (Tani et al, 2000), induce

IL-8 expression in lung epithelial cells (van Wetering et al, 1997), and promote IL-1β release through posttranslational processing (Perregaux et al, 2002).

With regard to the immunoregulatory effects of human β-defensins, hBD-1 and hBD-2 chemoattract immature dendritic cells and memory T-lymphocytes through a G-protein coupled chemokine receptor, i.e., CCR6, indicating the ability of these two β-defensins to bridge innate and acquired immunity (Yang et al, 1999). HBD-1 activates monocyte-derived dendritic cells and promotes the synthesis of several cytokines (Presicce et al, 2009). Moreover, hBD-1 up-regulates expression of CD91, a scavenger receptor that recognizes defensins, on the dendritic cell surface, indicating a positive feedback of dendritic cell activation (Presicce et al, 2009). However, hBD-2, but not hBD-1, enhances chemotaxis of mast cells (Niyonsaba et al, 2002b) and neutrophils treated with TNF-α (Niyonsaba et al, 2004), possibly via a CCR6 that mediates the signal through activation of phospholipase C. Furthermore, hBD-2 induces histamine release from mast cells and prostaglandin D synthesis (Niyonsaba et al, 2001). As with the dissociation of antimicrobial activities from the host immunostimulatory activities of LL-37 (Braff et al, 2005), it has recently been demonstrated that the chemoattractant and antimicrobial activities of β-defensins are exerted by distinct domains, and both of these activities do not rely on the intramolecular disulfide bridges of β-defensins (Taylor et al, 2008).

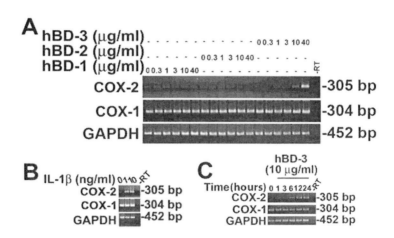

Figure 2. COX-2 mRNA up-regulation by hBD-3. Human gingival fibroblasts were treated for 18 hours with (A) various doses (0-40 μg/ml) of hBD-1, hBD-2, hBD-3, (B) IL-1β as a positive control, (C) 10 μg/ml of hBD-3 for various times (0-24 hours), or left untreated as a negative control. Total RNA was harvested and RT-PCR was conducted to analyze mRNA expression for cyclooxygenase-1 (COX-1), COX-2, and GAPDH. Note constitutive COX-1 mRNA expression, while COX-2 mRNA was up-regulated by hBD-3 treatment in dose- and time-dependent manners. This figure is reproduced from Chotjumlong and co-workers, 2010, with permission from the publisher, Wiley-Blackwell.

Regarding a potential role for human β-defensins in modulating host immune responses in periodontal disease, we have very recently shown that only hBD-3, but not hBD-1 or hBD-2, induces mRNA and protein expression of cyclooxygenase-2 (COX-2) in gingival fibroblasts in dose- and time-dependent fashions (Figures 2 and 3, respectively).

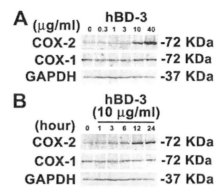

Figure 3. Up-regulation of COX-2 protein by hBD-3 in human gingival fibroblasts. Consistent with COX-2 mRNA up-regulation, COX-2 protein expression was up-regulated by hBD-3 treatment in (A) dose- and (B) time-dependent manners. Note constitutive COX-1 protein expression. This figure is reproduced from Chotjumlong and co-workers, 2010, with permission from the publisher, Wiley-Blackwell.

In comparison to up-regulation of COX-2 mRNA by 1-10 ng/ml of IL-1β, up-regulation by hBD-3 requires much higher concentrations (Figure 2), suggesting that epithelial-derived hBD-3 may act as a local immunomodulator on fibroblasts in adjacent connective tissue, where its concentration is sufficient to reach the low range of μg/ml. This concentration can probably be achieved by persistent inflammation in chronic periodontitis. Furthermore, up-regulated COX-2 expression by hBD-3 results in raised PGE_2 levels in cell-free culture supernatants (Table 1), which is confirmed by an experiment using a specific inhibitor of COX-2 activity, i.e., NS-398 (Figure 4). In summary, all of these findings suggest the potential role and ability of hBD-3 in initiating localized inflammation within periodontal tissues.

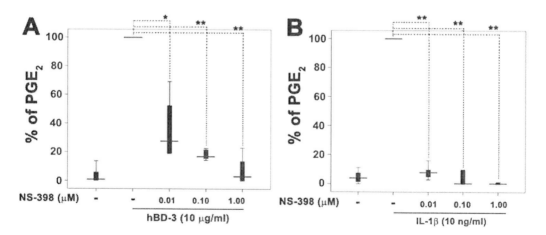

Figure 4. Elevated PGE_2 levels result from induced COX-2 expression. Human gingival fibroblasts were pretreated with indicated doses of NS-398, a specific COX-2 inhibitor, for 30 minutes prior to treatment with either (A) 10 μg/ml of hBD-3 or (B) 10 ng/ml of IL-1β for 18 hours. Cell-free culture supernatants were collected and analyzed for the PGE_2 levels by ELISA. Note a significant inhibition of elevated PGE_2 levels by NS-398 (*, $P < 0.05$; **, $P < 0.01$). This figure is reproduced from Chotjumlong and co-workers, 2010, with permission from the publisher, Wiley-Blackwell.

Table 1. HBD-3 treatment results in elevated PGE_2 levels in cell-free culture supernatants in a dose-dependent fashion. The cell-free culture supernatants from Figure 2 were collected and analyzed for PGE_2 concentrations (pg/ml) by ELISA. This table is modified from Chotjumlong and co-workers, 2010, with permission from the publisher, Wiley-Blackwell.

Concentration (µg/ml)		Median PGE_2 concentration (range)
Control		36.40 (34.49-38.32)
hBD-1	0.3	35.91 (33.74-38.08)
hBD-1	1.0	39.22 (36.28-42.16)
hBD-1	3.0	37.42 (34.99-39.85)
hBD-1	10.0	37.35 (34.96-39.73)
hBD-1	40.0	39.61 (35.43-43.78)
hBD-2	0.3	38.30 (35.70-40.89)
hBD-2	1.0	37.58 (35.00-40.16)
hBD-2	3.0	39.64 (34.86-44.42)
hBD-2	10.0	40.51 (38.37-42.66)
hBD-2	40.0	36.82 (32.94-40.69)
hBD-3	0.3	21.33 (20.00-23.00)
hBD-3	1.0	35.55 (22.64-48.31)
hBD-3	3.0	53.16 (48.31-58.00)
hBD-3	10.0	260.59[*] (260.56-266.03)
hBD-3	40.0	1934.00[*] (1824.20-2048.10)

[*] denotes statistically significant difference from untreated control cells at $P < 0.05$.

OTHER BIOLOGICAL ACTIVITIES

Besides the immunomodulation, LL-37 plays a role in tissue repair by stimulating airway epithelial cell proliferation and wound closure (Shaykhiev et al, 2005) and by activating keratinocyte proliferation and migration in the process of re-epithelialization (Heilborn et al, 2003) via transactivation of EGFR and phosphorylation of the signal transducers and activator of transcription 3 (STAT3) (Tokumaru et al, 2005). Consistent with these *in vitro* studies, the levels of LL-37 decrease in chronic ulcer epithelium (Heilborn et al, 2003), whereas adenoviral transfer of LL-37 to the wound in mice results in a significant improvement of wound healing by enhanced re-epithelialization and granulation tissue formation (Carretero et al, 2008). Furthermore, it has recently been shown that LL-37 can suppress keratinocyte apoptosis via a COX-2-dependent mechanism (Chamorro et al, 2009), which is in agreement with the function of LL-37 in promoting cell proliferation and tissue repair, as indicated above. Therefore, it is interesting to determine whether LL-37 plays any role in tissue repair and/or regeneration after periodontal surgery.

Interestingly, exogenously added LL-37 into the wound induces angiogenesis that corresponds to an *in vitro* study (Koczulla et al, 2003), which demonstrates endothelial cell proliferation and increased numbers of new blood vessel formation through FPRL1 on cultured endothelial cell membrane in response to LL-37 treatment. As in keratinocyte migration, LL-37 also induces migration of human corneal epithelial cells, as well as expression of IL-1β, IL-6, IL-8, and TNF-α (Huang et al, 2006). Moreover, it has been shown that LL-37 can internalize into human lung epithelial cells through endocytosis, and subsequently accumulates in the perinuclear region (Lau et al, 2005).

There are a number of reports that show other biological effects of neutrophil α-defensins and human β-defensins on various cell types. For instance, α-defensins enhance mitosis in some cell types (Murphy et al, 1993), promote tissue repair in airway epithelial cells via MAP kinase pathways (Aarbiou et al, 2002), regulate expression for adhesion molecules on endothelial cells (Chaly et al, 2000), control smooth muscle cell contraction via an α2-macroglobulin receptor (Nassar et al, 2002), induce proliferation of lung fibroblasts and collagen synthesis (Han et al, 2009), and induce expression of some mucin genes, i.e., *MUC5B* and *MUC5AC* (Aarbiou et al, 2004). As with the induction of mucin genes by neutropil α-defensins, it has lately been demonstrated that LL-37 also up-regulates *MUC2* and *MUC3* expression in intestinal epithelial cell lines (Otte et al, 2009). Furthermore, α-defensins affect histamine release from mast cell granules through a G-protein coupled receptor, suggesting their indirect role in vasodilatation (Befus et al, 1999).

Among human β-defensins, hBD-2 activates the differentiation of dental pulp mesenchymal cells into odontoblast-like cells, confirmed by up-regulation of dentin sialophosphoprotein (*DSPP*) gene expression (Shiba et al, 2003). In addition, stimulation of odontoblast-like cells with recombinant hBD-2 leads to increased mRNA expression of several inflammatory genes, including IL-6, IL-8, and cytosolic phospholipase A_2 (Dommisch et al, 2007). Consequently, it is probable that hBD-2 plays a role in reparative dentin formation, as well as immune regulation, in addition to its antimicrobial effect. Furthermore, like LL-37, hBD-2, hBD-3, and hBD-4 stimulate cell migration and proliferation, and production of cytokines and chemokines in skin keratinocytes (Niyonsaba et al, 2007).

DISEASE IMPLICATIONS

Several studies have shown the association between altered expression of epithelial-derived antimicrobial peptides, including LL-37 and human β-defensins, and various skin and epithelial diseases, e.g., acne vulgaris (Chronnell et al, 2001), oral lichen planus, leukoplakia (Nishimura et al, 2003), oral candidiasis (Abiko et al, 2002), condyloma acuminatum, verruca vulgaris (Conner et al, 2002), cholesteatoma (Jung et al, 2003), chronic nasal inflammatory disease (Kim et al, 2003), etc.

Due to space limitations, only one classic example of alteration in antimicrobial peptide expression is presented here to demonstrate the clinical significance of these antimicrobial peptides in the pathogenesis of inflammatory skin diseases. This example is described in some studies related to two well-characterized skin diseases, psoriasis and atopic dermatitis. In psoriatic lesions, expression of LL-37, hBD-2, and hBD-3 is up-regulated (Frohm et al, 1997; Harder et al, 1997a; Harder et al, 2001), whereas expression of these three peptides is significantly reduced in atopic dermatitis lesions (Ong et al, 2002). The difference in the levels of antimicrobial peptide expression between psoriasis and atopic dermatitis can be elaborated by different cytokine milieus between these two skin diseases, a Th1 versus a Th2 profile, respectively (Nomura et al, 2003). It has been demonstrated that enhanced production of IL-4 and IL-13, two cytokines categorized as a Th2 profile, in atopic dermatitis, can block expression of some antimicrobial peptides in skin keratinocytes (Nomura et al, 2003), which may then account for the reduction of antimicrobial peptide expression in this lesion.

It is known that one basic function of human skin is to form a natural barrier against microbial colonization and invasion, which leads to tissue homeostasis. To further enhance this function, the skin can also produce several antimicrobial peptides, which help control the number and types of microorganisms on the skin. If the production of antimicrobial peptides is impaired by dysfunction of the host immune system as a result of the pathogenesis of skin diseases, an increased risk of opportunistic infections from bacteria or viruses in the skin lesion ensues. Consequently, the deficiency of antimicrobial peptides, particularly LL-37, in atopic dermatitis lesions causes frequent infections from vaccinia virus (Howell et al, 2004). Similarly, a drastic reduction of LL-37 protein expression that results in increased susceptibility to infections has also been observed in patients with acute myeloid leukemia (An et al, 2005).

With respect to periodontal disease, data regarding the expression of β-defensin antimicrobial peptides in different types of periodontal diseases compared to healthy periodontal tissue are still contradictory and inconclusive. For example, the findings from one study (Dommisch et al, 2005) showed no significant differences in β-defensin mRNA expression in different clinical stages of periodontal disease as compared to that in normal tissue. Nevertheless, in the same study, hBD-2 expression was found to be significantly higher than hBD-1 expression in both gingivitis and periodontitis groups (Dommisch et al, 2005). In contrast, it was later shown in another study (Vardar-Sengul et al, 2007) that the levels of hBD-1 expression did not significantly differ from those of hBD-2 expression in patients with gingivitis. However, in patients with periodontitis, hBD-1 expression was significantly higher than hBD-2 expression in chronic periodontitis, whereas hBD-2 expression was significantly higher than hBD-1 expression in aggressive periodontitis (Vardar-Sengul et al, 2007). The reason behind these discrepancies may be due to a small number of patients and healthy volunteers, recruited in each study. Consequently, before any conclusions can be drawn for the relationship between β-defensin expression and periodontal disease, a larger study is required for assessing more accurate levels of β-defensin expression in both healthy and diseased tissues, obtained from different types of periodontal diseases.

It is noteworthy that significant up-regulation of both hBD-1 and hBD-2 expression is found in periodontal pocket epithelium as compared to the adjacent healthy epithelium from the same patient (Lu et al, 2004). In contrast, higher levels of hBD-3 expression are found in periodontally healthy tissues as compared to diseased tissues (Bissell et al, 2004). These may suggest differential functions between hBD-1/hBD-2 and hBD-3 in periodontal disease, and also a more protective role for hBD-3 in regulating host immune responses to microbial assaults, as mentioned under the previous headings.

To the best of our knowledge, there has been no report that shows the relationship between the deficiency of β-defensin expression in periodontal tissues and periodontal diseases. On the contrary, both LL-37, which is mainly derived from neutrophils, and neutrophil α-defensins show a direct link to the pathogenesis of a certain type of periodontitis. This is revealed by one study (Pütsep et al, 2002) that shows the deficiency in

LL-37 and the reduction of neutrophil α-defensins in patients with morbus Kostmann syndrome, a severe congenital neutropenia. These patients suffer from recurrent gingivitis and even severe periodontitis during early childhood that result from the lack of neutrophil-derived antimicrobial peptides. Furthermore, it has been demonstrated *in vitro* that several periodontal pathogens, e.g., *Aggregatibacter actinomycetemcomitans*, are sensitive to the bactericidal effects of LL-37 (Tanaka et al, 2000; Isogai et al, 2003), so it is likely that the defective antimicrobial function of neutrophils from patients with morbus Kostmann syndrome, who are deficient in LL-37, cannot eliminate *Aggregatibacter actinomycetemcomitams*, which is highly associated with early-onset periodontitis.

In this regard, it is interesting to further investigate whether the deficiency of these antimicrobial peptides is also implicated with other forms of periodontitis associated with a syndrome, for instance, juvenile periodontitis in Papillon-Lefèvre syndrome, whose abnormalities result from cathepsin C mutations (Hart et al, 1999; Toomes et al, 1999). Is it probable that some antimicrobial peptides are substrates for cathepsin C enzyme, and these peptides may become more active after enzymatic degradation? If the answer is positive, one can assume that impaired cathepsin C function may not yield sufficient amounts of active antimicrobial peptides to exert their antimicrobial effects on periodontal pathogens. The deficiency in active antimicrobial peptides finally leads to repeated periodontal infections.

CONCLUSIONS AND INTERESTING RESEARCH TOPICS

Substantial variations in expression of small cationic antimicrobial peptides, including LL-37 and defensins, in periodontal tissues, GCF, and saliva, exist and may be correlated with the pathogenesis of periodontal disease, as well as that of other oral inflammatory and infectious diseases. Therefore, the association between altered expression of antimicrobial peptides and some types of periodontitis, specifically the ones that are associated with syndromes, should be further explored in detail. Moreover, expression of some antimicrobial peptides and their clinical significance in other oral diseases should be further studied. Perhaps, it is possible that some peptides could be further developed as biomarkers for diagnosis and/or prognosis of oral diseases in the future.

Up to now, accumulated data gathered from *in vitro* and *in vivo* studies have exhibited a broad range of antimicrobial activities against oral microorganisms, especially some periodontal pathogens in a planktonic state. With respect to these data, it is interesting to further examine the microbicidal effects of antimicrobial peptides on dental plaque microorganisms. In addition, it is now becoming increasingly evident that the functions of antimicrobial peptides are not restricted to their antimicrobial activities, as was initially thought. It is, therefore, likely that other novel, but undiscovered, functions of these peptides will be unraveled in the near future. Consequently, additional studies into new biological activities of antimicrobial peptides are needed and will be beneficial for us to better understand and gain deep insight into the importance of these multifunctional molecules, particularly their essential roles in maintaining tissue homeostasis during the healthy and diseased states of the periodontium.

Furthermore, it is still necessary to continue regulation studies, involving cellular receptors and intracellular signaling pathways that mediate up-regulation of some inducible antimicrobial peptides, in order to understand the mechanisms used to enhance the expression of these peptides. In quest of new adjunctive treatment modalities against periodontitis, it is possible that enhancement of antimicrobial peptide expression by putative components of commensal periodontal bacteria that are not harmful to the human body, or by non-toxic agents, similar to vaccination, may be of significant interest in controlling the number of periodontopathic bacteria. Finally, we, as members of the health professions, should be constantly aware of the clinical significance of these antimicrobial peptides in the pathogenesis of oral infectious and inflammatory diseases, especially periodontal disease.

ACKNOWLEDGMENTS

The authors wish to thank Dr. M. Kevin O Carroll, Professor Emeritus of the University of Mississippi School of Dentistry, USA, and Faculty Consultant of Chiang Mai University Faculty of Dentistry, Thailand, for his critical reading of this chapter. We would also like to acknowledge support from the Thailand Research Fund (RMU5080035) and the Center of Excellence for Innovation in Chemistry (PERCH-CIC), Commission on Higher Education, Ministry of Education, Thailand.

REFERENCES

Aarbiou, J., Ertmann, M., van Wetering, S., van Noort, P., Rook, D., Rabe, K.F., Litvinov, S.V., van Krieken, J.H., de Boer, W.I. & Hiemstra, P.S. (2002). *Human neutrophil defensins induce lung epithelial cell proliferation in vitro.* J Leukoc Biol 72(1):167-174.

Aarbiou, J., Verhoosel, R.M., van Wetering, S., de Boer, W.I., van Krieken, J.H., Litvinov, S.V., Rabe, K.F. & Hiemstra, P.S. (2004). *Neutrophil defensins enhance lung epithelial wound closure and mucin gene expression in vitro.* Am J Respir Cell Mol Biol 30(2):193-201.

Abiko, Y., Jinbu, Y., Noguchi, T., Nishimura, M., Kusano, K., Amaratunga, P., Shibata, T. & Kaku, T. (2002). *Upregulation of human beta-defensin 2 peptide expression in oral lichen planus, leukoplakia and candidiasis. An immunohistochemical study.* Pathol Res Pract 198(8):537-542.

Abiko, Y., Saitoh, M., Nishimura, M., Yamazaki, M., Sawamura, D. & Kaku, T. (2007). *Role of beta-defensins in oral epithelial health and disease.* Med Mol Morphol 40(4):179-184.

Agerberth, B., Charo, J., Werr, J., Olsson, B., Idali, F., Lindbom, L., Kiessling, R., Jörnvall, H., Wigzell, H. & Gudmundsson, G.M. (2000). *The human antimicrobial and chemotactic peptides LL-37 and alpha-defensins are expressed by specific lymphocyte and monocyte populations.* Blood 96(9):3086-3093.

Agerberth, B., Gunne, H., Oderberg, J., Kogner, P., Boman, H.G. & Gudmundsson, G.H. (1995*). Fall-39, a putative human peptide antibiotic, is cysteine-free and expressed in bone marrow and testis.* Proc Natl Acad Sci USA 92(1):195-199.

Ali, R.S., Falconer, A., Ikram, M., Bissett, C.E., Cerio, R. & Quinn, A.G. (2001). *Expression of the peptide antibiotics human beta defensin-1 and human beta defensin-2 in normal human skin.* J Invest Dermatol 117(1):106-111.

An, L.L., Ma, X.T., Yang, Y.H., Lin, Y.M., Song, Y.H. & Wu, K.F. (2005). *Marked reduction of LL-37/hCAP-18, an antimicrobial peptide, in patients with acute myeloid leukemia.* Int J Haematol 81(1):45-47.

Bachrach, G., Altman, H., Kolenbrander, P.E., Chalmers, N.I., Gabai-Gutner, M., Mor, A., Friedman, M. & Steinberg, D. (2008). *Resistance of Porphyromonas gingivalis ATCC33277 to direct killing by antimicrobial peptides is protease independent.* Antimicrob Agents Chemother 52(2):638-642.

Bals, R., Wang, X., Zasloff, M. & Wilson, J.M. (1998). *The peptide antibiotic LL-37/hCAP-18 is expressed in epithelia of the human lung where it has broad antimicrobial activity at the airway surface.* Proc Natl Acad Sci USA 95(16):9541-9546.

Becker, M.N., Diamond, G., Verghese, M.W. & Randell, S.H. (2000). *CD14-dependent lipopolysaccharide-induced beta-defensin-2 expression in human tracheobronchial epithelium.* J Biol Chem 275(38):29731-29736.

Befus, A.D., Mowat, C., Gilchrist, M., Hu, J., Solomon, S. & Bateman, A. (1999). *Neutrophil defensins induce histamine secretion from mast cells: mechanisms of action.* J Immunol 163(2):947-953.

Belas, R., Manos, J. & Suvanasuthi, R. (2004). *Proteus mirabilis ZapA metalloprotease degrades a broad spectrum of substrates, including antimicrobial peptides.* Infect Immun 72(9):5159-5167.

Bensch, K.W., Raida, M., Mägert, H.J., Schulz-Knappe, P. & Forssmann, W.G. (1995). *hBD-1: a novel beta-defensin from human plasma.* FEBS Lett 368(2):331-335.

Bevins, C.L., Jones, D.E., Dutra, A., Schaffzin, J. & Muenke, M. (1996). *Human enteric defensin genes: chromosomal map position and a model for possible evolutionary relationships.* Genomics 31(1):95-106.

Bissell, J., Joly, S., Johnson, G.K., Organ, C.C., Dawson, D., McCray, P.B.Jr. & Guthmiller, J.M. (2004*). Expression of beta-defensins in gingival health and in periodontal disease.* J Oral Pathol Med 33(5):278-285.

Blomqvist, M., Bergquist, J., Westman, A., Hâkansson, K., Hâkansson, P., Fredman, P. & Ekman, R. (1999). *Identification of defensins in human lymphocyte nuclei.* Eur J Biochem 263(2):312-318.

Bollag, W.B., Zhong, X., Dodd, M.E., Hardy, D.M., Zheng, X. & Allred, W.T. (2005). *Phospholipase D signaling and extracellular signal-regulated kinase-1 and -2 phosphorylation (activation) are required for maximal phorbol ester-induced transglutaminase activity, a marker of keratinocyte differentiation.* J Pharmacol Exp Ther 312(3):1223-1231.

Bonass, W.A., High, A.S., Owen, P.J. & Devine, D.A. (1999). *Expression of beta-defensin genes by human salivary glands.* Oral Microbiol Immunol 14(6):371-374.

Bowdish, D.M., Davidson, D.J., Speert, D.P. & Hancock, R.E. (2004). *The human cationic peptide LL-37 induces activation of the extracellular signal-regulated kinase and p38 kinase pathways in primary human monocytes.* J Immunol 172(16):3758-3765.

Braff, M.H., Hawkins, M.A., Di Nardo, A., Lopez-Garcia, B., Howell, M.D., Wong, C., Lin, K., Streib, J.E., Dorschner, R., Leung, D.Y. & Gallo, R.L. (2005). *Structure-function relationships among human cathelicidin peptides: dissociation of antimicrobial properties from host immunostimulatory activities.* J Immunol 174(7):4271-4278.

Brissette, C.A. & Lukehart, S.A. (2002). *Treponema denticola is resistant to human β-defensins.* Infect Immun 70(7):3982-3984.

Brissette, C.A. & Lukehart, S.A. (2007). *Mechanisms of decreased susceptibility to beta-defensins by Treponema denticola.* Infect Immun 75(5):2307-2315.

Brissette, C.A., Pham, T.-T.T., Coats, S.R., Darveau, R.P. & Lukehart, S.A. (2008). *Treponema denticola does not induce production of common innate immune mediators from primary gingival epithelial cells.* Oral Microbiol Immunol 23(6):474-481.

Carlisle, M.D., Srikantha, R.N. & Brogden, K.A. (2009). *Degradation of α- and β-defensins by culture supernatants of Porphyromonas gingivalis strain 381.* J Innate Immun 1(2):118-122.

Carretero, M., Escámez, M.J., García, M., Duarte, B., Holguín, A., Retamosa, L., Jorcano, J.L., Río, M.D. & Larcher, F. (2008). *In vitro and in vivo wound healing-promoting activities of human cathelicidin LL-37.* J Invest Dermatol 128(1):223-236.

Chaly, Y.V., Paleolog, E.M., Kolesnikova, T.S., Tikhonov, I.I., Petratchenko, E.V. & Voitenok, N.N. (2000). *Neutrophil alpha-defensin human neutrophil peptide modulates cytokine production in human monocytes and adhesion molecule expression in endothelial cells.* Eur Cytokine Netw 11(2):257-266.

Chamorro, C.I., Weber, G., Grönberg, A., Pivarcsi, A. & Ståhle, M. (2009). *The human antimicrobial peptide LL-37 suppresses apoptosis in keratinocytes.* J Invest Dermatol 129(4):937-944.

Chertov, O., Michiel, D.F., Xu, L., Wang, J.M., Tani, K., Murphy, W.J., Longo, D.L., Taub, D.D. & Oppenheim, J.J. (1996). *Identification of defensin-1, defensin-2, and CAP37/azurocidin as T cell chemoattractant proteins released from interleukin-8-stimulated neutrophils.* J Biol Chem 271(6):2935-2940.

Chotjumlong, P., Khongkhunthian, S., Ongchai, S., Reutrakul, V. & Krisanaprakornkit, S. (2010). *Human β-defensin-3 up-regulates cyclooxygenase-2 expression and prostaglandin E_2 synthesis in human gingival fibroblasts.* J Periodontal Res (doi:10.1111/j.1600-0765.2009.01259.x).

Chronnell, C.M., Ghali, L.R., Ali, R.S., Quinn, A.G., Holland, D.B., Bull, J.J., Cunliffe, W.J., McKay, I.A., Philpott, M.P. & Müller-Röver, S. (2001). *Human beta defensin-1 and -2 expression in human pilosebaceous units: upregulation in acne vulgaris lesions.* J Invest Dermatol 117(5):1120-1125.

Chung, W.O., Hansen, S.R., Rao, D. & Dale, B.A. (2004). *Protease-activated receptor signaling increases epithelial antimicrobial peptide expression.* J Immunol 173(8):5165-5170.

Ciornei, C.D., Egesten, A. & Bodelsson, M. (2003). *Effects of human cathelicidin antimicrobial peptide LL-37 on lipopolysaccharide-induced nitric oxide release from rat aorta in vitro.* Acta Anaesthesiol Scand 47(2):213-220.

Conner, K., Nern, K., Rudisill, J., O'Grady, T. & Gallo, R.L. (2002). *The antimicrobial peptide LL-37 is expressed by keratinocytes in condyloma acuminatum and verruca vulgaris.* J Am Acad Dermatol 47(3):347-350.

Cowland, J.B., Johnsen, A.H. & Borregaard, N. (1995). *hCAP-18, a cathelin/pro-bactenecin-like protein of human neutrophil specific granules.* FEBS Lett 368(1):173-176.

Dale, B.A. & Fredericks, L.P. (2005). *Antimicrobial peptides in the oral environment: expression and function in health and disease.* Curr Issues Mol Biol 7(2):119-133.

Dale, B.A., Kimball, J.R., Krisanaprakornkit, S., Roberts, F., Robinovitch, M., O'Neal, R., Valore, E.V., Ganz, T., Anderson, G.M. & Weinberg, A. (2001). *Localized antimicrobial peptide expression in human gingiva.* J Periodontal Res 36(5):285-294.

Darveau, R.P., Belton, C.M., Reife, R.A. & Lamont, R.J. (1998). *Local chemokine paralysis, a novel pathogenic mechanism for Porphyromonas gingivalis.* Infect Immun 66(4):1660-1665.

Davidson, D.J., Currie, A.J., Reid, G.S., Bowdish, D.M., MacDonald, K.L., Ma, R.C., Hancock, R.E. & Speert, D.P. (2004). *The cationic antimicrobial peptide LL-37 modulates dendritic cell differentiation and dendritic cell-induced T cell polarization.* J Immunol 172(2):1146-1156.

De Yang, Chen, Q., Schmidt, A.P., Anderson, G.M., Wang, J.M., Wooters, J., *Oppenheim, J.J. & Chertov, O. (2000). LL-37, the neutrophil granule- and epithelial cell-derived cathelicidin, utilizes formyl peptide receptor-like 1 (FPRL1) as a receptor to chemoattract human peripheral blood neutrophils, monocytes, and T cells.* J Exp Med 192(7):1069-1074.

den Hertog, A.L., van Marle, J., van Veen, H.A., van't Hof, W., Bolscher, J.G., Veerman, E.C. & Nieuw Amerongen, A.V. (2005). *Candidacidal effects of two antimicrobial peptides: Histatin 5 causes small membrane defects, but LL-37 causes massive disruption of the cell membrane.* Biochem J 388(Pt 2):689-695.

Di Nardo, A., Vitiello, A. & Gallo, R.L. (2003). *Cutting edge: mast cell antimicrobial activity is mediated by expression of cathelicidin antimicrobial peptide.* J Immunol 170(5):2274-2278.

Diamond, D.L., Kimball, J.R., Krisanaprakornkit, S., Ganz, T. & Dale, B.A. (2001). *Detection of beta-defensins secreted by human oral epithelial cells.* J Immunol Methods 256(1-2):65-76.

Dommisch, H., Açil, Y., Dunsche, A., Winter, J. & Jepsen, S. (2005). *Differential gene expression of human beta-defensins (hBD-1, -2, -3) in inflammatory gingival disease.* Oral Microbiol Immunol 20(3):186-190.

Dommisch, H., Winter, J., Willebrand, C., Eberhard, J. & Jepsen, S. (2007). *Immune regulatory functions of human beta-defensin-2 in odontoblast-like cells.* Int Endod J 40(4):300-307.

Dunsche, A., Açil, Y., Siebert, R., Harder, J., Schröder, J.M. & Jepsen, S. (2001). *Expression profile of human defensins and antimicrobial proteins in oral tissues.* J Oral Pathol Med 30(3):154-158.

Dunsche, A., Açil, Y., Dommisch, H., Siebert, R., Schröder, J.M. & Jepsen, S. (2002). *The novel human beta-defensin-3 is widely expressed in oral tissues.* Eur J Oral Sci 110(2):121-124.

Edfeldt, K., Agerberth, B., Rottenberg, M.E., Gudmundsson, G.H., Wang, X.B., Mandal, K., Xu, Q. & Yan, Z.Q. (2006*). Involvement of the antimicrobial peptide LL-37 in human atherosclerosis.* Arterioscler Thromb Vasc Biol 26(7):1551-1557.

Exton, J.H. (1999). *Regulation of phospholipase D.* Biochim Biophys Acta 1439(2):121-133.

Feucht, E.C., DeSanti, C.L. & Weinberg, A. (2003). *Selective induction of human beta-defensin mRNAs by Actinobacillus actinomycetemcomitans in primary and immortalized oral epithelial cells.* Oral Microbiol Immunol 18(6):359-363.

Filewod, N.C., Pistolic, J. & Hancock, R.E. (2009). *Low concentrations of LL-37 alter IL-8 production by keratinocytes and bronchial epithelial cells in response to pro-inflammatory stimuli.* FEMS Immunol Med Microbiol 56(3):233-240.

Frohm, M., Agerberth, B., Ahangari, G., Stâhle-Bäckdahl, M., Lidén, S., Wigzell, H. & Gudmundsson, G.H. (1997). *The expression of the gene coding for the antibacterial peptide LL-37 is induced in human keratinocytes during inflammatory disorders.* J Biol Chem 272(24):15258-15263.

Frohm Nilsson, M., Sandstedt, B., Sørensen, O., Weber, G., Borregaard, N. & Stâhle-Bäckdahl, M. (1999). *The human cationic antimicrobial protein (hCAP-18), a peptide antibiotic, is widely expressed in human squamous epithelia and colocalizes with interleukin-6.* Infect Immun 67(5):2561-2566.

Frye, M., Bargon, J. & Gropp, R. (2001). *Expression of human beta-defensin-1 promotes differentiation of keratinocytes.* J Mol Med 79(5-6):275-282.

Fukumoto, K., Nagaoka, I., Yamataka, A., Kobayashi, H., Yanai, T., Kato, Y. & Miyano, T. (2005). *Effect of antibacterial cathelicidin peptide CAP18/LL-37 on sepsis in neonatal rats.* Pediatr Surg Int 21(1):20-24.

Ganz, T., Selsted, M.E., Szklarek, D., Harwig, S.S., Daher, K., Bainton, D.F. & Lehrer, R.I. (1985). *Defensins, natural peptide antibiotics of human neutrophils.* J Clin Invest 76(4):1427-1435.

Ganz, T. (2003). *Defensins: antimicrobial peptides of innate immunity.* Nat Rev Immunol 3(9): 710-720.

García, J.R., Jaumann, F., Schulz, S., Krause, A., Rodríguez-Jiménez, J., Forssmann, U., Adermann, K., Klüver, E., Vogelmeier, C., Becker, D., Hedrich, R., Forssmann, W.G. & Bals, R. (2001). *Identification of a novel, multifunctional beta-defensin (human beta-defensin 3) with specific antimicrobial activity. Its interaction with plasma membranes of Xenopus oocytes and the induction of macrophage chemoattraction.* Cell Tissue Res 306(2):257-264.

Ghosh, D., Porter, E., Shen, B., Lee, S.K., Wilk, D., Drazba, J., Yadav, S.P., Crabb, J.W., Ganz, T. & Bevins, C.L. (2002). *Paneth cell trypsin is the processing enzyme for human defensin-5.* Nat Immunol 3(6):583-590.

Goldman, M.J., Anderson, G.M., Stolzenberg, E.D., Kari, U.P., Zasloff, M. & Wilson, J.M. (1997). *Human beta defensin 1 is a salt sensitive antibiotic in lung that is inactivated in cystic fibrosis.* Cell 88(4):553-560.

Grigat, J., Soruri, A., Forssmann, U., Riggert, J. & Zwirner, J. (2007*). Chemoattraction of macrophages, T lymphocytes, and mast cells is evolutionarily conserved within the human α-defensin family.* J Immunol 179(6):3958-3965.

Han, W., Wang, W., Mohammed, K.A. & Su, Y. (2009). *α-defensins increase lung fibroblast proliferation and collagen synthesis via the β-catenin signaling pathway.* FEBS J 276(22):6603-6614.

Harder, J., Bartels, J., Christophers, E. & Schröder, J.M. (1997a). *A peptide antibiotic from human skin.* Nature 387(6636):861.

Harder, J., Siebert, R., Zhang, Y., Matthiesen, P., Christophers, E., Schlegelberger, B. & Schröder, J.M. (1997b). *Mapping of the gene encoding human beta-defensin-2 (DEFB2) to chromosome region 8p22-p23.1.* Genomics 46(3):472-475.

Harder, J., Meyer-Hoffert, U., Teran, L.M., Schwichtenberg, L., Bartels, J., Maune, S. & Schröder, J.M. (2000). *Mucoid Pseudomonas aeruginosa, TNF-alpha, and IL-1beta, but not IL-6, induce human beta-defensin-2 in respiratory epithelia.* Am J Respir Cell Mol Biol 22(6):714-721.

Harder, J., Bartels, J., Christophers, E. & Schröder, J.M. (2001). *Isolation and characterization of human beta-defensin-3, a novel human inducible peptide antibiotic.* J Biol Chem 276(8):5707-5713.

Hart, T.C., Hart, P.S., Bowden, D.W., Michalec, M.D., Callison, S.A., Walker, S.J., Zhang, Y. & Firatli, E. (1999). *Mutations of the cathepsin C gene are responsible for Papillon-Lefèvre syndrome.* J Med Genet 36(12):881-887.

Hase, K., Murakami, M., Iimura, M., Cole, S.P., Horibe, Y., Ohtake, T., Obonyo, M., Gallo, R.L., Eckmann, L. & Kagnoff, M.F. (2003). *Expression of LL-37 by human gastric epithelial cells as a potential host defense mechanism against Helicobacter pyroli.* Gastroenterology 125(6):1613-1625.

Heilborn, J.D., Nilsson, M.F., Kratz, G., Weber, G., Sørensen, O., Borregaard, N. & Ståhle-Bäckdahl, M. (2003). *The cathelicidin anti-microbial peptide LL-37 is involved in re-epithelialization of human skin wounds and is lacking in chronic ulcer epithelium.* J Invest Dermatol 120(3):379-389.

Hill, C.P., Yee, J., Selsted, M.E. & Eisenberg, D. (1991). *Crystal structure of defensin HNP-3, an amphiphilic dimer: mechanisms of membrane permeabilization.* Science 251(5000):1481-1485.

Hosokawa, I., Hosokawa ,Y., Komatsuzawa, H., Goncalves, R.B., Karimbux, N., Napimoga, M.H., Seki, M., Ouhara, K., Sugai, M., Taubman, M.A. & Kawai, T. (2006). *Innate immune peptide LL-37 displays distinct expression pattern from beta-defensins in inflamed gingival tissue.* Clin Exp Immunol 146(2):218-225.

Howell, M.D., Jones, J.F., Kisich, K.O., Streib, J.E., Gallo, R.L. & Leung, D.Y. (2004). *Selective killing of vaccinia virus by LL-37: implications for eczema vaccinatum.* J Immunol 172(3):1763-1767.

Huang, L.C., Petkova, T.D., Reins, R.Y., Proske, R.J. & McDermott, A.M. (2006). *Multifunctional roles of human cathelicidin (LL-37) at the ocular surface.* Invest Ophthalmol Vis Sci 47(6):2369-2380.

Isogai, E., Isogai, H., Matuo, K., Hirose, K., Kowashi, Y., Okumuara, K. & Hirata, M. (2003). *Sensitivity of genera Porphyromonas and Prevotella to the bactericidal action of C-terminal domain of human CAP18 and its analogues.* Oral Microbiol Immunol 18(5):329-332.

Ji, S., Kim, Y., Min, B.-M., Han, S.H. & Choi, Y. (2007a). *Innate immune responses of gingival epithelial cells to nonperiodontopathic and periodontopathic bacteria.* J Periodontal Res 42(6):503-510.

Ji, S., Hyun, J., Park, E., Lee, B.-L., Kim, K.-K. & Choi, Y. (2007b). *Susceptibility of various oral bacteria to antimicrobial peptides and to phagocytosis by neutrophils.* J Periodontal Res 42(5):410-419.

Jia, H.P., Schutte, B.C., Schudy, A., Linzmeier, R., Guthmiller, J.M., Johnson, G.K., Tack, B.F., Mitros, J.P., Rosenthal, A., Ganz, T. & McCray, P.B.Jr. (2001). *Discovery of new human beta-defensins using a genomics-based approach.* Gene 263(1-2):211-218.

Joly, S., Maze, C., McCray, P.B.Jr. & Guthmiller, J.M. (2004). *Human β-defensin-2 and -3 demonstrate strain-selective activity against oral microorganisms.* J Clin Microbiol 42(3):1024-1029.

Joly, S., Organ, C.C., Johnson, G.K., McCray, P.B.Jr. & Guthmiller, J.M. (2005). *Correlation between β-defensin expression and induction profiles in gingival keratinocytes.* Mol Immunol 42(9):1073-1084.

Jones, D.E. & Bevins, C.L. (1992). *Paneth cells of the human small intestine express an antimicrobial peptide gene.* J Biol Chem 267(32):23216-23225.

Jones, D.E. & Bevins, C.L. (1993). *Defensin-6 mRNA in human Paneth cells: implications for antimicrobial peptides in the host defense of the human bowel.* FEBS Lett 315(2):187-192.

Jung, H.H., Chae, S.W., Jung, S.K., Kim, S.T., Lee, H.M. & Hwang, S.J. (2003). *Expression of a cathelicidin antimicrobial peptide is augmented in cholesteatoma.* Laryngoscope 113(3):432-435.

Karlsson, C., Andersson, M.L., Collin, M., Schmidtchen, A., Björck, L. & Frick, I.M. (2007). *SufA--a novel subtilisin-like serine proteinase of Finegoldia magna.* Microbiology 153(Pt12):4208-4218.

Kim, S.T., Cha, H.E., Kim, D.Y., Han, G.C., Chung, Y.S., Lee, Y.J., Hwang, Y.J. & Lee, H.M. (2003). *Antimicrobial peptide LL-37 is upregulated in chronic nasal inflammatory disease.* Acta Otolaryngol 123(1):81-85.

Koczulla, R., von Degenfeld, G., Kupatt, C., Krötz, F., Zahler, S., Gloe, T., Issbrücker, K., Unterberger, P., Zaiou, M., Lebherz, C., Karl, A., Raake, P., Pfosser, A., Boekstegers, P., Welsch, U., Hiemstra, P.S., Vogelmeier, C., Gallo, R.L., Clauss, M. & Bals, R. (2003). *An angiogenic role for the human peptide antibiotic LL-37/hCAP-18.* J Clin Invest 111(11):1665-1672.

Kopitar, M., Ritonja, A., Popovic, T., Gabrijelcic, D., Krizaj, I. & Turk, V. (1989). *A new type of low-molecular mass cysteine proteinase inhibitor from pig leukocytes.* Biol Chem Hoppe Seyler 370(10):1145-1151.

Krisanaprakornkit, S., Weinberg, A., Perez, C.N. & Dale, B.A. (1998). *Expression of the peptide antibiotic human beta-defensin 1 in cultured gingival epithelial cells and gingival tissue.* Infect Immun 66(9):4222-4228.

Krisanaprakornkit, S., Kimball, J.R., Weinberg, A., Darveau, R.P., Bainbridge, B.W. & Dale, B.A. (2000). *Inducible expression of human beta-defensin 2 by Fusobacterium nucleatum in oral epithelial cells: multiple signaling pathways and role of commensal bacteria in innate immunity and the epithelial barrier.* Infect Immun 68(5):2907-2915.

Krisanaprakornkit, S., Kimball, J.R. & Dale, B.A. (2002). *Regulation of human beta-defensin-2 in gingival epithelial cells: the involvement of mitogen-activated protein kinase pathways, but not the NF-kappaB transcription factor family.* J Immunol 168(1):316-324.

Krisanaprakornkit, S., Jotikasthira, D. & Dale, B.A. (2003). *Intracellular calcium in signaling human β-defensin-2 expression in oral epithelial cells.* J Dent Res 82(11):877-882.

Krisanaprakornkit, S., Chotjumlong, P., Kongtawelert, P. & Reutrakul, V. (2008). *Involvement of phospholipase D in regulating expression of anti-microbial peptide human β-defensin-2.* Int Immunol 20(1):21-29.

Lau, Y.E., Rozek, A., Scott, M.G., Goosney, D.L., Davidson, D.J. & Hancock, R.E. (2005). *Interaction and cellular localization of the human host defense peptide LL-37 with lung epithelial cells.* Infect Immun 73(1):583-591.

Laube, D.M., Dongari-Bagtzoglou, A., Kashleva, H., Eskdale, J., Gallagher, G. & Diamond, G. (2008). *Differential regulation of innate immune response genes in gingival epithelial cells stimulated with Aggregatibacter actinomycetemcomitans.* J Periodontal Res 43(1):116-123.

Liu, L., Zhao, C., Heng, H.H. & Ganz, T. (1997). *The human beta-defensin-1 and alpha-defensins are encoded by adjacent genes: two peptide families with differing disulfide topology share a common ancestry.* Genomics 43(3):316-320.

Liu, L., Wang, L., Jia, H.P., Zhao, C., Heng, H.H., Schutte, B.C., McCray, P.B.Jr. & Ganz, T. (1998). *Structure and mapping of the human beta-defensin HBD-2 gene and its expression at sites of inflammation.* Gene 222(2):237-244.

Lu, Q., Jin, L., Darveau, R.P. & Samaranayake, L.P. (2004). *Expression of human beta-defensin-1 and -2 peptides in unresolved chronic periodontitis.* J Periodontal Res 39(4):221-227.

Lu, Q., Samaranayake, L.P., Darveau, R.P. & Jin, L. (2005). *Expression of human beta-defensin-3 in gingival epithelia.* J Periodontal Res 40(6):474-481.

Lundy, F.T., Orr, D.F., Shaw, C., Lamey, P.-J. & Linden, G.J. (2005). *Detection of individual human neutrophil α-defensins (human neutrophil peptides 1, 2 and 3) in unfractionated gingival crevicular fluid-A MALDI-MS approach.* Mol Immunol 42(5):575-579.

Malm, J., Sørensen, O., Persson, T., Frohm-Nilsson, M., Johansson, B., Bjartell, A., Lilja, H., Ståhle-Bäckdahl, M., Borregaard, N. & Equesten, A. (2000). *The human cationic antimicrobial protein (hCAP-18) is expressed in the epithelium of the human epididymis, is present in seminal plasma at high concentrations, and is attached to spermatozoa.* Infect Immun 68(7):4297-4302.

Mars, W.M., Patmasiriwat, P., Maity, T., Huff, V., Weil, M.M. & Saunders, G.F. (1995). *Inheritance of unequal numbers of the genes encoding the human neutrophil defensins HP-1 and HP-3.* J Biol Chem 270(51):30371-30376.

Mathews, M., Jia, H.P., Guthmiller, J.M., Losh, G., Graham, S., Johnson, G., Tack, B.F. & McCray, P.B.Jr. (1999). *Production of beta-defensin antimicrobial peptides by the oral mucosa and salivary glands.* Infect Immun 67(6):2740-2745.

McKay, M.S., Olson, E., Hesla, M.A., Panyutich, A., Ganz, T., Perkins, S. & Rossomando, E.F. (1999). *Immunomagnetic recovery of human neutrophil defensins from the human gingival crevice.* Oral Microbiol Immunol 14(3):190-193.

Midorikawa, K., Ouhara, K., Komatsuzawa, H., Kawai, T., Yamada, S., Fujiwara, T., Yamazaki, K., Sayama, K., Taubman, M.A., Kurihara, H., Hashimoto, K. & Sugai, M. (2003). *Staphylococcus aureus susceptibility to innate antimicrobial peptides, beta-defensins and CAP18, expressed by human keratinocytes.* Infect Immun 71(7):3730-3739.

Mizukawa, N., Sugiyama, K., Yamachika, E., Ueno, T., Mishima, K., Takagi, S. & Sugahara, T. (1999). *Presence of defensin in epithelial Langerhans cells adjacent to oral carcinoma and precancerous lesions.* Anticancer Res 19(4B):2969-2971.

Mizukawa, N., Sugiyama, K., Kamio, M., Yamachika, E., Ueno, T., Fukunaga, J., Takagi, S. & Sugahara, T. (2000). *Immunohistochemical staining of human alpha-defensin-1 (HNP-*

1), in the submandibular glands of patients with oral carcinomas. Anticancer Res 20(2B):1125-1127.

Mookherjee, N., Brown, K.L., Bowdish, D.M., Doria, S., Falsafi, R., Hokamp, K., Roche, F.M., Mu, R., Doho, G.H., Pistolic, J., Powers, J.-P., Bryan, J., Brinkman, F.S. & Hancock, R.E. (2006). *Modulation of the TLR-mediated inflammatory response by the endogenous human host defense peptide LL-37.* J Immunol 176(4):2455-2464.

Murakami, M., Ohtake, T., Dorschner, R.A. & Gallo, R.L. (2002a). *Cathelicidin antimicrobial peptides are expressed in salivary glands and saliva.* J Dent Res 81(12):845-850.

Murakami, M., Ohtake, T., Dorschner, R.A., Schittek, B., Garbe, C. & Gallo, R.L. (2002b). *Cathelicidin antimicrobial peptide expression in sweat, an innate defense system for the skin.* J Invest Dermatol 119(5):1090-1095.

Murphy, C.J., Foster, B.A., Mannis, M.J., Selsted, M.E. & Reid, T.W. (1993). *Defensins are mitogenic for epithelial cells and fibroblasts.* J Cell Physiol 155(2):408-413.

Nagaoka, I., Hirota, S., Yomogida, S., Ohwada, A. & Hirata, M. (2000). *Synergistic actions of antibacterial neutrophil defensins and cathelicidins.* Inflamm Res 49(2):73-79.

Nassar, T., Akkawi, S., Bar-Shavit, R., Haj-Yehia, A., Bdeir, K., Al-Mehdi, A.B., Tarshis, M. & Higazi, A.A. (2002). *Human alpha-defensin regulates smooth muscle cell contraction: a role for low-density lipoprotein receptor-related protein/alpha 2-macroglobulin receptor.* Blood 100(12):4026-4032.

Nishimura, E., Eto, A., Kato, M., Hashizume, S., Imai, S., Nisizawa, T. & Hanada, N. (2004). *Oral Streptococci exhibit diverse susceptibility to human beta-defensin-2: antimicrobial effects of hBD-2 on oral streptococci.* Curr Microbiol 48(2):85-87.

Nishimura, M., Abiko, Y., Kusano, K., Yamazaki, M., Saitoh, M., Mizoguchi, I., Jinbu, Y., Noguchi, T. & Kaku, T. (2003). *Localization of human beta-defensin 3 mRNA in normal oral epithelium, leukoplakia, and lichen planus: an in situ hybridization study.* Med Electron Microsc 36(2):94-97.

Niyonsaba, F., Someya, A., Hirata, M., Ogawa, H. & Nagaoka, I. (2001). *Evaluation of the effects of peptide antibiotics human beta-defensins-1/-2 and LL-37 on histamine release and prostaglandin D(2) production from mast cells.* Eur J Immunol 31(4):1066-1075.

Niyonsaba, F., Iwabuchi, K., Someya, A., Hirata, M., Matsuda, H., Ogawa, H. & Nagaoka, I. (2002a). *A cathelicidin family of human antibacterial peptide LL-37 induces mast cell chemotaxis.* Immunology 106(1):20-26.

Niyonsaba, F., Iwabuchi, K., Matsuda, H., Ogawa, H. & Nagaoka, I. (2002b). *Epithelial cell-derived human beta-defensin-2 acts as a chemotaxin for mast cells through a pertussis toxin-sensitive and phospholipase C-dependent pathway.* Int Immunol 14(4):421-426.

Niyonsaba, F., Ogawa, H. & Nagaoka, I. (2004). *Human beta-defensin-2 functions as a chemotactic agent for tumor necrosis factor-alpha-treated human neutrophils.* Immunology 111(3):273-281.

Niyonsaba, F., Ushio, H., Nakano, N., Ng, W., Sayama, K., Hashimoto, K., Nagaoka, I., Okumura, K. & Ogawa, H. (2007). *Antimicrobial peptides human β-defensins stimulate epidermal keratinocyte migration, proliferation, and production of proinflammatory cytokines and chemokines.* J Invest Dermatol 127(3):594-604.

Noguchi, T., Shiba, H., Komatsuzawa, H., Mizuno, N., Uchida, Y., Ouhara, R., Asakawa, R., Kudo, S., Kawaguchi, H., Sugai, M. & Kurihara, H. (2003). *Synthesis of prostaglandin E$_2$*

and E-cadherin and gene expression of β-defensin-2 by human gingival epithelial cells in response to Actinobacillus actinomycetemcomitans. Inflammation 27(6):341-349.

Nomura, I., Goleva, E., Howell, M.D., Hamid, Q.A., Ong, P.Y., Hall, C.F., Darst, M.A., Gao, B., Boguniewicz, M., Travers, J.B. & Leung, D.Y. (2003). *Cytokine milieu of atopic dermatitis, as compared to psoriasis, skin prevents induction of innate immune response genes.* J Immunol 171(6):3262-3269.

Ohgami, K., Ilieva, I.B., Shiratori, K., Isogai, E., Yoshida, K., Kotake, S., Nishida, T., Mizuki, N. & Ohno, S. (2003). *Effect of human cationic antimicrobial protein 18 peptide on endotoxin-induced uveitis in rats.* Invest Ophthalmol Vis Sci 44(10):4412-4418.

Ong, P.Y., Ohtake, T., Brandt, C., Strickland, I., Boguniewicz, M., Ganz, T., Gallo, R.L. & Leung, D.Y. (2002). *Endogenous antimicrobial peptides and skin infections in atopic dermatitis.* N Engl J Med 347(15):1151-1160.

Oren, A., Ganz, T., Liu, L. & Meerloo, T. (2003). *In human epidermis, beta-defensin 2 is packaged in lamellar bodies.* Exp Mol Pathol 74(2):180-182.

Otte, J.M., Zdebik, A.E., Brand, S., Chromik, A.M., Strauss, S., Schmitz, F., Steinstraesser, L. & Schmidt, W.E. (2009). *Effects of the cathelicidin LL-37 on intestinal epithelial barrier integrity.* Regul Pept 156(1-3):104-117.

Ouhara, K., Komatsuzawa, H., Yamada, S., Shiba, H., Fujiwara, T., Ohara, M., Sayama, K., Hashimoto, K., Kurihara, H. & Sugai, M. (2005). *Susceptibilities of periodontopathogenic and cariogenic bacteria to antibacterial peptides, (beta)-defensins and LL-37, produced by human epithelial cells.* J Antimicrob Chemother 55(6):888-896.

Ouhara, K., Komatsuzawa, H., Shiba, H., Uchida, Y., Kawai, T., Sayama, K., Hashimoto, K., Taubman, M.A., Kurihara, H. & Sugai, M. (2006). *Actinobacillus actinomy cetemcomitans outer membrane protein 100 triggers innate immunity and production of β-defensin and the 18-kilodalton cationic antimicrobial protein through the fibronectin-integrin pathway in human gingival epithelial cells.* Infect Immun 74(9):5211-5220.

Perregaux, D.G., Bhavsar, K., Contillo, L., Shi, J. & Gabel, C.A. (2002). *Antimicrobial peptides initiate IL-1 beta posttranslational processing: a novel role beyond innate immunity.* J Immunol 168(6):3024-3032.

Presicce, P., Giannelli, S., Taddeo, A., Villa, M.L. & Della Bella, S. (2009). *Human defensins activate monocyte-derived dendritic cells, promote the production of proinflammatory cytokines, and up-regulate the surface expression of CD91.* J Leukoc Biol 86(4):941-948.

Puklo, M., Guentsch, A., Hiemstra, P.S., Eick, S. & Potempa, J. (2008). *Analysis of neutrophil-derived antimicrobial peptides in gingival crevicular fluid suggests importance of cathelicidin LL-37 in the innate immune response against periodontogenic bacteria.* Oral Microbiol Immunol 23(4):328-335.

Pütsep, K., Carlsson, G., Boman, H.G. & Andersson, M. (2002). *Deficiency of antibacterial peptides in patients with morbus Kostmann: an observation study.* Lancet 360(9340):1144-1149.

Ritonja, A., Kopitar, M., Jerala, R. & Turk, V. (1989). *Primary structure of a new cysteine proteinase inhibitor from pig leucocytes.* FEBS Lett 255(2):211-214.

Romeo, D., Skerlavaj, B., Bolognesi, M. & Gennaro, R. (1988). *Structure and bactericidal activity of an antibiotic dodecapeptide purified from bovine neutrophils.* J Biol Chem 263(20):9573-9575.

Sahasrabudhe, K.S., Kimball, J.R., Morton, T.H., Weinberg, A. & Dale, B.A. (2000). *Expression of the antimicrobial peptide, human beta-defensin 1, in duct cells of minor salivary glands and detection in saliva.* J Dent Res 79(9):1669-1674.

Schauber, J., Svanholm, C., Termén, S., Iffland, K., Menzel, T., Scheppach, W., Melcher, R., Agerberth, B., Lührs, H. & Gudmundsson, G.H. (2003). *Expression of the cathelicidin LL-37 is modulated by short chain fatty acids in colonocytes: relevance of signaling pathways.* Gut 52(5):735-741.

Schibli, D.J., Hunter, H.N., Aseyev, V., Starner, T.D., Wiencek, J.M., McCray, P.B.Jr., Tack, B.F. & Vogel, H.J. (2002). *The solution structure of the human beta-defensins lead to a better understanding of the potent bactericidal activity of HBD3 against Staphylococcus aureus.* J Biol Chem 277(10):8279-8289.

Schmidtchen, A., Frick, I.M., Andersson, E., Tapper, H. & Björck, L. (2002). *Proteinases of common pathogenic bacteria degrade and inactivate the antibacterial peptide LL-37.* Mol Microbiol 46(1):157-168.

Schnapp, D., Reid, C.J. & Harris, A. (1998). *Localization of expression of human beta defensin-1 in the pancreas and kidney.* J Pathol 186(1):99-103.

Schutte, B.C., Mitros, J.P., Bartlett, J.A., Walters, J.D., Jia, H.P., Welsh, M.J., Casavant, T.L. & McCray, P.B.Jr. (2002). *Discovery of five conserved beta-defensin gene clusters using a computational search strategy.* Proc Natl Acad Sci USA 99(4):2129-2133.

Scott, M.G., Davidson, D.J., Gold, M.R., Bowdish, D. & Hancock, R.E. (2002). *The human antimicrobial peptide LL-37 is a multifunctional modulator of innate immune responses.* J Immunol 169(7):3883-3891.

Semple, C.A., Rolfe, M. & Dorin, J.R. (2003). *Duplication and selection in the evolution of primate beta-defensin genes.* Genome Biol 4(5):R31.

Shaykhiev, R., Beisswenger, C., Kändler, K., Senske, J., Püchner, A., Damm, T., Behr, J. & Bals, R. (2005). *Human endogenous antibiotic LL-37 stimulates airway epithelial cell proliferation and wound closure.* Am J Physiol Lung Cell Mol Physiol 289(5):L842-L848.

Shiba, H., Mouri, Y., Komatsuzawa, H., Ouhara, K., Takeda, K., Sugai, M., Kinane, D.F. & Kurihara, H. (2003). *Macrophage inflammatory protein-3alpha and beta-defensin-2 stimulate dentin sialophosphoprotein gene expression in human pulp cells.* Biochem Biophys Res Commun 306(4):867-871.

Sørensen, O., Cowland, J.B., Askaa, J. & Borregaard, N. (1997). *An ELISA for hCAP-18, the cathelicidin present in human neutrophils and plasma.* J Immunol Methods 206(1-2): 53-59.

Sørensen, O.E., Follin, P., Johnsen, A.H., Calafat, J., Tjabringa, G.S., Hiemstra, P.S. & Borregaard, N. (2001). *Human cathelicidin, hCAP-18, is processed to the antimicrobial peptide LL-37 by extracellular cleavage with proteinase 3.* Blood 97(12):3951-3959.

Sørensen, O.E., Cowland, J.B., Theilgaard-Mönch, K., Liu, L., Ganz, T. & Borregaard, N. (2003). *Wound healing and expression of antimicrobial peptides/polypeptides in human keratinocytes, a consequence of common growth factors.* J Immunol 170(11):5583-5589.

Sparkes, R.S., Kronenberg, M., Heinzmann, C., Daher, K.A., Klisak, I., Ganz, T. & Mohandas, T. (1989). *Assignment of defensin gene(s) to human chromosome 8p23.* Genomics 5(2):240-244.

Taggart, C.C., Greene, C.M., Smith, S.G., Levine, R.L., McCray, P.B.Jr., O'Neill, S. & McElvaney, N.G. (2003). *Inactivation of human beta-defensin 2 and 3 by elastolytic cathepsins.* J Immunol 171(2):931-937.

Taguchi, Y. & Imai, H. (2006). *Expression of β-defensin-2 in human gingival epithelial cells in response to challenge with Porphyromonas gingivalis in vitro.* J Periodontal Res 41(4): 334-339.

Tanaka, D., Miyasaki, K.T. & Lehrer, R.I. (2000). *Sensitivity of Actinobacillus actinomycetemcomitans and Capnocytophaga spp. to the bactericidal action of LL-37: a cathelicidin found in human leukocytes and epithelium.* Oral Microbiol Immunol 15(4):226-231.

Tani, K., Murphy, W.J., Chertov, O., Salcedo, R., Koh, C.Y., Utsunomiya, I., Funakoshi, S., Asai, O., Herrmann, S.H., Wang, J.M., Kwak, L.W. & Oppenheim, J.J. (2000). *Defensins act as potent adjuvants that promote cellular and humoral immune responses in mice to a lymphoma idiotype and carrier antigens.* Int Immunol 12(5):691-700.

Tao, R., Jurevic, R.J., Coulton, K.K., Tsutsui, M.T., Roberts, M.C., Kimball, J.R., Wells, N., Berndt, J. & Dale, B.A. (2005). *Salivary antimicrobial peptide expression and dental caries experience in children.* Antimicrob Agents Chemother 49(9):3883-3888.

Taylor, K., Clarke, D.J., McCullough, B., Chin, W., Seo, E., De Yang, Oppenheim, J., Uhrin, D., Govan, J.R.W., Campopiano, D.J., MacMillan, D., Barran, P. & Dorin, J.R. (2008). *Analysis and separation of residues important for the chemoattractant and antimicrobial activities of β-defensin 3.* J Biol Chem 283(11):6631-6639.

Tjabringa, G.S., Aarbiou, J., Ninaber, D.K., Drijfhout, J.W., Sørensen, O.E., Borregaard, N., Rabe, K.F. & Hiemstra, P.S. (2003). *The antimicrobial peptide LL-37 activates innate immunity at the airway epithelial surface by transactivation of the epidermal growth factor receptor.* J Immunol 171(12):6690-6696.

Tjabringa, G.S., Ninaber, D.K., Drijfhout, J.W., Rabe, K.F. & Hiemstra, P.S. (2006). *Human cathelicidin LL-37 is a chemoattractant for eosinophils and neutrophils that acts via formyl-peptide receptors.* Int Arch Allergy Immunol 140(2):103-112.

Tokumaru, S., Sayama, K., Shirakata, Y., Komatsuzawa, H., Ouhara, K., Hanakawa, Y., Yahata, Y., Dai, X., Tohyama, M., Nagai, H., Yang, L., Higashiyama, S., Yoshimura, A., Sugai, M. & Hashimoto, K. (2005). *Induction of keratinocyte migration via transactivation of the epidermal growth factor receptor by the antimicrobial peptide LL-37.* J Immunol 175(7):4662-4668.

Tollin, M., Bergman, P., Svenberg, T., Jörnvall, H., Gudmundsson, G.H. & Agerberth, B. (2003). *Antimicrobial peptides in the first line defence of human colon mucosa.* Peptides 24(4): 523-530.

Toomes, C., James, J., Wood, A.J., Wu, C.L., McCormick, D., Lench, N., Hewitt, C., Moynihan, L., Roberts, E., Woods, C.G., Markham, A., Wong, M., Widmer, R., Ghaffar, K.A., Pemberton, M., Hussein, I.R., Temtamy, S.A., Davies, R., Read, A.P., Sloan, P., Dixon, M.J. & Thakker, N.S. (1999). *Loss-of-function mutations in the cathepsin C gene result in periodontal disease and palmoplantar keratosis.* Nat Genet 23(4):421-424.

Tsutsumi-Ishii, Y. & Nagaoka, I. (2002). *NF-kappa B-mediated transcriptional regulation of human beta-defensin-2 gene following lipopolysaccharide stimulation.* J Leukoc Biol 71(1):154-162.

Türkoğlu, O., Emingil, G., Kütükçüler, N. & Atilla, G. (2009). *Gingival crevicular fluid levels of cathelicidin LL-37 and interleukin-18 in patients with chronic periodontitis.* J Periodontol 80(6):969-976.

Valore, E.V. & Ganz, T. (1992). *Posttranslational processing of defensins in immature human myeloid cells.* Blood 79(6):1538-1544.

Valore, E.V., Park, C.H., Quayle, A.J., Wiles, K.R., McCray, P.B.Jr. & Ganz, T. (1998). *Human beta-defensin-1: an antimicrobial peptide of urogenital tissues.* J Clin Invest 101(8):1633-1642.

van Wetering, S., Mannesse-Lazeroms, S.P., van Sterkenburg, M.A., Daha, M.R., Dijkman, J.H. & Hiemstra, P.S. (1997). *Effect of defensins on interleukin-8 synthesis in airway epithelial cells.* Am J Physiol 272(5 Pt 1):L888-L896.

Vardar-Sengul, S., Demirci, T., Sen, B.H., Erkizan, V., Kurulgan, E. & Baylas, H. (2007). *Human beta defensin-1 and -2 expression in the gingiva of patients with specific periodontal diseases.* J Periodontal Res 42(5):429-437.

Weber, G., Heilborn, J.D., Chamorro Jimenez, C.I., Hammarsjo, A., Törmä, H. & Stahle, M. (2005). *Vitamin D induces the antimicrobial protein hCAP-18 in human skin.* J Invest Dermatol 124(5):1080-1082.

Wilde, C.G., Griffith, J.E., Marra, M.N., Snable, J.L. & Scott, R.W. (1989). *Purification and characterization of human neutrophil peptide 4, a novel member of the defensin family.* J Biol Chem 264(19):11200-11203.

Yang, D., Chertov, O., Bykovskaia, S.N., Chen, Q., Buffo, M.J., Shogan, J., Anderson, M., Schröder, J.M., Wang, J.M., Howard, O.M. & Oppenheim, J.J. (1999). *Beta-defensins: linking innate and adaptive immunity through dendritic and T cell CCR6.* Science 286(5439):525-528.

Yang, D., Chen, Q., Chertov, O. & Oppenheim, J.J. (2000). *Human neutrophil defensins selectively chemoattract naïve T and immature dendritic cells.* J Leukoc Biol 68(1):9-14.

Yu, J., Mookherjee, N., Wee, K., Bowdish, D.M., Pistolic, J., Li, Y., Rehaume, L. & Hancock, R.E. (2007). *Host defense peptide LL-37, in synergy with inflammatory mediator IL-1β, augments immune responses by multiple pathways.* J Immunol 179(11):7684-7691.

Zaiou, M., Nizet, V. & Gallo, R.L. (2003). *Antimicrobial and protease inhibitory functions of the human cathelicidin (hCAP-18/LL-37) prosequence.* J Invest Dermatol 120(5):810-816.

Zanetti, M., Gennaro, R. & Romeo, O. (1995). *Cathelicidins: a novel protein family with a common proregion and a variable C-terminal antimicrobial domain.* FEBS Lett 374(1):1-5.

Zasloff, M. (2002). *Antimicrobial peptides of multicellular organisms.* Nature 415(6870):389-395.

Zhao, C., Wang, I. & Lehrer, R.I. (1996). *Widespread expression of beta-defensin hBD-1 in human secretory glands and epithelial cells.* FEBS Lett 396(2-3):319-322.

Zuyderduyn, S., Ninaber, D.K., Hiemstra, P.S. & Rabe, K.F. (2006). *The antimicrobial peptide LL-37 enhances IL-8 release by human airway smooth muscle cells.* J Allergy Clin Immunol 117(6):1328-1335.

In: Periodontitis Symptoms, Treatment and Prevention   ISBN: 978-1-61668-836-3
Editor: Rosemarie E. Walchuck, pp. 105-139   ©2010 Nova Science Publishers, Inc.

Chapter 4

PROGNOSIS: PREDICTABILITY REDEFINED

M.V. Jothi [*1], *K.M. Bhat*[2], *P.K.Pratibha*[3] *and G.S. Bhat*[4]

Assistant Professor, Department of Periodontics, Manipal college of Dental Sciences,
Manipal, Karnataka, India[1]
Professor, Department of Periodontics & Implantology, Manipal college of Dental
Sciences, Manipal, Karnataka, India[2]
Associate professor, Department of Periodontics, Manipal college of Dental Sciences,
Karnataka, India[3]
Professor & Head, Department of Periodontics, Manipal college of Dental Sciences,
Manipal, Karnataka, India[4]

ABSTRACT

This comprehensive review highlights a detailed overview related to devising
a periodontal prognosis. A precise predictability of the results of a disease is
profound and crucial for proper treatment planning. Since the understanding of
periodontal disease has progressed to include the influence of risk factors,
assigning a prognosis has become more perplexing to the clinician. Various
factors that influence the overall and individual tooth prognosis have been
enumerated. The classification systems required to assign a prognosis has also
been included. The potential adverse influences of both local and systemic
factors have also been discussed. An experienced clinician should analyze all
these factors, along with the patients attitude towards dental therapy, prior to
arriving at a judgment for a single tooth or teeth. With newer trends in treatment
modalities, patients can seek better options for treatment, thus improving the long
term prognosis.

*Corresponding author : Dr M.V. Jothi, Assistant Professor, Department of Periodontics, Manipal College of Dental
Sciences, Manipal – 576104, Karnataka, India. Telephone: +91-0820-4292352, Email:jothimv@gmail.com
Fax: 0091-0820-2570061

INTRODUCTION

Prognosis simply means "forecast". The term derives its origin from the Greek words "pro" which means "before" and "gignoskein" which means "know". It is the art of foretelling the duration, course, result and termination of disease [1]. A precise predictability of the results of a disease is both essential and profound in the treatment plan.

In earlier days, when only fewer periodontal diseases had been identified both diagnosis and prognosis were easier. But with discovery of complex forms of the disease, prognosis became more complex. To further complicate matters, periodontal diseases have predilection for individual teeth rather than the complete dentition or even a segment of the entire dentition. The ability to prognosticate accurately for the entire dentition or an individual tooth is important for many reasons. The patient uses this information to determine whether the treatment seems worthwhile. It would benefit the patient for insurance purposes and lastly, the clinician uses these factors to determine which treatment modality would be most effective to develop restorative recommendations.

Periodontal literature have considered many factors which judge whether a tooth should be retained or not, but since the understanding of periodontal diseases has progressed to include the influences of risk factors such as genetics, smoking, stress etc in the occurrence and severity of periodontal diseases, assigning a prognosis has become even more perplexing to the clinician.

This compilation provides a detailed overview on the various factors that determine prognosis and highlights its relevance in predicting the newer treatment modalities.

VARIOUS TERMINOLOGIES RELATED TO PERIODONTAL PROGNOSIS

Provisional prognosis : a provisional or tentative prognosis is that which allows the clinician to initiate treatment of teeth that have a doubtful outlook in the hope that a favorable response may tip the balance and allow teeth to be retained.[1]

Guarded prognosis : The prognosis is graded as Guarded, if plaque or calculus control is poor or if resolution of inflammation is inadequate. If increasing attachment loss, radiographic evidence of increasing bone loss, increasing mobility, or persistent third-degree mobility is found 1 to 3 months after anti-infective and initial occlusal therapy, the prognosis may be assigned as guarded or poor.[2]

Diagnostic prognosis: It is an evaluation of the course of disease without treatment. It answers the queries, on the current status of the teeth and the anticipated future of these teeth. [3]

Therapeutic prognosis: refers to the effect of periodontal treatment on the course of the disease. Information of a prognosis, the clinician may be dealt with various circumstances which require skillful therapeutic judgment. For example: the clinician may find situations in which teeth have ample support but are mobile and teeth that have little support but are firm or incases with two walled defects that are narrow and deep, that can be successfully treated with techniques that aim at new attachment and bone regeneration than deep horizontal defects which lack regenerative capacity.[3]

Prosthetic prognosis: Once the anticipated result of periodontal treatment and periodontal health status is obtained for the patient, the following queries arise regarding the forecast for success of prosthetic restoration, whether the prosthesis is therapeutic or detrimental and dictating the necessity of the prosthesis. [3]

PROGNOSIS AND RISK

Prognosis and risk are terms used interchangeably and often creates a certain degree of confusion. Risk is the probability that an individual will get a specific disease at a given period or an unwanted outcome may occur in the future [4]. Risk factors are objective findings that indicate a strong probability of developing unwanted outcomes in people who have not been subjected to the given disease.

Many times, the factors associated with a poor prognosis are the same as those associated with increased risk. Specifically, if factors that increase the risk of acquiring the disease are present while the patient has the disease, they can worsen its prognosis. Knowledge about certain measurable factors may provide information about future disease onset and / or disease progression. Genetic susceptibility to disease in patients with juvenile periodontitis is an example of a factor that predisposes to both disease onset and progression.

In contrast, prognostic factors are characteristics or factors that predict the outcome of a disease once a disease is present. The process of using prognostic factors to predict a course of a disease is called Prognosis Assessment [5]. In some cases risk factors and prognostic factors are the same. For example some factors such as smoking may be both risk factor and prognostic factor .Thus once a person has a disease, two processes may be considered that is, reducing the risk in healthy sites and increasing the risk of a positive prognosis in the sites with the disease.

Prognostic Indicators

These are factors which are found to be associated with further disease progression. The mere co-existence of the indicators in subjects or sites exhibiting an ongoing periodontal destruction does not necessarily suggest a cause and effect relationship. In order to determine if a prognostic indicator is a true prognostic factor, it is necessary to follow untreated periodontitis patients longitudinally, and determine an association between the disease progression and the presence / absence of the marker in question. [4]

Individual tooth prognostic factors such as type of bone loss, probing depth, mobility including whether or not, one or more sites are undergoing an episode of active periodontal disease are important. Some patients may have active disease at multiple sites, and other patients may be in remission. [6]

Machtei EE et al [7] in a longitudinal study examined the clinical, microbiological and immunological indicators to determine whether the presence or combination of these parameters would correlate positively with true prognostic factors. The results showed that the overall mean attachment loss and bone loss were almost identical. They concluded that past periodontal destruction, smoking habits, Bacteriodes forsythus, Prevotella intermedia and

Porphyromonas gingivalis at baseline are prognostic factors for further periodontal breakdown.

Factors to be Considered when Determining a Prognosis

The assignment of prognosis is one of the most important functions involved in clinical practice. It involves an examiner identifying one or more commonly taught parameters as they uniquely apply to the tooth.

Glickman (1973) considered two aspects to the determination of prognosis in patients with periodontal disease: The *overall prognosis* and the *prognosis of individual teeth*.

Carranza [4] considered some factors that may be more important in determining a prognosis [refer Table 1]. Consideration of each factor may be beneficial to the clinician. In most cases, analysis of these factors allows the clinician to assign a prognosis.

Table I. Factors to be considered for determining prognosis [4].

Overall Clinical Factors	Systemic / Environmental Factors	Local Factors	Prosthetic/ Restorative Factors
Patient age	Smoking	Plaque / calculus	Abutment selection
Disease severity	Systemic disease / condition	Subgingival restorations	Caries
Plaque control	Genetic factors	Anatomic factors:	Nonvital teeth
Patient compliance	Stress	Short, tapered roots Cervical enamel projections Enamel pearls Bifurcation ridges Root concavities Developmental grooves Root proximity Furcation involvement Tooth mobility	Root resorption

Prognosis for Patients with Gingival Diseases

Gingival diseases are diverse group of complex and distinct pathological entities found within the gingiva resulting from a variety of etiologies. A classification system consisting of four main types were developed. The common form is plaque induced gingivitis resulting from dental plaque only [refer Table II] The other three types of plaque-associated gingival diseases are those modified by: 1) systemic factors 2) medications 3) malnutrition [refer Table III]

**Table II. Classification for dental plaque-induced gingival diseases
and their prognosis [4].**

Plaque induced gingival diseases	Prognosis
1. Gingivitis associated with dental plaque only a) Without other local contributing factors b) With local contributing factors	Prognosis of gingivitis associated with dental plaque is considered as good, provided 1. all local irritants are eliminated, 2. other local factors contributing to plaque retention are eliminated 3. gingival contours conducive to the preservation of health are attained, 4. the patient cooperates by maintaining good oral hygiene.

2. Gingival disease modified by systemic factors
a) Associated with the endocrine system
  1) Puberty-associated gingivitis
  2) Menstrual cycle-associated gingivitis
  3) Pregnancy-associated
a) Gingivitis
b) Pyogenic granuloma
  4) Diabetes mellitus- associated gingivitis
a) Associated with blood dyscrasias
  1) Leukemia- associated gingivitis
  2) Other
	The long-term prognosis for these patients depends not only on control of bacterial plaque, but also on control or correction of the systemic factor(s).

3) Gingival diseases modified by medications
a) drug-induced gingival diseases
  1) drug-induced gingival enlargements
  2) drug-induced gingivitis
b) Oral contraceptive-associated gingivitis
	Reductions in dental plaque can limit the severity of the lesions. The long-term prognosis is dependent on whether the patient's systemic problem can be treated with an alternative medication that does not have gingival enlargement as a side effect.
	
	Long-term prognosis in these patients is dependent not only on the control of bacterial plaque, but also on the likelihood of continued use of the oral contraceptives.

4. Gingival diseases modified by malnutrition a) Ascorbic acid-deficiency gingivitis b) Others	The prognosis in these cases may be dependent on the severity and duration of deficiency and on the likelihood of reversing the deficiency through dietary supplementation.

Table III. Classification for Non-plaque induced gingival lesions and their prognosis[4].

1. Gingival diseases of specific bacterial origin a) Neisseria Gonorrhea – associated lesions b) Treponema Pallidum-associated lesions c) Streptococcal species-associated lesions d) Other	Prognosis is dependent on elimination of the source of the infectious agent.

2. Gingival diseases of viral origin
a) Herpesvirus infections
  i) herpetic primary gingivostomatitis
  ii) recurrent oral herpes
  iii)varicella-zoster infection
b) Others
	Prognosis is dependent on elimination of the source of the infectious agent

3. Gingival diseases of fungal origin a) Candida- species infections b) Linear gingival erythema c) Histoplasmosis d) Others	Prognosis is dependent on elimination of the source of the infectious agent

4. Gingival manifestations of systemic conditions
a) Mucocutaneous disorders
  1) Lichen planus
  2) Pemphigoid
  3) Pemphigus vulgaris
  4) Erythema multiforme
  5) Lupus erythematosis
  6) Drug- induced
  7) others
b) Allergic reactions
  1) Dental restorative materials
a) Mercury
b) Nickel
c) Acrylic
d) others
  2) Reactions attributable to
a) toothpastes/dentifrices
b) mouthrinses/mouthwashes
c) chewing gum additives
d) food and additives
  3) Others
	Prognosis for these patients is linked to management of the associated dermatologic disorder
	Prognosis for these cases is dependent on avoidance of causative agent

5.Traumatic lesions (factitious, iatrogenic, accidental) a) Chemical injury b) Physical injury c) Thermal injury	Prognosis for these cases is dependent on avoidance of causative agent
6. Foreign body reactions	Prognosis for these cases is dependent on elimination of the causative agent.

Prognosis for Patients with Periodontal Diseases

Two main aspects are considered for determination of prognosis in patients with Periodontitis:

1) Overall prognosis: refers to the dentition as a whole. Many specific dental conditions can affect the overall prognosis of the dentition. [Table 1]

Factors Influencing Overall Prognosis in Periodontitis Patients

1) Types of Periodontitis

   a) Chronic periodontitis

It is the most common form of periodontitis,that can present in a localized or generalized form. It is a slow progressive disease associated with well-known local environmental factors that generally influences the normal host bacterial interaction. In cases of slight to moderate periodontitis, the prognosis is generally good; provided good oral hygiene is maintained and local plaque retentive factors are eliminated. In patients with severe form of chronic periodontitis, as evidenced by furcation involvement and increasing clinical mobility or non-compliant patients, the prognosis may be fair to questionable[4]. In cases, where the etiology is as a result of smoking or stress, elimination of these factors can lead to favourable prognosis.

   b) Aggressive Periodontitis

Aggressive periodontitis comprises a group of rare, often severe, rapidly progressive forms of periodontitis, characterized by an early age of clinical manifestation and a distinctive susceptibility for cases to aggregate in families[8]. Since this disease usually occurs at early age, it implies that etiologic agents have been able to cause clinically detectable levels of disease over a relatively short time. Diagnosis of aggressive periodontitis requires exclusion of the presence of systemic diseases that may severely impair host defenses and lead to premature tooth loss.

The prognosis for patients with aggressive periodontitis depends on whether the disease is generalized or localized and on the degree of destruction present at the time of examination. In general, the treatment of patients with generalized forms of aggressive periodontitis should be very similar to that of patients with refractory forms of the disease. The generalized forms, which are usually associated with some systemic disease, have a worse prognosis than the localized forms. The rate of disease progression may be faster in these younger individuals, and therefore the clinician should monitor such patients more often.

Flare-ups of proliferative gingival inflammation can be observed early when the patient is on a frequent monitoring cycle. Currently, monitoring every 3 weeks or less is suggested while the disease is in an active phase. Aggressive periodontitis rarely undergoes spontaneous remission. It is important to obtain earlier radiographs to assess the stage of the disease. In case of localized aggressive periodontitis, a number of treatment modalities have been attempted in the past with varying degrees of success. However, the response has been unpredictable[4].

Patients who are diagnosed as having an early form of aggressive periodontitis may respond to standard periodontal therapy. In general, the earlier the disease is diagnosed (as determined by less destruction), the more conservative the therapy may be and the more predictable the outcome.

c)   Periodontitis as a manifestation of systemic diseases

Periodontitis as a manifestation of systemic diseases can be divided into two categories. (1) Those associated with hematological disorders such as leukemia and acquired neutropenias and (2) those associated with genetic disorders such as familial and cyclic neutropenia, Down syndrome, Papillon-Lefevre syndrome and hypophosphastasia. Although the primary etiologic factor in periodontal diseases is bacterial plaque, systemic diseases alter the prognosis. For example, decreased numbers of circulating neutrophils (as in acquired neutropenias) may contribute to widespread destruction of the periodontium. Unless the neutropenia can be corrected, these patients present with a fair-to-poor prognosis. Similarly, genetic disorders that alter the way the host responds to bacterial plaque (as in leukocyte adhesion deficiency syndrome) also can contribute to the development of periodontitis. Because these disorders generally manifest early in life, the impact on the periodontium may be clinically similar to generalized aggressive periodontitis. The prognosis in these cases will be fair to poor. [4]

d)   Necrotizing Periodontal Diseases

Necrotizing periodontal diseases can be divided into necrotic diseases that affect the gingival tissues exclusively that is, necrotizing ulcerative gingivitis (NUG) and necrotic ulcerative periodontitis (NUP) that affect deeper tissues of the periodontium. In necrotizing ulcerative gingivitis the main predisposing factor is bacterial plaque. However, this disease is usually complicated by the presence of secondary factors such as acute psychological stress, smoking and poor nutrition, all of which can contribute to immune suppression.Therefore superimposition of these secondary factors on a preexisting gingivitis can result in painful, necrotic lesions characteristic of necrotizing ulcerative gingivitis. With control of both the bacterial plaque and the secondary factors, prognosis for such patients is good.

In systemically healthy patients, this progression may have resulted from multiple episodes of necrotizing ulcerative gingivitis or the necrotizing disease may occur at a site previously affected with periodontitis. In these cases the prognosis is dependent on alleviating the plaque and secondary factors associated with necrotizing ulcerative gingivitis. However, many patients presenting with necrotic ulcerative periodontitis are immune compromised through systemic conditions, such as HIV infection. In these cases, the prognosis is dependent on not only reducing local and secondary factors, but also on dealing with the systemic problem. Prognosis in these cases is unfavourable. [4]

2) Overall Clinical Factors

   (i) Age

Many of the studies confirm that older age groups have consistently more destruction compared to the younger [9,10].This is attributed to the chronicity of the disease process. However aging, per se is not likely to be a predisposing factor for periodontal disease.

The classical work carried out by Loe et al, on experimental gingivitis was studied in the young (20-24 year old) and the old (65-78 year old) age groups, gingival inflammation was considerably more rapid and more severe in the elderly groups [11].

The strong association between age and periodontal destruction reported in cross-sectional studies is mostly due to effect of age as surrogate for the length of exposure to etiologic factors.

Limited information suggests that increased age may be associated with slower bone healing after extractions, placement of intraosseous implants and bone grafting [12].

Although aging does not appear to affect the outcome of periodontal therapy, it is a very important factor that should always be considered when assessing patient susceptibility.

   (ii) Disease severity

Knowledge of past dental health status is a good predictor for future oral health status of the dentition. Steady progression implies a poorer prognosis that does arrest disease, even at an advanced stage. Rapid progression about many teeth, simultaneously or sequentially, carries a poorer prognosis than does a rapid destruction of the periodontal tissues of a single tooth. The severity of the disease might be slight, moderate or severe.It can be determined by clinical or radiographic examination. Severity depends on pocket depth, level of attachment,degree of bone loss, tooth mobility, and crown-root ratio. The determination of the level of clinical attachment reveals the approximate extent of root surface that is devoid of periodontal ligament.

Loe et al [13] conducted a study on the attachment loss in 480 male labourers at two tea plantations in Sri Lanka. Based on the inter-proximal loss of attachment and tooth mortality rates, three sub populations were identified: 1) individuals with rapid progression of periodontal disease (8%), 2) individuals with moderate progression (81%), 3) individuals who exhibited no progression of periodontal disease beyond gingivitis (11%). It was noted that at the age of 35 years, the mean loss of attachment in the rapid progression group was around 9mm, the moderate periodontitis group showed around 4mm attachment loss and no progression group had less than 1mm loss of attachment. Ten years later, the mean loss of attachment in the rapid progression group was 13mm, moderate group was around 7mm. the annual rate of destruction in the rapid progression group varied between 0.1-1mm, in the moderate progression group between 0.05-0.5mm and in the no progression group between 0.05-0.09mm. Since this population was caries free, essentially all missing teeth were lost due to periodontal disease. In moderate progression group, the tooth mortality started after 30 years of age and increased throughout the decade. At 45 years of age the mean loss of teeth in this group was 7 teeth. The no progression group did not show any tooth loss.

(iii) Patient Compliance / Cooperation

The most important determinant of treatment outcomes in clinical practice is patient compliance. Regardless of the type of initial periodontal therapy rendered, patients with poor oral hygiene who fail to comply with recommended recall schedules are more likely to have less favorable results. The prognosis for patients with gingival and periodontal disease is critically dependent on the patient's attitude; desire to retain the natural teeth, and willingness to maintain good oral hygiene [14]. Patients should be clearly informed of the important role they must play for treatment to succeed.

Dental literature covers two principal areas: compliance with oral hygiene regimens and utilization of dental care by the public. The reasons for non-compliance are highly variable but include lack of pertinent information, fear, economics and the patient's perception of lack of compassion on the part of the dental therapist. In general, it has been found that patients comply better when they are positively reinforced and when barriers to treatment are reduced.[15]

Chace [16] retrospectively studied data from 166 fairly compliant patients who were seen for periodontal maintenance therapy every 3 months for 40 years. Only 12% of teeth initially classified as having a questionable prognosis were extracted during the follow-up period. The average survival rate for the teeth extracted was 8.8 years. These data suggest that when patients comply with recommended program of periodontal maintenance care, they have an excellent chance of retaining most of their teeth.

(iv) Plaque control

Bacterial plaque is the prime etiologic factor associated with periodontal disease. Therefore effective removal of plaque on a regular basis by the patient is critical to the success of periodontal therapy and to the prognosis. The patient who does not have the motivation, dexterity, and discipline to keep the plaque score at baseline levels will definitely have a poorer prognosis. Some patients have more viscous saliva than others, which provides for a more rapid plaque accumulation. Others accumulate plaque slowly and in scanty amounts,hence, they have a better prognosis. Persons with high caries rates may exhibit a relatively poor prognosis.

3) Systemic / Environmental Factors

(i) Smoking

Smoking is related to periodontal disease in a dose related manner and appears to exert its most hazardous effects on areas in direct contact with smoke, such as lingual aspect of maxillary teeth. This deleterious relationship between smoking and periodontal disease is seen in smokers regardless of their overall levels of plaque accumulation. However, the specific microbial flora in smokers may shift to a more pathogenic profile[17]. These findings suggest that tobacco smoking may itself promote the development of local environments that favor growth of such pathogenic species, in addition; substances in smoke such as cotinine may also promote the pathogenic activites of periodontal flora.

A series of epidemiological studies[18,19] was done to compare the periodontal destruction in current smokers, former smokers and non smokers. The results from these studies indicate: (i) level of periodontal destruction in former smoker's lies somewhere between the level of periodontal destruction of current smokers and nonsmokers. (ii) The progressive damage seen in smokers can be retarded or halted with smoking cessation. (iii) The clinical response to flap surgery is poorer in smokers when compared to non smokers; the clinical response of former smokers is similar to nonsmokers as long as the former smokers do not resume their smoking habit. These types of studies demonstrate that smoking cessation can markedly improve the prognosis and outcomes of periodontal treatment [20].Therefore the prognosis in patients who smoke and have slight-to-moderate periodontitis is generally fair to poor. In patients with severe periodontitis, the prognosis may be poor to hopeless.

However, it should be emphasized that smoking cessation can affect the treatment outcome and therefore the prognosis. Patient's with slight to moderate periodontitis who stop smoking can often be upgraded to a good prognosis, whereas those with severe periodontitis who stop smoking may be upgraded to a fair prognosis.

(ii) Systemic background

Although the relationship of general health status and systemic disorders to periodontal disease has been studied extensively, there is no conclusive evidence that they are primary etiologic factors in periodontal disease. It is more accurate to consider systemic diseases as contributing factors in the pathogenesis of periodontal disease. The patient's systemic background affects overall prognosis in several ways. In patients with known systemic disorders that could affect the periodontium (for example, nutritional deficiency, hyperthyroidism, and hyperparathyroidism) prognosis improves with the correction of systemic problem.

Diabetes: Of all the systemic diseases that are relatively common, diabetes has emerged in recent years as the one with the strongest potential influence on periodontal diseases. In well-controlled diabetics, clinical responses to both surgical and nonsurgical periodontal therapy produced similar results to those observed in non-diabetics [21]. In general, poorly controlled diabetes appears to be associated with an increased risk of loss of attachment by gingival inflammation ranging from marginal gingivitis to periodontitis. With control of the diabetes, this group of symptoms may be expected to decrease in severity and occasionally subside [22]. The controlled diabetic exhibits a more favorable prognosis.

Immunodeficiency states: HIV-infected patients may also present with common forms of periodontal disease such as chronic periodontitis. Because of their severely compromised immune system, AIDS patient generally have poor prognosis. An Epidemiologic survey have shown a higher prevalence of bone loss and attachment loss in HIV-infected patients accompanied by a greater degree of gingival recession and shallower probing depths compared to control populations[23]. However, the effects of HIV infection on the long-term prognosis of the dentition in chronic periodontitis remain unresolved. On the one hand, a more rapid progression of bone loss and attachment loss in a HIV-infected periodontal patient may imply a poorer prognosis for the dentition when compared to the HIV-negative patient. With the advent of highly active retroviral drugs and proteinase inhibitor, long term prognosis turns out to be good.

The prognosis is guarded, when surgical periodontal treatment is required but cannot be provided because of patient's health incapacitating conditions that limit patient's performance of oral hygiene procedures (Parkinson's disease) also adversely affects the prognosis. Newer automated oral hygiene devices such as electric tooth brushes may be helpful for these patients and improve the prognosis.

(iii) Assessment of the past bone response

The past response of the alveolar bone to local factors is a useful guide for predicting the bone response to treatment and the likelihood of arresting the bone destructive process. This entails consideration of severity and distribution of the periodontal bone loss in terms of the following: the patient's age; the distribution, severity, and duration of local irritants such as plaque, calculus, food impaction, occlusal abnormalities and habits[24].

If the amount of bone loss can be accounted for by the local factors, conventionall treatment can be expected to arrest the bone destruction; then the overall prognosis for the dentition is good.

If the bone loss is more severe than one would ordinarily expect at the patient's age in the presence of local factors of comparable severity and duration, factors other than those in the oral cavity are contributing to the bone destruction. The overall prognosis is then poor, because of the difficulty generally encountered in determining the responsible systemic factors. The prognosis is not necessarily hopeless without systemic therapy, provided the disease is detected early and sufficient bone remains to support the teeth. In such cases, local treatment often can retain the dentition in useful function for many years by eliminating local destructive factors and limiting the bone destruction to that caused by the systemic conditions.

(iv) Genetic Factors

An important problem related to research in the hereditary of periodontitis is that, whatever the etiology of the disease, the symptoms are same, such as deepening of pocket, loss of attachment, bone loss. In most of cases, the development of periodontitis at an individual level depends probably on the collective presence of a number of environmental risk factors in conjunction with number of susceptibility factors at a given time during life. Literature search suggests genetic polymorphisms in certain genes involved in immune response(eg. IL-1, IL-10, Fc-gamma receptors) may be associated with susceptibility to severe periodontitis in some populations.

Familial aggregation studies support the idea that both aggressive and chronic periodontitis tends to cluster within families and single/major locus autosomal dominant gene is involved in the disease [25]. This supports the use of family background of periodontitis as a risk factor for the development of future periodontal disease. Tumor necrosis factor-α polymorphisms, HLA antigens, and FcγR genotypes have been evaluated for their association with chronic periodontitis. But results have been equivocal [4]. The genetic susceptibility test for severe chronic periodontitis that is commercially available is the Periodontal Susceptibility Test (PST). This test evaluates the simultaneous occurrence of allele 2 at the IL-1A +4845 and IL-1B +3954 loci.A patient with allele 2 at both of these loci is considered "genotype- positive" and therefore more susceptible to developing chronic periodontitis [26].

The rationale for this association is that persons with this combination of alleles tend to produce more 1L-1 in response to bacterial challenge and therefore will be predisposed to have more inflammation and tissue-damage. The influence of genetic factors on prognosis is not simple. Although microbial and environmental factors can be altered through conventional periodontal therapy and patient education, genetic factors currently cannot be altered. However, detection of genetic variation that are linked with periodontal disease can potentially influence the prognosis in several ways. First, early detection of patients at risk due to genetic factors can lead to early implementation of preventive and treatment measures. Second, identification of genetic risk factors later in the disease and / or during the course of treatment can influence treatment recommendations, such as the use of adjunctive antibiotic therapy or increased frequency of maintenance visits. Finally, identification of young individuals who have not been evaluated for periodontitis, but who are recognized as being at risk can lead to the development of early intervention strategies. In each of these cases, early diagnosis, intervention and / or alterations in the treatment regimen may lead to an improved prognosis for the patient.

   (v) Stress

   Physical and emotional stress as well as substance abuse may alter the patient's ability to respond to the periodontal therapy performed. Stress, distress and coping behavior are regarded as important risk indicators for periodontal disease[27].

   A deleterious effect of stress and psychosocial factors on health was extensively elucidated by Selye (1946) [28]. He established the term "General Adaptation Syndrome", describing the sum of all non-specific, systemic reactions of the body that ensue upon long, continued exposure to stress. The type of tissue response to irritation and infection influences prognosis.

   High stress / low coping patients have more susceptibility to periodontal breakdown as elevated systemic levels of cortisol can suppress several host response mechanisms such as T-helper cell function, antibody production and neutrophil function. Reducing psychological depression and improving coping strategies for stressful life events may improve periodontal prognosis and treatment outcomes [29]. There are also studies which do not agree to the above results [30].

   4) Economic considerations

   Periodontal disease is more severe in individuals of lower socio-economic status and poorer education. However, when periodontal status is adjusted for oral hygiene and smoking, the associations between low socio-economic and educational status and severe periodontal disease are not seen. Thus socio economic and educational status does not appear to directly affect disease progression.

   Gamonal JA, Lopez NJ, Aranda W [31] conducted a survey involving 1150 Chileans aged 35-44 and 65-74 years. Prevalence of chronic inflammatory periodontal disease was 90% in subjects aged 35 – 44 years and 100% in subjects aged 65-74 years. A total prevalence for both age cohorts were 92%. A significant association between socio-economic status and periodontal health was found. Prevalence was 56% in subjects of high status, 98% in subjects of low-socio economic status. An association between educational level and periodontal health was apparent. The only subjects who were periodontally healthy were in the group with university education. There was also a significant association between educational level and loss of teeth. Thus their study shows that periodontal health is better in the educated and also people belonging to higher socio-economic status.

5)   Oral habits and compulsions

Habit is an important factor in the initiation and progression of periodontal disease. Habits of significance in the etiology of periodontal disease include:

1)   Neuroses
2)   Occupational habits
3)   Miscellaneous

Recognition and elimination of a habits detrimental to periodontal health (like tongue thrusting, mouth-breathing, bruxism) are of utmost importance in the treatment of the periodontal manifestation. Unless the dentist understands the damage that can or does occur due to a deleterious habit and the need for eliminating it, he will find himself hindered in periodontal therapy. Therefore, the prognosis depends on the degree of destruction caused by the habits on the periodontium. If the underlying etiology is corrected, then the prognosis will be favorable[32].

Chewing habits: betel quid and tobacco chewing may result in increase in prevalence of chronic gingivitis, acute necrotizing ulcerative gingivitis as well as periodontitis. Increased accumulation of plaque and calculus formation has been observed in smokers. Gingivitis toxica, characterized by the destruction of gingival and the underlying bone, has been attributed to the chewing of tobacco.The magnitude of the occlusal forces placed on teeth can vary from patient to patient and affect the prognosis. If the patient has a habit of clenching or grinding the teeth, the bone support for the teeth will have to be greater than for a person who does not have these parafunctional habits. If the occlusal forces are excessive, the prognosis is often limited [32].

6)   Malocclusion

Irregularly aligned teeth, malformations of the jaws and abnormal occlusal relationships may be important factors in the etiology of periodontal disease, as they may interfere with plaque control or produce occlusal interferences. A frequently encountered situation is, when tooth migrates or tips mesially, that surface of the teeth can become inaccessible for self performed oral hygiene. This can lead to clinical attachment loss and bone loss at the mesial tooth sites, which might pose some risk for development of periodontal inflammation that could lead to loss of support.

The overall prognosis is poor, for occlusal discrepancies that cannot be corrected. The distribution of teeth is also important. Having teeth on both sides of a mouth is more favourable than having all the teeth on one side of the mouth. It is usually favourable to have all the remaining teeth either in the posterior part of the mouth or in both the anterior and posterior parts of the mouth. If all the remaining teeth are in the anterior part of the mouth, prognosis is usually less favourable.

7)   Prosthetic / Restorative Factors

The overall prognosis requires a general consideration of bone levels (evaluated radiographically) and attachment levels (determined clinically) to establish whether enough teeth can be saved either to provide a functional and aesthetic dentition or to serve as abutments for a useful prosthetic replacement of the missing teeth. When a tooth is lost, the structural integrity of the dental arch is disrupted, and there is subsequent realignment of teeth as a new state of equilibrium is achieved. Teeth adjacent to or opposing the edentulous space frequently moves into it. At this point, the overall prognosis and the prognosis for individual teeth overlap because the prognosis for key individual teeth may affect the overall prognosis for prosthetic rehabilitation. When few teeth remain, the prosthodontic needs become more important, and sometimes periodontally treatable teeth may have to be extracted if they are not compatible with the design of the prosthesis. [4]

Selection of the Type of Prosthesis

Missing teeth may be replaced by one of three prosthesis types, a removable partial denture, a tooth supported fixed partial denture, or an implant supported fixed partial denture. Several factors must be weighed when choosing the type of prosthesis to be used in any given situation.

Abutment Evaluation

Teeth that serve as abutments are subjected to increased functional demands. This is of particular significance when designing and fabricating a fixed partial denture, since the forces that would normally be absorbed by the missing tooth are transmitted, through the pontic, connectors, and retainers to the abutment teeth. More rigid standards are required when evaluating the prognosis of teeth adjacent to edentulous areas [33]. A tooth that has undergone endodontic treatment that has a post is more likely to fracture when serving as a distal abutment supporting a distal removable partial denture. However, the tooth should have some sound, surviving coronal tooth structure to ensure longevity. Even then some compensation must be made for the coronal tooth structure that has been lost.

This is accomplished through the use of dowel core or pin-retained amalgam or composite resin core. Teeth that have been pulp capped should not be used as fixed partial denture abutments unless they are endodontically treated. There is a risk that they will require endodontic treatment later, with the resultant destruction of retentive tooth structure and of the retainer itself.

The supporting tissues surrounding the abutment teeth must be healthy and free from inflammation before any prosthesis can be contemplated. Normally, abutment teeth should not exhibit mobility, since they will be carrying an extra load. The roots and their supporting tissues should be evaluated for three factors:

(i) Crown-root ratio

The ratio is a measure of the length occlusal to the alveolar crest of the bone compared with the length of root embedded in the bone. As the level of the alveolar bone moves apically, the lever arm of the portion of bone increases and the chances for harmful lateral forces is increased. The optimum crown-root ratio for a tooth to be utilized as a fixed partial denture abutment is 2:3. A ratio of 1:1 is the minimum ratio that is acceptable for a prospective abutment under normal circumstances [33].

(ii) Root configuration

This is an important point in the assessment of an abutment's suitability from a periodontal standpoint. Roots that are broader labiolingually than they are mesiodistally are preferable to roots that are round in cross-section. Multirooted posterior teeth with widely separated roots will offer better periodontal support than roots that converge, fuse, or generally present a conical configuration. The tooth with conical roots can be used as an abutment for a short span fixed partial denture if all other factors are optimal. A single rooted tooth with evidence of irregular configuration or with some curvature in the apical third of the root is preferable to the tooth that has nearly perfect taper [33].

(iii) Periodontal ligament area

Larger teeth have a greater surface area and are better able to bear added stresses. When supporting bone has been lost because of periodontal disease, the involved teeth have a lessened capacity to serve as abutments [33] The length of the pontic span can be successfully restored, in part, by the abutment teeth and their ability to accept the additional load. In a statement designated as "Ante's law" by Johnson et al [34] the root surface area of the abutment teeth had to equal or surpass that of the teeth being replaced by pontics. As a clinical guideline, there is some validity in this concept .Fixed partial dentures with short pontic spans have a better prognosis than do those with excessively long spans. It would be an oversimplification to attribute this merely to the overstressing of the periodontal ligament. Failures from abnormal stresses have been attributed to leverage and torque rather than overload.

FACTORS INFLUENCING PROGNOSIS OF INDIVIDUAL TEETH

Individual Tooth Prognosis

The prognosis for individual teeth is determined after the overall prognosis and is often affected by it. [35] In periodontal procedures, the main goal is the preservation of the entire dentition as a functioning unit. This means that individual components are not as vital as the overall function of the entire unit. The loss of single tooth or several teeth does not destroy the dentition, if the teeth can be restored to function and esthetics. For example, in a patient with a poor overall prognosis the dentist likely would not attempt to retain a tooth that has a questionable prognosis because of local conditions. Many of the factors listed under local factors and prosthetic / restorative factors have a direct effect on the prognosis for individual teeth in addition to any overall systemic or environmental factors that may be present [11].

1) Bone topography

The single most important factor in the prognosis of an individual tooth affected by periodontal disease is the topography of the bone surrounding it. Other factors that are considered are morphology of the bony deformity, surgical accessibility for correction of the defect, anatomy of the root/s, and the functional demands to which the tooth is subjected. If the tooth is supported adequately with bone and the osseous defect can be corrected by surgical intervention, then the pocket can be eliminated,resulting in a favourable prognosis [1]. All pockets are not amenable to surgical correction; the regional anatomy frequently makes pocket elimination impossible and the long term prognosis unfavourable.

2) Percentage of bone loss

Greater the bone loss, poorer the prognosis. The depth of a pocket is relatively equivalent to the amount of bone loss seen in radiographs. Gingival (pseudo) pockets do not generally have accompanying bone destruction, and hence can be treated and restored to health, for the prognosis to be graded fair to good. When greater bone loss has occurred on one surface of a tooth, the bone height on the less involved surfaces should be taken into consideration. Because of the greater height of bone in relation to other surfaces, the center of rotation of the tooth will be nearer the crown, resulting in a more favourable distribution of forces to the periodontium and less tooth mobility. If the bone loss occurs as a result of acute infectious disease like a periodontal abscess, prognosis is generally favorable as the resultant angular defects are more amenable to regenerative procedures. A similar bony deformity caused by a chronic process induces horizontal bone loss making prognosis less favourable. Progressive bone resorption may also lower the prognosis but the deciding factor should be the etiology of the progressive bone loss and the probability of its correction [3].

Janson L et al [36] in his 10 year follow up study found the annual marginal bone loss to be approximately 0.09 mm. Prognosis was graded favourable as the bone level remained in relatively stationary position after initial bone loss.

3) Probing depth and pocket formation

Evaluation of pocket probing depth has been the most critical marker for determining prognosis. It remains the most reliable indicator of past periodontal destruction [37]. Longitudinal clinical observations of probing depths that increase over time are associated with future loss of attachment. The pocket depth, level of attachment, and type of pocket are most important for determination of prognosis. These are determined by probing and radiographic evaluation. Prognosis is adversely affected, if the base of the pocket (level of attachment) is close to the root apex. The injurious bacterial products may reach the pulp through the apical foramina. Root canal therapy is necessary in such cases to obtain optimal results from periodontal treatment. When the periodontal pocket extends to involve the apex, the prognosis is generally poor. The presence of apical disease as a result of endodontic involvement also worsens the prognosis. However, good apical and lateral bone repair can sometimes be obtained by combining endodontic and periodontal procedures.

The location of the pocket is important. Some deep infrabony pockets on the proximal surfaces respond by fill and reattachment, others do not: a deep infrabony proximal pocket that does not respond will result in reverse architecture and will have a poor prognosis. Shallow defects can be treated by either fill or elimination. Pockets made deeper by inflammatory hyperplasia (pseudopockets) have a good prognosis[1].

4) Presence and severity of furcation

The anatomical location of the molar, makes the tooth vulnerable to periodontal destruction and eventual loss. The concavities and convexities of the furcal aspects of molar roots and of the maxillary first bicuspid are potential sites for plaque retention[1].

The presence of furcation involvement does not indicate hopeless prognosis. However, when the lesion reaches the furcation, it causes two additional problems; it causes difficulty of access to the areas both for scaling, root planing and performing surgery. The second is the inaccessibility of the area to plaque removal by the patient. If both these problems can be solved, then prognosis is similar to or even better than that of single rooted teeth with similar degree of bone loss.

Prognosis for teeth with furcation invasions depends on: [1]

1) Extent of bone destruction horizontally and vertically in the interradicular space.
2) Number of roots and their morphology.
3) Morphology of the inter-radicular space
    a) Width
    b) Depth
4) Condition of the periodontal attachment as determined by clinical mobility tests and percussion.
5) Access for surgical correction of the deformity.
6) Patient's access for oral hygiene after therapy.

Mandibular molars: These molars with furca involvement usually have a more favorable prognosis than maxillary molars with furca because of better access for oral hygiene. Mandibular first molars with bone loss in the furca have a favourable prognosis if the roots are reasonably long and interrradicular space is wide. Root caries is often a greater threat to the longevity of mandibular first molars with furcation invasion than periodontal disease.

Mandibular second molars: These teeth with furcation invasions usually have a less favorable prognosis than first molars since their roots are shorter and the interradicular space is constricted. The proximity of the ascending ramus of the mandible on the distal aspect and the position of the external oblique ridge and muscle attachments on the buccal aspect of the second molar often makes it impossible, even with modern techniques, to obtain an adequate zone of attached gingival for a favorable long term prognosis. These anatomic restrictions often make it impossible to create a gingival papilla in the furca because a selective recession cannot be secured that will place the gingival margin apical to the furca. In this event, the pocket will be eliminated and the long range prognosis is poor.

Maxillary bicuspids: Maxillary first bicuspids often have two roots-buccal and palatal. Joseph I et al [38] examined the furcation anatomy of 100 of these teeth. In 62% of the bifurcated teeth, a furcal concavity was seen on the palatal aspect of the buccal root. The mean furcation width was 0.71mm; less than the diameter of a curette. Concavities were found on the proximal surfaces of all teeth with deeper concavity on the mesial than the distal aspect. Maxillary bicuspids may also display a V-shaped groove on the proximal surfaces. These often persist towards the apical region and are associated with greater loss of attachment than that found around non-grooved teeth.

Maxillary molars: Maxillary first molar with furcation invasion usually have a favourable prognosis if the septal bone is still present in the interfurca. The position of the furcation entrance, particularly in maxillary molars is important [39]. Furcation involvement on the mesial aspect or buccal aspect has a favourable prognosis since they are accessible for surgical reconstruction that makes oral hygiene possible. Furca invasion on distal aspect of these teeth are generally hopeless because of inaccessibility. Prognosis of the maxillary second molar with a furca invasion is less favourable than for a similar invasion of the first molar because of the second molar's smaller root structure, restricted inter-radicular space, and more distal position in the arch.

As seen from the classic observations of Hirschfeld and Wasserman, the teeth with minimal(class I) or no furcation invasions generally have good prognosis. The greater the amount of attachment loss in the furcation, the worse the long term prognosis.The teeth with complete loss of bone in the coronal aspect of the furcation(class III) generally have a poor prognosis[40].

5) Mobility and clinical crown-to-clinical root ratio

Tooth mobility and clinical crown-to-clinical root ratio, influence prognosis and are important factors in determining the number of teeth that must be used as abutments if missing teeth are to be replaced [41].

The prognosis for reducing tooth mobility through periodontal therapy is related to the etiology of mobility. Increased tooth movement may be related to inflammation in the gingival and / or periodontal ligament, the presence of occlusal trauma, loss of periodontal support or a combination of any of these factors.

If extreme mobility is detectable but pocket depth is not, it can be presumed that the loosening is due to trauma from occlusion or from oral habits and compulsions. This can be determined by the clinical examination and dental history. It can be presumed that such looseness will be co-related with widening of periodontal ligament space around the teeth as seen in radiographs. If these findings are confirmed, the prognosis can be considered as favourable and the mobility can be resolved by selective tooth grinding, use of night guards and/or fixed splinting [42]. However, if mobility is related to occlusal trauma and / or loss of attachment, occlusal adjustment and/or splinting may be indicated as part of the therapy and the long-range results are less predictable.

The root form and length should be compared with the degree of mobility and the amount of bone loss, pocket depth. Teeth with bulky, long rooted teeth with extreme mobility in which only the apical third of the bone is present will have a better chance of survival following periodontal therapy and splinting, thus favouring prognosis. Teeth with spindly roots and advanced mobility in which only the apical third of the bone remains have very poor prognosis.

6) Root Anatomy

The amount of cemental surface available for periodontal ligament attachment varies with the length, shape, and circumference of each root. Root circumference is usually greatest at the cervix. As it tapers toward the apex, the circumference decreases and less surface area are available for attachment. Root contour must be considered as well as the clinical-crown-to-clinical-root ratio. Prognosis for a tooth with a rectangular-shaped root is more favorable than for a tooth of the same length with a cone-shaped root. Scaling and root planing of root surfaces are fundamental, if successful treatment is to be attained and anything that decreases the efficiency of this procedure, such as bizarre root morphology can decrease the prognosis.[14]

Good oral hygiene is also essential for maintaining the healthy state obtained after therapy. This too can be made difficult by various root morphologies. Determination of prognosis and proper treatment planning is based on recognition of these diverse root forms.

7) Local Factors

(i) Plaque / calculus

A unifying concept emerged in 1965, when the cause and effect relationship between plaque and gingival inflammation was demonstrated in a classic study by Loe et al [11]

The principal concept was that plaque was the primary and essential disease initiator from health to gingivitis and if the gingivitis were untreated it might progress to adult periodontitis.

Plaque retentive factors are important in the development and progression of chronic periodontitis because they retain plaque microorganisms in close proximity to the periodontal tissues, providing an ecologic niche for plaque growth and maturation. Calculus is considered the most important plaque retentive factor because of its ability to harbor plaque bacteria on its rough surface. As a result, calculus removal is essential for the maintenance of a healthy periodontium.

(ii) Subgingival Restoratons

Subgingival margins, in addition to influencing the progression of periodontitis, can have other effects on the attachment apparatus.

a) Effects of subgingival margins

The area between the depth of a healthy gingival sulcus and the alveolar crest is described as the biologic width. This constitutes the junctional epithelium and the supracrestal connective tissue.

Schatzle et al [43] in a 26 year prospective cohort study analysed the gingival indices and attachment level and compared between those who did and those who did not have restorative margins greater than 1 mm from the gingival margin. After 10 years, the cumulative mean loss of attachment was 0.5 mm more for the group with sub gingival margins, which was statistically significant.

b)   Overhanging margins

Overhanging margins of dental restorations contribute to the development of periodontal disease by changing the ecologic equilibrium of the gingival sulcus to an area that favours the growth of disease – associated organisms (predominantly gram negative anaerobic species) at the expense of health – associated organisms (gram positive facultative species) and by inhibiting the patients access to remove accumulated plaque. A highly significant statistical relationship has been reported between marginal defects and reduced bone height [44]. Removal of overhangs permits more effective plaque control, resulting in reduction of gingivitis and a small increase in radiographic alveolar bone support [45]. Overhangs can also impinge on the interproximal embrasure space, making cleansing with floss difficult and cause displacement of the gingiva. Violation of the biologic width by overhanging restorations is another possible mechanism by which they may damage the periodontium [46].

The sub gingival zone is composed of the margin of the restoration, the luting material, and prepared as well as the unprepared tooth surface. Sources of marginal roughness include (1) grooves and scratches in the surface of carefully polished acrylic resin, porcelain restoration (2) separation of the restoration margin and luting material from the cervical finish line, thereby exposing the rough surface of the prepared tooth. (3) dissolution and disintegration of the luting material between the preparation and the restoration, leaving a space (4) inadequate marginal fit of the restoration.

c)   Contour

The facial and lingual contours of restorations are also important in the preservation of gingival health. The most common error in recreating the contours of tooth in dental restorations is overcontouring of the facial and lingual surfaces. It generally occurs in the gingival third of the crown and results in an area in which oral hygiene procedures are unable to control plaque [47].   Consequently, leading to plaque accumulation and gingival inflammation. Apparently, undercontoured preparation is not nearly as damaging to the gingiva as over-contouring.In patients in whom periodontal disease causes the gingival margin to be in a more apical position than it was in health, the facial and lingual contours become even more significant. In these cases, the bulge on the facial contour of the crown, which normally would be subgingival appears supragingival. If the furcation has been exposed by periodontal surgical procedure or by gingival recession, it is important that the restoration be contoured in such a way as to facilitate access for oral hygiene. Occlusal surfaces should be designed to direct masticatory forces along the long axis of the teeth. The anatomy of the occlusal surface should provide well formed marginal ridges and occlusal sluiceways to prevent interproximal food impaction. [48]

d) Restorative materials

Surface textures of restorative materials differ in their capacity to retain plaque. All can be adequately cleaned if they are polished and accessible to oral hygiene measures. Damage to the periodontal tissue might occur during the preparation and fabrication of the restoration; the materials used might contain components that irritate tissue; and the physical or chemical properties of the restorations may cause retention of bacterial plaque in the long term, thus affecting prognosis[48].

e) The effect of surface finish of restorative materials on the periodontium

The surface of restorations should be as smooth as possible to limit plaque accumulation. Roughened tooth and restoration surfaces in the subgingival region result in increased plaque accumulation and increased gingival inflammation. There is evidence that the amount of plaque that accumulates in patients with relatively poor oral hygiene is not affected to a significant degree by minor changes in root surface configuration. All restorative materials placed in the gingival environment should have the highest possible polish to avoid plaque accumulation and to give a favourable prognosis[49].

(iii) Anatomic Factors

Anatomic factors that may predispose the periodontium to disease and therefore affect the prognosis include short, tapered roots with large crowns, cervical enamel projections (CEPs) and enamel pearls, intermediate bifurcation ridges, root concavities, and developmental grooves. The clinician must also consider root proximity and the location and anatomy of furcations when developing a prognosis[4].

a) Short tapered roots: Prognosis is poor for teeth with short, tapered roots and relatively large crowns. Because of the disproportionate crown-to-root ratio and the reduced root surface available for periodontal support, the periodontium may be more susceptible to injury by occlusal forces.

b) Cervical enamel projections (CEP), Enamel pearls: CEP's are flat, ectopic extensions of enamel that extend beyond the normal contours of the cementoenamel junction. They extend into the furcation of 28.6% of mandibular molars and 17% of maxillary molars[50]. They are most likely to be found on buccal surfaces of maxillary second molars. Enamel pearls are larger, round deposits of enamel that can be located in furcations or other areas on the root surface.These projections can affect plaque removal and should be removed to facilitate maintenance.

c) Furcation Ridge: The anatomy of the furcation is complex. The presence of bifurcational ridges, a concavity in the dome, and possible accessory canals complicates not only conventional and surgical therapy, but also periodontal maintenance.These ridges run from one root to the other, and in some maxillary molars continue apically. In mandibular molars there may be a central bifurcational ridge that forms distinct pits in the roof of the furcation.

Hou and Tsai [51] determined that these ridges are strongly associated with attachment loss in furcations. These reports emphasize the complexity of the furcation topography of molars that has to be taken into consideration when debriding teeth with furcal attachment loss.

d) Root Concavities / Proximities: Root concavities exposed through loss of attachment can vary from shallow flutings to deep depressions. They appear more marked on maxillary first premolars, the mesiobuccal root of the maxillary first molar, both roots of mandibular first molars, and the mandibular incisors. Any tooth, however, can have a proximal concavity. Although these concavities increase the attachment area and produce a root shape that may be more resistant to torquing forces, they also create areas that can be difficult for both the dentist and the patient to clean. Access to the furcation area is usually difficult to obtain. Maxillary first premolars offer the greatest difficulties, and therefore their prognosis is usually poor when the lesion reaches the mesial-distal furcation. Maxillary molars also offer some degree of difficulty because of their furcation width. Sometimes their prognosis can be improved by resecting one of the buccal roots, thereby improving access to the area. When mandibular first molars or buccal furcations of maxillary molars offer good access to the furcation area, their prognosis is usually fair [4].

e) Developmental Grooves: Other anatomic considerations that present accessibility problems are developmental grooves. Developmental grooves, which sometimes appear in the maxillary lateral incisors (palatogingival groove) or in the lower incisors, create an accessibility problem. They initiate on enamel and can extend a significant distance on the root surface, providing a plaque-retentive area that is difficult to instrument. These palatogingival grooves are found on 5.6% of maxillary lateral incisors and 3.4% of maxillary central incisors. Treatment consists of odontoplasty of the groove, placing bone substitutes, and surgical management of the soft tissue and underlying bone. Radicular grooves can result in self-sustaining infrabony pockets and therefore scaling and root planing will not suffice. Although the acute nature of the problem may be alleviated initially, the source of the chronic or acute inflammation must be eradicated by a surgical approach. Occasionally, the tooth needs to be extracted due to a poor prognosis.[4]

Leknes KN, Lie T, Selvig KA [52] did a retrospective study on 103 extracted teeth with grooves, to evaluate the effect of proximal root grooves as a risk factor in periodontal attachment loss. Following staining, the teeth were examined under light microscopy. On each tooth, loss of attachment was measured along the long axis of the root from the cemento-enamel junction to the most coronal level of the stained periodontal ligament remnants on mesial as well as on distal surfaces. For both groups, a statistically significant greater loss of attachment was present on grooved than on non-grooved surfaces. Generally, there was a direct relationship between groove location and maximum loss of attachment. The results indicate that proximal root grooves should be considered in periodontal diagnosis, prognosis, and treatment planning.

8) Caries, Nonvital Teeth, and Root Resorption

For teeth mutilated by extensive caries, the feasibility of adequate restoration and endodontic therapy should be considered before undertaking periodontal treatment. Extensive idiopathic root resorption or root resorption that has occurred as a result of orthodontic therapy, jeopardizes the stability of teeth and adversely affects the response to periodontal treatment. The periodontal prognosis of treated nonvital teeth is not different from that of vital teeth. Caries destroys tooth structure, creating open contacts, poor embrasure form and plunger cusps, all of which encourage food impaction, plaque formation and periodontal disease. In the presence of debris and decay, the adjacent gingival soft tissue can become more inflamed and caries can extend deep into periodontal pockets, especially around defective restorations that suffer from recurrent caries. The removal of dental caries and the restorations of sound tooth structure are necessary components of early treatment of a patient with periodontal disease. The re-establishment of marginal integrity with normal interproximal contacts and proper embrasure space will facilitate oral hygiene, prevent plaque accumulation, and create a local environment conducive to health. Restoration of dental caries should be as conservative as possible to maintain natural tooth structure and provide for gingival margins that are able to be kept plaque free by the patient, which will improve prognosis[4].

9) Pulpal involvement

The relationship that exists between the pulp of a tooth and the surrounding periodontium is undisputed. Healthy periodontal tissue provides nourishment and support for the roots. Unhealthy pulpal tissue or an infected pulpal space can contribute to loss of the periodontal attachment. Direct communication exists between the pulp and periodontal ligament by way of dentinal tubules, lateral and / or accessory canals and the apical foramina[2]. While pulp vitality may not often be affected by periodontal disease, evidence exists that periodontal disease can affect the health of the pulp. For example, in the presence of long-standing periodontal disease, the pulp may exhibit degenerative changes such as internal resorptions, calcifications and infarctions. Lesions affecting the periodontium may be the result of inadequate or incomplete root canal treatment, perforations, fractures, resorptions, or coronal leakage, in addition to an unhealthy or necrotic pulp. Treatment may involve nonsurgical treatment and/or surgical management. When the etiology is removed, the potential for healing exists. The greater the periodontal involvement, the poorer the prognosis. The healing potential should dictate the course of treatment [53].

10) Strategic value

Ultimately, one of the first decisions that must be made is the strategic value of a tooth. This will have a bearing on whether the tooth is retained or extracted. For example, a third molar in an arch with many missing teeth may need to be saved so that it can be used as an abutment for a partial denture.
This same decision process can be made for other strategic abutment teeth. A full denture is a poor substitute for natural teeth; however, an average patient is usually satisfied with a

maxillary complete denture after some period of adjustment. The same cannot be said for many mandibular complete dentures. A mandibular complete denture is much more difficult to adapt to and every effort should be made to maintain strategic abutment teeth as long as possible to provide retention for a partial denture. This is especially true if the patient is a poor candidate for a dental implant.

A few strategically placed teeth can serve as abutments for a fixed prosthesis and can have a favorable prognosis than an implant. Drifting of teeth often occurs following failure to replace missing teeth. It often creates conditions that lead to initial periodontal disease. The pattern of changes that may follow due to failure to replace missing first molar is characteristic[32]

(i)   The drifting of second and third molars often result in a decrease of the vertical dimension.
(ii) The premolars drift distally and the mandibular incisors tilt or drift lingually. The mandibular premolars while moving distally lose their intercuspating relationship with the maxillary teeth and may tilt distally.
(iii) Anterior overbite is increased, the mandibular incisors strike the maxillary incisors near the gingiva or traumatize the gingiva.
(iv) Diastemata are created by the separation of anterior teeth.

The disturbed proximal contact relationships lead to gingival inflammation, food impaction and pocket formation followed by tooth loss and mobility. Occlusal disharmonies created by altered tooth positions traumatize the supporting tissues of the periodontium and aggravate the destruction caused by inflammation [54]. Reduction in periodontal support leads to migration of teeth and occlusal problems.

(i)   Teeth adjacent to edentulous area

Teeth that serve as abutments are subjected to increased functional demands. More rigid standards are required in evaluating the prognosis of teeth adjacent to edentulous areas [1].

(ii) Relation to adjacent teeth

In dealing with a tooth with questionable prognosis, the chances of successful treatment should be weighed against the benefits that would accrue to the adjacent teeth, if the tooth under consideration were extracted. An attempt to retain hopelessly involved teeth jeopardizes the adjacent teeth. Extraction of the questionable tooth is followed by partial restoration of the bone support of the adjacent teeth [48].

(iii) Location of remaining bone in relation to the individual tooth surfaces

When greater bone loss has occurred on one surface of a tooth, the bone height on the less involved surfaces should be taken into consideration, when determining a prognosis. Because of greater height of bone in relation to other surfaces, the center of rotation of the tooth will be nearer the crown. This will result in a more favourable distribution of forces to the periodontium and less tooth mobility [48].

11) Therapist's knowledge and skill

Although precise and well directed treatment planning is important, skillful and efficient performance is just as important. Needless trauma to flaps, dehydration of the tissues and imprecise closure of the wound are all crucial contributions to the therapeutic failures. Such errors make the difference between success and failure of the therapy. Restorative skill is every bit as important as periodontal skills. Good therapy is ineffective in the face of poor restorative sequelae. [1]

12) Trauma from Occlusion

Occlusal trauma has been associated with periodontal disease for many years. Various animal studies[55,56] were conducted to demonstrate this relationship and controversial results were obtained. Some investigators did not support the concept that excessive occlusal forces were causative agent of periodontal destruction. Further, Glickman and co-workers summarized all their work and concluded that excessive occlusal forces were a co-destructive force in the presence of gingival inflammation and could lead to vertical osseous defects. Only a few studies have evaluated the effects of excessive occlusal forces on the periodontium. These studies have indicated that treating occlusal discrepancies may lead to better results following periodontal treatment[55].

The outlook for retaining teeth that are affected in periodontal occlusal trauma depends on the degree of control the dentist has over the etiological factors and the severity of the periodontal tissue loss.If the occlusal trauma is related to a restoration that was placed in supraocclusion, the prognosis is favorable because the dentist has control over the occlusal contours of restorations. Also, if the occlusal trauma is related to reduced periodontal support, splinting and replacement of missing teeth can often control the occlusal trauma for long periods.

13) Mucogingival deformities

Assessment of the mucogingival status of a patient is an essential part of an oral examination, particularly if there are major restorative or orthodontic work planned. Mucogingival status refers to the quality and quantity of keratinized gingival tissue, the amount of gingival recession, the presence of aberrant frena and the depth of the vestibule.

Gingival recession can be a problem for patients for esthetic reasons, dentinal hypersensitivity or interference with normal hygiene procedures. A number of factors have been implicated in the etiology of gingival recession. An extreme buccal or lingual positioning of the tooth in the dental arch, whether natural or due to orthodontic movement, can lead to thinning of the alveolar plate and associated gingival tissues. This makes the area more susceptible to recession, either from trauma or inflammation. Trauma is usually the result of vigorous tooth brushing. Plaque-induced disease can also cause recession, particularly in patients with a thin periodontium. [57]

The outlook for preventing further loss of tissue in areas of gingival recession depends primarily on maintaining the tissues free of inflammation along with the severity and etiology of the recession. In general, if the recession is not too extensive and the etiological factors can be identified and corrected,then the prognosis for preventing further recession is favourable.

The restoration of gingiva on root surfaces previously denuded by recession is possible and is indicated when gingival health cannot be established because of a mucogingival defect or for esthetic reasons. If an adequate zone of attached gingiva is present on an adjacent tooth, a pedicle flap can be positioned over the exposed root, and the outlook for covering, it is quite good. If a suitable donor site is not located on an adjacent tooth, a free autogenous soft-tissue graft must be used. While the coverage of denuded root surfaces with this method is possible, it is not as favourable as with the pedicle graft.

When a high frenum or muscle attachment is involved, a frenectomy or detachment of the muscle is done in conjunction with the procedures just mentioned.

Prognosis may improve when the following treatment is instituted

- Root demineralization with citric acid
- Orthodontic movement or recontouring of the tooth to place it within the alveolar housing.
- Replacement of overcontoured restorations, improper prosthetic appliances.

PROGNOSIS AND RADIOGRAPHS

The radiograph is a valuable aid in the diagnosis of periodontal disease, determination of patient prognosis, and the evaluation of the outcome of the treatment. However it is an adjunct to the clinical examination, not a substitute for it. [1]

Radiographic evaluation of bone changes in periodontal disease is based mainly on the appearance of the inter-dental septa because the relatively dense root structure obscures the facial and lingual bony plates. The width and the shape of the interdental septum and the angle of the crest normally vary according to the convexity of the proximal surfaces of the teeth at the level of the cemento-enamel junctions of the approximating teeth. The angulations of the crest of the interdental septum are generally parallel to a line between the cemento-enamel junctions of the approximating teeth. When there is a difference in the levels of the cemento-enamel junctions, the crest of the inter-dental bone appears angulated rather than horizontal.

- The alveolar bone, the alveolar process and the periodontal space on the mesial, distal, apical aspects of the root are recorded on the x-ray in a single plane.
- The clinical crown to root ratio is recorded
- Dense deposits of calculus and margins of metallic restoration may be observed on the proximal surfaces of the teeth.

Radiographic Appearance of Bone Destruction in Periodontal Disease

The radiograph does not reveal minor destructive changes in bone, therefore slight radiographic changes in the periodontal tissues mean that the disease has progressed beyond its earlier stages. Atleast 40% of bone reduction should be present to be seen in the radiograph. The radiographic image tends to show less severe bone loss than is actually present. The difference between the actual alveolar crest height and the height as it appears on the radiograph ranges from 0 to 1.6mm, most of which can be accounted for x-ray angulations. It is an indirect method for determining the amount, distribution and pattern of bone loss. [1]

PROGNOSIS OF IMPLANTS

The replacement of missing teeth in partially or fully edentulous patients has conventionally involved fixed or removable and partial or full prostheses supported by natural teeth, soft tissues or both. Prosthetic reconstructions were often limited by the number or distribution of abutment teeth, the morphology of the alveolar ridges, the periodontal health or the remaining hard tissue structures of the abutment teeth. The possibility of adding abutments by the insertion of oral implants has been a treatment goal desired by practitioners. However, until the early 1980s, dental implants lacked sufficient long-term evaluation [58]

Among the earlier implant designs, only the mandibular transosteal staples demonstrate sufficient long-term efficacy. Although subperiosteal and blade implants improved the functional and aesthetic comfort of patients, the overall long-term assessment of such implants did not fulfill the requirements for long-term success. Long-term success rates from several studies of blade implants healing by fibro-osseous integration range from 42% to 83% over 5 years. Although improvements with biomaterials and designs have been claimed, the installation of such implants is still accompanied by a high number of long-term complications.The type of dental implants widely used today as a result of their high predictability is endosseous root form implants healing with direct bone-to-implant contact (osseointegration). This high level of predictability could finally be achieved by applying new basic knowledge of biomaterials and the study of the reactions by the adjacent tissues to the design of a new generation of implants. Additionally, important surgical and restorative concepts necessary for implant survival were recognized.

Based on the predictability in fully edentulous jaws, implants have more and more been used in partially edentulous patients to another single crowns or fixed partial dentures. Data in the literature indicate that the implant survival rates may be expected to be as high as in the treatment of fully edentulous ridges. However, not all of these studies have been designed in a prospective format, as described. A prospective trial with non-submerged implants including a 5-year life-table analysis demonstrates that implants do not have to be submerged under the mucosa to achieve osseointegration and survival rates comparable to submerged implants.

- For implants with a relatively smooth surface, lower success rates have to be expected in bone of lesser quality (density) and quantity.

- For this type of implant, shorter fixtures (<8 mm) have had higher failure rates in fully edentulous arches than longer implants (> 7mm). This difference was, however, not found when implants were used to support fixed partial dentures.
- Implants with a rough or porous surface do not show that difference between mandibular and maxillary survival rates.

A controversy exists regarding the use of hydroxyapatite coating. Despite the lack of adequate long-term clinical data in the literature, coated implants are very popular in clinical practice. The enthusiasm about hydroxyapatite-coated implants is the results of their osteoinductive capacity, leading to a higher number of bone-to-implant contacts, which may influence implant survival in spongy bone positively. However, a number of long-term problems have been reported with hydroxyapatite-coated implants[58]. The long-term prognosis of acid-etched implant strongly depends on the degree of tissue integration during the first year following implantation[59, 60].

CASE SELECTION FOR IMPLANT SURGERY

1) Primary judgement (prosthetic level)

When patients are referred seeking implant treatment, initial oral prophylaxis and any specific oral problems must first be identified by the clinician, after which different treatment alternatives can be presented. If patient has any oral problems and if healing is delayed, this can lead unfavourable prognosis [61].

2) Secondary assessment (surgical level)

In this stage, the medical condition of the patient as well as the local health and bone morphology of the future implant sites is analyzed. The medical state of the patient should be taken into consideration prior to any surgical treatment. So far, no specific condition has been identified which would exclusively prevent implant surgery. Factors like gender, age do not seem to have much influence on the outcome. Still, it should be remembered that elderly patients are more susceptible to infections and/or slow healing, and therefore may constitute potential risks for problems pre-operatively and post-operatively. Patients with history of any disease should be thoroughly examined prior to posting for implant surgery, thus favouring prognosis.

Intraoral health and bone morphology: It is also important to examine the intaoral health status of the soft and hard tissues as well as of the bone morphology in future implant areas. This is mainly done using both clinical and radiographic parameters. Any defects should thereby be identified and treated prior to implant procedure. Furthermore, the clinical examination should include a judgement of interarch and interdental spaces to see if that there is accessibility for the instruments as well as for the future prosthetic construction. It is also important to study the jaw relation, as that will have influence on the implant direction [61].

3)   Treatment planning (combined surgical-prosthetic level)

Based on clinical and radiographic data collected, a final treatment planning is carried out by the clinician. As the placement of the implants is an important part of the strategy, the clinician should take part in detailed planning regarding implant location, that is participate in team approach. In order to create acceptable function and esthetics, the best position and direction of the implants must be identified together with the number and type of implants that can be inserted.

Implant placement: The main purpose of the implant surgery is to establish the anchorage for the future fixed prosthetic construction. In order to create a favorable and lasting result, it is first of all important to understand that the jawbone is living tissue that cannot be violated during surgery. Other factors are which should be considered during placement are flap design, bone drilling, implant position, implant direction, abutment selection and implant selection [62]. All these factors can influence the long term prognosis.

ASSIGNING PROGNOSIS

According to McGuire and Nunn [63] following the initial phase of periodontal therapy and prior to placing the patient on maintenance recall, each tooth is assigned a prognosis. [refer Table IV]. Excellent, good and hopeless are the only prognoses that can be established with a reasonable degree of accuracy. Fair, poor and even questionable prognoses depend on a large number of factors that can interact in an unpredictable number of ways. In many of these cases, it is advisable to establish a provisional prognosis until phase I therapy is completed and evaluated [4].

Table IV. Assigning prognosis according to Mcguire and Nunn[63].

Excellent prognosis: No bone loss, excellent gingival condition, good patient cooperation, no systematic environmental factors.
Good prognosis (one or more of the following): Control of the etiologic factors and adequate periodontal support as measured clinically and radiographically to assure the tooth would be relatively easy to maintain by the patient and clinician, assuming proper maintenance.
Fair prognosis (one or more of the following): Approximately 25% attachment loss as measured clinically and radiographically and / or class I furcation involvement. The location and depth of the furcation would allow proper maintenance with good patient compliance.
Poor prognosis (one or more of the following): 50% attachment loss with class II furcations. The location and depth of the furcations would allow proper maintenance, but with difficulty.
Questionable prognosis (one or more of the following): Greater than 50% attachment loss resulting in poor crown-to-root ratio. Poor root form Class II furcations not easily accessible to maintenance care or class III furcations. 2 + mobility or greater. Significant root proximity.
Hopeless prognosis: Inadequate attachment to maintain the tooth. Extraction performed and suggested.

Recently, Kwok and Caton [64] designed a periodontal prognostication system based on the probability of disease progression. The individual tooth prognosis relies on the prediction of future stability of the periodontal supporting tissues. Basically comprises of four classifications [refer Table V].The classification system comprises primarily of favorable, questionable, unfavorable and hopeless prognosis.

Table V. A Periodontal Prognostication System by Kwok and Caton [64].

Favorable Prognosis: local and/or systemic factors can be controlled and the periodontal status of the tooth can be obtained with comprehensive periodontal therapy and maintenance.
Questionable Prognosis: Local and/or systemic factors may or may not be controlled. However, periodontal stability is achieved through comprehensive periodontal therapy and maintenance, provided, these factors are controlled. Otherwise, future breakdown may occur.
Unfavorable Prognosis: Local and/or systemic factors cannot be controlled. Periodontal breakdown is likely to occur even with comprehensive periodontal therapy and maintenance.
Hopeless Prognosis: Extraction is the only therapy

Prognosis of Dentition

All branches of dentistry strive at the ultimate goal, that is preservation of teeth/tooth. In periodontal procedures, the prime consideration is the functioning unit. This means that the individual components are not as vital as overall function of the entire organ. In most cases, one should consider removing the tooth with poor prognosis, especially in patients with systemic conditions that compromise the overall prognosis. Teeth with good periodontal prognosis should be maintained, provided the patient is capable of maintaining oral hygiene and follows the recall appointments [65].

CONCLUSION

Prognostication is a skill not easily acquired and is highly dependent upon the experience and skill of the clinician. The ability to predict the response of the dentition to periodontal therapy is essential in developing a definitive periodontal maintenance and restorative treatment plan. It is generally agreed that a tooth with a hopeless prognosis is one that despite the patients and clinicians best efforts is not going to improve. In such situations, it is difficult to arrest the disease process and restore periodontal health.

In this review, the potential adverse influences of a variety of factors (local and systemic) on prognosis have been discussed. While each of these factors alone may have a detrimental effect on prognosis and treatment outcomes, it should be kept in mind that the presence of any of these factors alone or in combination does not imply poorer outcomes.

In order to reduce the likelihood of developing the disease and improving prognosis, patients are encouraged to control as many of these factors which include smoking cessation, stress reduction, microbiological testing etc. With recent advances in microbiological and radiographical diagnostic methods, the clinician can utilize these aids to monitor the recurrence of on going periodontal disease and predict the outcome. Also considerable amount of work has to be done on possible genetic disposition of certain individuals to periodontal diseases.

All in all, prognosis is dependent on the experience of the operator, his ability to examine and interpret findings, his judgement concerning the healing capacity of the patient and his technical ability all combined with the patients co-operation.

REFERENCES

[1]   Prichard J. *Prognosis.* In: Advanced Periodontal Disease, 2nd edition, W. B. Saunders, 1972: 165.

[2]   Genco R, Goldman H, Cohen W. *Anti-infective and adjunctive management of periodontal diseases.* Contemporary Periodontics, Part II. C.V Mosby co. Philadelphia 1990:356

[3]   Grant, Stern, Listgarten. *Prognosis* In: Periodontics, in the tradition of Gottlieb and Orban, 6th edition, C.V. Mosby Co, 1979: 541-573.

[4]   Newman M, Takei H, Carranza F. *Determination of Prognosis.* In: Goodman S and Novak K. Clinical Periodontology, 9th edition, Saunders Co. 2003; 33: 475.

[5]   Newman M, Takei H, Carranza F. Determination of Prognosis. In: Goodman S and Novak K. Clinical Periodontology, 9th edition, Saunders Co. 2003: 79.

[6]   Goldman H, Cohen W. Prognosis. Periodontal Therapy, 6th edition, C.V. Mosby Co., 1973; 403-411.

[7]   Machtei EE, Dunford R, Hausmann E et al. Longitudinal study of prognostic factors in established periodontitis patients. J Clin Periodontol 1997; 24: 102-109.

[8]   Lindhe J, Karring T, Lang N. Aggressive Periodontitis. In: Tonetti M and Mombelli A. Clinical Periodontology and Implant dentistry,4th edition, Blackwell Publishing Co. 2003: 217.

[9]   Miller AJ et al. Oral health of United States Adult: National Findings. NIDR, Bethesda Md., 1987.

[10] Schei O, Waerhaug J et al. Alveolar bone loss as related to oral hygiene and age. J Periodontol 1959;30:7-16

[11] Loe H, Theilade E, Jensen SB. Experimental gingivitis in man. J. Periodontol 1965; 36:177.

[12] Schwartz Z, Somers A, Mellonig JT, Carnes DL Jr. Ability of commercial demineralized freeze-dried bone allograft to induce new bone formation is dependent on donor age but not gender. J Periodontol 1998; 69:470-478.

[13] Loe H, Anerud A, Boysen H, Morrison E. Natural history of periodontal disease in man. Rapid, moderate and no loss of attachment in Sri Lankan laborers 14 to 46 years of age. J Clin Periodontol 1986; 13:431-440.

[14] Prichard J. The diagnosis and treatment of periodontal disease, W B Saunders Co. 1979: 130.

[15] Mendonza AR, Newcomb GM, Nixon KC. Compliance with supportive periodontal therapy. J Periodontol 1991; 62:731-736.

[16] Chace R, Low S. Survival characteristics of periodontally involved teeth. A 40 years study. J Periodontol 1993; 64: 701-705.

[17] Haffajee AD, Socransky S, Goodson JM. Clinical parameters as predictors of destructive periodontal disease activity. J Clin Periodontol 1983; 10: 257-265.

[18] Bostrom L, Linder LE, Bergstrom J. Influence of smoking on the outcome of periodontal surgery, a 5 year follow-up. J Clin Peridontol 1998; 25:194-200.

[19] Kaldahl WB, Kalkwarf KL, Patil KD, Molvar MP, Dyer JK. A review of longitudinal studies that compared periodontal therapies. J Periodontol 1993; 64:243-253.

[20] Van der Weijden GA, de Slegte C, Timmerman MF, van der Velden U. Periodontitis in smokers and non-smokers: intra oral distribution of pockets. J Clin Periodontol 2001; 28: 955-960.

[21] Grossi SG. Treatment of periodontal disease and control of diabetes: an assessment of the evidence and need for future research. Ann Periodontol 2001; 6: 138-145.

[22] Soskolne WA, Klinger A. The relationship between periodontal diseases and diabetes: an overview. Ann Periodontol 2001; 6: 91-98.

[23] Barr C, Lopez MR, Rua-Dobles A. Periodontal changes by HIV serostatus in a cohort of homosexual and bisexual men. J Clin Periodontol 1992; 19: 794-801.

[24] Glickman I. The "bone factor" concept of periodontal disease. Clinical periodontology, prevention, diagnosis and treatment of periodontal disease in practice of general dentistry, 4th edn, W.B. Saunders Co. Philadelphia 1973: 332.

[25] Vander velden, Abbas F, De Graaff J,Timmerman MF,Winkelhoff AJ. The effect of sibling relationship on the periodontal condition. J Clin Periodontol 1993;20:683-690.

[26] Kornman KS, Crane A, Wang HY, Newman MJ, Wilson TG Jr. The interleukin-1 genotype as a severity factor in periodontal disease. J Clin Periodontol 1997;24:72-77.

[27] Genco RJ, Ho A, Grossi SG, Dunford RG, Tedescco LA. Models to evaluate the role stress in periodontal disease Ann Periodontol 1998; 3:288-302

[28] Selye H. The general adaptation syndrome and the disease of adaptation .J Clin Periodontol 1946;6:117.Cited in Periodontal abstracts 2000;3:48.

[29] Elter JR, White BA, Gaynes BN. Relationship of clinical depression to periodontal treatment outcome. J Periodontol 2002; 73: 441-449.

[30] Solis AC, Lotufo RF, Pannuti CM, Brunheiro EC, Marques AH. Association of periodontal disease to anxiety and depression symptoms and pschysocial stress factors. J Clin Periodontol 2004; 31:633-638.

[31] Gamonal JA, Lopez NJ, Aranda W. Periodontal conditions and treatment needs, by CPITN in the 34-44 and 65-74 years old population in Santiago, Chile. J Int Dent 1998; 48:96-103.

[32] Glickman I. Food impaction, habits and other local factors. Clinical periodontology, prevention, diagnosis and treatment of periodontal disease in practice of general dentistry, 4th edn, W.B. Saunders Co. Philadelphia 1973: 355.

[33] Nallaswamy D, Ramalingam K, Bhatt V. Text book of Prosthodontics. First edition. Jaypee Brothers medical Publishers Ltd. 2003;13:219-237.

[34] Johnson JF, Philips RW, Dykema RW. Modern practice in crown and bridge prosthodontics, 3 edition, Philadelphia, WB Saunders co, 1971.

[35] McGuire MK. Prognosis versus actual outcome :a long term survey of 100 treated periodontal patients under maintenance care. J Periodontol 1991; 62:51

[36] Janson L, Lavstedt S, Zimmerman M. Prediction of marginal boneloss and toothloss-a prospective study over 20 years. J Clin Periodontol 2002; 29: 672-678.

[37]   Listgarten MA. Periodontal probing, what does it mean? J Clin Periodontol 1980; 7: 165.

[38]   Joseph I, Varma BRR, Bhat KM. Clinical significance of furcation anatomy of the maxillary first bicuspid: a biometric study on extracted teeth. J Periodontol 1996; 67: 386-389.

[39]   Svardstrom G, Wennstrom JL. Furcation topography of mandibular and maxillary first molar. J Clin Periodontol 1988; 15: 271-275.

[40]   Hirschfeld I, Wasserman B. A long term survey of tooth loss in 600 treated periodontal patients.J Periodontol 1978;49:225-237

[41]   Prichard J. The diagnosis and treatment of periodontal disease. W B Saunders Co. 1979: 130.

[42]   Beube F. Correlation of degree of alveolar bone loss with other factors for determining the removal or retention of teeth. Dent Clin North Am 1969; 13: 801-806.

[43]   Schatzle M, Lang NP, Anerud A, Boysen H, Burgin W, Loe H. The influence of margins of restorations of the periodontal tissues over 26 years. J Clin Periodontol 2001; 28(1): 57-64.

[44]   Hakkarainen K, Ainamo J. Influence of overhanging posterior tooth restorations on alveolar bone height in adults. J Clin Periodontol 1980; 7: 114.

[45]   Jeffcoat M, Howell T. Alveolar bone destruction due to overhanging amalgam in periodontal disease. J Periodontol 1980; 51:599.

[46]   De Waal H, Castellucci G. The importance of restorative margin placement to the biologic width and periodontal health. Part I. Int J Periodontics Restorative Dent 1993; 13: 461-471.

[47]   Blieden TM. Tooth related issues. Ann Periodontol 1999; 4: 91-95.

[48]   Carranza F, Newman M. Determination of prognosis. In: Fermin Carranza. Clinical Periodontology, 8th edition, Saunders Co. 1996; 31:338.

[49]   Highfield J, Rowell R. Effects of removal of posterior overhanging metallic margins of restorations upon the periodontal tissues. J Clin Periodontol 1978; 5: 169.

[50]   Grewe JM, Meskin LH, Miller T. Cervical enamel projections: prevalence, location and extent with associated periodontal implications. J. Periodontal 1965; 36: 460-465.

[51]   Hou GL, Tsai CC. Cervical enamel projection and intermediate bifurcational ridge correlated with molar furcation involvements. J Periodontol 1997; 68: 687-693.

[52]   Leknes KN, Lie T, Selvig KA. Root grooves: a risk factor in periodontal attachment loss. J Periodontol 1994; 65:859-863.

[53]   Kenneth S, Kornman K, Paul B. Fundamental principles affecting the outcomes of therapy for osseous lesions. Periodontology 2000 2000; 22: 22 – 41.

[54]   Muhlemann HR, Herzog H, Rateitschak KH. Quantitative evaluation of the therapeutic effect of selective grinding. J Periodontol 1957; 28:11. Cited in Hoag P. Occlusal Treatment. Proceedings of the World Workshop in Clinical Periodontics, 1989; 1.

[55]   Philstrom BL, Ramfjord SP. Periodontal effect of non-function in monkeys. J Periodontol 1971; 42:748-756.

[56]   Burgett FG, Ramfjord SP, Nissle RR, Morrison EC, Charbeneau TD, Caffesse RG. Randomized trial of occlusal adjustment in the treatment of periodontitis patient. J Clin Periodontol 1992;19:381-387.

[57]   Paterson JR. The etiology of gingival recession. Review of Literature.Cited in Ann Periodontol 1999;4:91-96.

[58]   Joseph P, Hans P. Clinical trials on the prognosis of dental implants. Periodontology 2000 1994; 4: 498 – 108.

[59]   Khang W, Feldman S, Hawley C and Gunsolley J. A multicentrer study comparing dual acid etched and machine-surface implants in various bone qualities. J Periodontol 2001;72:1384-1390.

[60]   Adell R, Lekholm U, Rockler B et al. Marginal tissue reactions at osseointegrated titanium fixatures(1):A 3 year longitudinal prospective study.Int J Oral Maxillofac Implants 1986;1:39-52.

[61]   Sennerby L, Rasmusson L. Osseointegration surgery; Host determinants and outcome criteria. In : Zarb G, Lekholm U, Albrekesson T, Tenenbaum H, eds Aging, Osteoporosis and Dental Implants. Quitessence, 2001:55-66. Cited in: Lindhe J, Karring T, Lang N. Clinical Periodontology and Implant dentistry, 4th edition, the surgical site. ULF Lekholm: 853.

[62]   Branemark PI, Zarb GA, Albrektsson T. Tissue integrated prostheses. Osseointegration in clinical dentistry.Quintessence 1985.Cited in: Lindhe J, Karring T, Lang N. Clinical Periodontology and Implant Dentistry,4th edition, the surgical site. ULF Lekholm:853

[63]   McGuire M, Nunn M. Prognosis versus Actual Outcome III. The effectiveness of clinical parameters in accurately predicting tooth survival. J Periodontol 1996; 67:666-674.

[64]   Kwok V, Caton J. Prognosis revisited: A system for assigning periodontal prognosis. J Periodontol 2007;78:2063-2071.

[65]   Schonfeld S. The art and science of periodontal prognosis. Cda journal 2008;36:175-179.

In: Periodontitis Symptoms, Treatment and Prevention   ISBN: 978-1-61668-836-3
Editor: Rosemarie E. Walchuck, pp. 141-166   ©2010 Nova Science Publishers, Inc.

Chapter 5

BIOLUMINESCENT *LUX* GENE BIOSENSORS IN ORAL STREPTOCOCCI: DETERMINATION OF COMPLEMENTARY ANTIMICROBIAL ACTIVITY OF MINOCYCLINE HYDROCHLORIDE WITH THE ANESTHETIC LIDOCAINE/PRILOCAINE OR THE ANTISEPTIC CHLORHEXIDINE

Viet Ton That[1]*, Sarah Nguyen[1]*, David Poon[2]*,
W. Shawn Monahan[5], Rebecca Sauerwein[2], Dan C. Lafferty[2],
Lindsey Marie Teasdale[2], Amanda L. Rice[5],
Winthrop Carter[1], Tom Maier[2,3], and Curtis A. Machida[2,4]+

Departments of Periodontology[1], Integrative Biosciences[2], Oral Pathology
and Radiology[3], and Pediatric Dentistry[4] and Academic DMD Program[5], Oregon Health
& Science University School of Dentistry, 611 SW Campus Drive,
Portland, Oregon 97239, USA
*Equal contributors to this work

ABSTRACT

Background: Plaque-induced periodontitis is gingival inflammation at sites undergoing loss of connective tissue, apical migration of junctional epithelium and loss of alveolar bone. Non-surgical treatment of plaque-induced periodontitis typically involves removal of biofilm conducted through mechanical scaling and root planing (SRP) procedures. The antibiotic minocycline hydrochloride, delivered as a sustained-release product[1] used for professional subgingival administration into periodontal pockets, has been shown to be beneficial as an adjunct to conventional SRP. Use of chlorhexidine rinse is also a typical adjunct therapy to SRP procedures for chemical

+Corresponding Author: Curt Machida, PhD, Department of Integrative Biosciences, OHSU School of Dentistry, 611 SW Campus Drive, Portland, OR 97239, 503-494-0034, FAX: 503-494-8554, machidac@ohsu.edu
[1]Brand name for minocycline hydrochloride used as a sustained release product is Arestin

control of supragingival plaque. Lidocaine (2.5%) and prilocaine (2.5%)[2] provides localized anesthesia for SRP. The objective of this study is to develop and use bioluminescent recombinants of oral streptococci in determining the potential antibacterial activity of minocycline hydrochloride used either alone or in combination with the anesthetic lidocaine/prilocaine, or with the antiseptic chlorhexidine.

Methods: Recombinant plasmids containing the bioluminescence-generating *lux* gene from *Photorhabdus luminescens* were transformed into the oral bacterium *Streptococcus mutans*, strains UA159 and ATCC 25175. Transformants were verified as *S. mutans* derivatives by selection and growth on mitis salivarius agar supplemented with bacitracin, in addition to an antibody test directed specifically against *S. mutans* cell wall proteins and polymerase chain reaction experiments targeting sequences in the *S. mutans* glucosyltransferase (*gtf*) gene. *S. mutans* transformants were then subjected to growth analysis for comparison of absorbance and bioluminescence activity. Minocycline hydrochloride and lidocaine/prilocaine, or minocycline hydrochloride and chlorhexidine, were used in combination to determine the potential interactive effects of these agents on the antibacterial activity of minocycline hydrochloride.

Results: Using two distinct *S. mutans* transformants representing both strains UA159 and ATCC 25175, we observed rapid and pronounced bacteriostatic activity when using high doses of minocycline hydrochloride (≥ 1 µg/ml), which were statistically distinct from untreated cultures (p=0.000058) when measured at the peak of metabolic activity. Reduced bacteriostatic activity was seen using lower doses. When lidocaine/prilocaine at doses >100 µg/ml is used in conjunction with minocycline hydrochloride, we observed an additive antibacterial effect. The *S. mutans* transformant strain UA159, when treated with chlorhexidine (0.01%) in conjunction with either high (1 µg/ml) or low (0.1 µg/ml) doses of minocycline hydrochloride, displayed reduced levels of cell mass accumulation, as measured by absorbance, that were additive when both antimicrobial agents were deployed. Bioluminescence determinations, which are a direct measure of metabolic activity and an indirect measure of cell number when cells are in logarithmic stage of growth, displayed similar reductions when cultures were treated with minocycline hydrochloride and chlorhexidine used singularly or in combination.

Conclusions: The *S. mutans* lux transformants serve as sensitive biosensors in the determination of antimicrobial activity, and can rapidly monitor inhibition of bacterial metabolism. We conclude that the anesthetic lidocaine/prilocaine does not interfere with the potent bacteriostatic activity of minocycline hydrochloride, and actually has an additive antibacterial effect. The potent bacteriostatic activity of minocycline hydrochloride can also be complemented with the addition of chlorhexidine. The application of the *lux* biosensor system in the assessment of minocycline hydrochloride and lidocaine/prilocaine, or minocycline hydrochloride and chlorhexidine, represents its first use in examining antimicrobial drug interactions in periodontology.

Keywords: *lux* biosensors, Minocycline hydrochloride-Lidocaine/prilocaine interactions, *Streptococcus mutans*, minocycline hydrochloride, lidocaine/prilocaine, chlorhexidine

INTRODUCTION

Plaque-induced periodontitis is gingival inflammation at sites where there has been loss of connective tissue, apical migration of junctional epithelium and loss of alveolar bone [1]. The subgingival plaque linked with chronic periodontitis is usually associated with Gram-

---

[2] Brand name for the lidocaine (2.5%) and prilocaine (2.5%) anesthetic is Oraqix.

negative anaerobes that coexist with hundreds of other species of bacteria in a highly organized biofilm [2,3]. Biofilms are natural communal aggregations of microbes that form on a wide range of surfaces, including teeth [4]. Plaque is a highly organized biofilm [5] that possesses several features that help to protect and increase the nutritional advantages for bacteria [6] and provide competitive advantages over free-floating bacteria. Bacteria in biofilms produce a matrix, or glycocalyx, that encloses and shelters the microbial community from harmful effects of the surrounding environment. These bacterial matrixes form slimy, insoluble coatings that promote retention of bacteria, and inhibit removal by surrounding fluids, such as saliva and crevicular fluid [6]. In active periodontitis, biofilm removal and resultant healing of periodontal tissues can often only be achieved by clinical means, such as scaling and root planing (SRP) procedures [7,8].

SRP becomes substantially more difficult as pocket depths increase [9], with periodontal pockets > 4 mm retaining up to 66% of the plaque and calculus on root surfaces following non-surgical therapy [10-12]. Despite an improvement in periodontal status, periodontal pathogens remain subgingivally within the residual biofilm, in the remaining calculus, and within the exposed dentin tubules [7,8,13,14,15]. With the probability of pocket re-infection under these circumstances being high, additional means to decrease microbial load should be considered with non-surgical therapy [8].

USE OF MINOCYCLINE HYDROCHLORIDE ANTIBIOTIC AS ADJUNCT THERAPY FOR SRP

Minocycline hydrochloride (Arestin, OraPharma, Inc., Warminster, PA) is a sustained-release product for professional subgingival administration into periodontal pockets, and has been shown to be beneficial as an adjunct to conventional SRP in the treatment of periodontal disease [16-19]. Each unit-dose cartridge delivers product equivalent to 1 mg of minocycline free-base that is transported via microspheres. The minocycline free-base is slowly hydrolyzed and liberated over a 2-3 week period upon contact with moisture, with concentrations > 300 micrograms per ml being released into the gingival crevicular fluid [16]. Minocycline hydrochloride is a member of the tetracycline class of antibiotics and has a broad spectrum of activity. It is bacteriostatic and exerts its antimicrobial activity by inhibiting protein synthesis. *In vitro* susceptibility testing has shown that many putative periodontal pathogens, such as *Porphyromonas gingivalis*, *Prevotella intermedia*, and *Aggregatibacter actinomycetemcomitans*, are susceptible to minocycline hydrochloride at concentrations ≤ 8 micrograms per ml [20].

The typical indication for use of minocycline hydrochloride is in a pocket of >5 mm with bleeding on probing. Minocycline hydrochloride has been demonstrated to more effectively decrease the red complex periodontal pathogens as compared to SRP alone, and also act to block collagenases, which are involved in host tissue breakdown [21]. Increased benefits have been shown in patients that have advanced periodontal disease and in smokers [22,23]. Likely explanations for these observations are that there are more susceptible pathogens in these sites since SRP is not as effective in the deeper periodontal pockets, and that smokers may exhibit higher proportions of periodontal pathogens. Additionally, minocycline hydrochloride retains anti-metalloproteinase properties that may counteract the increased protease activity exhibited in smokers [24].

In addition to the beneficial effects of minocycline hydrochloride with SRP [21,25-27], recent studies have suggested that this antibiotic may also be used as an adjunct for surgical therapy [28] and for treatment of peri-implantitis [29-31].

USE OF CHLORHEXIDINE ANTISEPSIS AS AN ADJUNCT THERAPY FOR SRP

Chlorhexidine diglucanate (0.12%) has been used in the treatment of periodontitis for over 40 years and has well-documented success as an anti-plaque and anti-gingivitis mouthrinse [32,33]. Chlorhexidine is a cationic bisbiguanide that has a broad-spectrum antimicrobial effect due to its ability to bind to the negative charge of the cell walls of Gram-positive and Gram-negative bacteria, causing rupture of the membrane through alteration of the osmotic equilibrium [34,35]. This antiseptic agent has demonstrated effectiveness due to its ability to absorb onto cationic substrates, such as pellicle and salivary glycoproteins, and subsequent release over an 8-12 hour period [34,36]. Combined, these properties have demonstrated chlorhexidine to be highly effective for the treatment and prevention of gingivitis [37,38]. However, in the case of periodontal disease, chlorhexidine has decreased effectiveness due to difficulty in delivery of the drug to the depth of deep pockets [39] as well as difficulty in penetrating structured biofilm. Thus chlorhexidine has been shown to be more effective in conjunction with mechanical removal of the biofilm [40]. The clinician has several choices for mode of delivery, as chlorhexidine can be used as a mouth rinse, a supra- or subgingival irrigant, or as a locally delivered antimicrobial in the form of a bioabsorbable chip.

As a mouth rinse, typical dosing with chlorhexidine is to rinse with one-half fluid ounce for 30 seconds after brushing and flossing, with no eating or drinking for the following 30 minutes. Because chlorhexidine is poorly absorbed in the gastrointestinal tract, it has a high margin of safety [34]. Additionally, antibiotic resistance to chlorhexidine has not been demonstrated as with systemic antibiotics [41]. Although chlorhexidine rinse provides many benefits, it also has several reversible side effects. Chlorhexidine use may cause extrinsic staining of teeth, restorations, and tongue, as well as an altered or decreased taste perception [42,43]. Patients may also exhibit increased calculus formation [44-46]. In rare instances, gingival desquamation and painful mucosa have been also reported [33,42].

Due to its side effects, chlorhexidine should not be considered for long-term use in every periodontal patient. Indications for use may include treatment of gingivitis or peri-implantitis [47], or post-surgically to prevent infection [48,49] or to enhance healing [50]. Chlorhexidine can also be used to prevent infections in patients who are immunocompromised, as in the case of cancer or transplantation [49]. Some clinicians use local chlorhexidine application as part of a daily oral hygiene regimen for implants. It has even been advocated for improved fixed prosthetic restoration impressions [51].

In 1998, a locally delivered, sustained-released chlorhexidine chip was developed for use as an adjunct therapy for SRP. The advantages to the use of the chlorhexidine chip include its reliable effect on subgingival sites, continued release, and lack of visible staining of teeth [26]. The PerioChip (Perio Products Ltd.) is supplied in the form of a bioabsorbable 5 x 4 x 0.35 mm hydrolyzed gelatin chip which contains 2.5 mg of chlorhexidine gluconate. In the process of dissolving over the 7-10 days following placement, chlorhexidine is released at an average drug concentration >125 micrograms per ml in the gingival crevicular fluid [52], which is higher than the minimal inhibitory concentration (MIC) for more than 99% of the subgingival microorganisms from periodontal pockets [53].

USE OF LIDOCAINE/PRILOCAINE PERIODONTAL GEL AS ANESTHETIC DURING SRP

Lidocaine/prilocaine, a composite of 2.5% lidocaine and 2.5% prilocaine (Oraqix, DENTSPLY Pharmaceutical, York, PA), is applied directly to the periodontal pocket to provide effective, non-invasive localized anesthesia during SRP procedures [54,55]. The anesthetic mixture contains poloxamers that allows reversible temperature-dependent gelation. Therefore, lidocaine/prilocaine exists as a low-viscosity fluid at room temperature and as an elastic gel in the periodontal pocket. Once gelation occurs in the periodontal pocket, the anesthetics, lidocaine and prilocaine, are released to provide sufficient anesthesia for SRP.

Potential Interactions between Minocycline Hydrochloride and Lidocaine/ Prilocaine and Between Minocycline Hydrochloride and Chlorhexidine

Because both minocycline hydrochloride and lidocaine/prilocaine may be applied subgingivally in the same periodontal pocket, with the anesthetic applied prior to SRP and the antibiotic applied following SRP, an interaction seems plausible. The purpose of this study is to test the efficacy of minocycline hydrochloride, when used in conjunction with the anesthetic lidocaine/prilocaine periodontal gel. We will also test the interactions of minocycline hydrochloride and chlorhexidine, which is commonly used for treatment of periodontal patients. To begin developing an understanding of these interactions, we transformed oral mutans streptococci with the luminescence (*lux*) gene from *Photorhabdus luminescens* for use as biosensors for antibiotic or drug sensitivity tests. Streptococci were selected as biosensors since they are among the most common colonizers in plaque biofilm, which will reform following SRP. These bacterial species will influence the ultimate biofilm composition, including the numbers and types of periodontopathogens present [56]. Mutans streptococci have also been found in the subgingival plaque of patients with periodontitis, and may be important in the development of root caries [57]. The *lux* biosensors will allow rapid and uniform determination of *in vitro* drug sensitivity experiments, either singular or in combination with test agents, and provide measurements of inhibition. Thus, these biosensors will assess potential effects of the lidocaine/prilocaine anesthetic, or chlorhexidine antiseptic, on the bactericidal activity of the minocycline hydrochloride antibiotic.

MATERIALS AND METHODS

Lux Recombinant and Oral Streptococci Strains

The *lux* recombinant contains the *lux* operon (*A-E*) from *Photorhabdus luminescens* modified for expression in *Streptococcus pneumoniae* [58,59]. The recombinant *lux A-E* operon reconstitutes an aldehyde-recycling pathway [60], and allows for continual build-up of substrate (long chain aliphatic aldehyde) to drive the generation of measureable light. The *lux* recombinant also contains an *Escherichia coli* origin of replication and erythromycin-resistance gene, used for recombinant plasmid generation in *E. coli* and selection of transformants, respectively. *Streptococcus mutans* strains UA159 (also known as ATCC 700610), ATCC 25175 and ATCC 35668, in addition to *Streptococcus sobrinus* (ATCC 33478) and *Streptococcus salivarius* (ATCC 25975), were obtained from the American Type Culture Collection (ATCC; Manassas, VA).

Transformation of Oral Bacteria with *Lux* Recombinants and Validation of *Streptococcus Mutans* Strains

Cultures of oral streptococci were prepared by inoculating 10 ml of THYE broth (Todd Hewitt broth supplemented with 0.3% yeast extract) and incubating overnight at 37°C with 5% CO_2. Cultures were then diluted 1:20 in pre-warmed THYE broth and incubated until reaching an A_{600} of 0.1. *Lux* recombinant plasmid DNA (200 ng) was added to 0.5 ml of cells, and incubated for an additional 2.5 hours. Transformation mixes were then plated on THYE agar plates, containing either 250 µg/ml or 500 µg/ml of erythromycin, for selection of transformants. Mutans streptococci transformed with the *lux* recombinant include *Streptococcus mutans* UA159 and *Streptococcus mutans* ATCC 25175. These transformants were validated as being *S. mutans* derivatives with the subsequent growth and selection on mitis salivarius agar (MSA) supplemented with bacitracin (10 U /ml) and affirmed positive reaction on the Saliva-Check Mutans antibody test (GC America; Alsip, IL), which uses monoclonal antibodies against *S. mutans* cell wall components.

Polymerase Chain Reaction (PCR) and Acidification Reactions

Additional validation of the transformants as *S. mutans* derivatives was obtained with PCR using specific primers directed against *S. mutans* or *S. sobrinus* gene targets. We developed primers recognizing sequences from the glucosyltransferase genes in *S. mutans* UA159 (Genbank accession numbers AE014133 [complete genome] and NC 004350 [*gtfB* gene], position of *gtfB* gene in *S. mutans* genome [951112 – 955542]) and in *S. sobrinus* (Genbank accession number D63570, *gtfI* gene [position 1 – 6368]). Specific primer sets include: 1) mutans *gtfB* forward primer 793 (position in *gtfB* gene; 85 -> 106) and mutans *gtfB* reverse primer 1309 (position in *gtfB* gene; 601 -> 580) and 2) sobrinus *gtfI* forward primer 871 (position in *gtfI* gene; 1723 -> 1744) and sobrinus *gtfI* reverse primer 1582 (position in *gtfI* gene; 2434 -> 2413). PCR was conducted with an initial denaturation step at 94°C for 5 minutes followed by 30 cycles of denaturation at 94°C for 30 seconds, annealing at 57°C for 30 seconds, and extension at 72°C for 30 seconds, with final extension at 72°C for 5 minutes followed by 4°C soak. GoTaq Green Master Mix (Promega, Madison, WI) was used in all amplifications.

Acidification reactions (D-ribose, L-arabinose, D-mannitol, D-sorbitol, D-lactose, D-trehalose, inulin, D-raffinose, amidon, and glycogen; derived from API-20 Strep kit, Biomurieux SA) using the two transformants were compared against *S. mutans* strains

UA159, ATCC 25175 and ATCC 35668, and *S. salivarius*. Acidification reactions discriminating *S. mutans* strains include the use of D-mannitol, D-sorbitol and D-raffinose. Validated transformants were grown in TYYE broth supplemented with erythromycin and tested for bioluminescent activity.

Minocycline Hydrochloride and Lidocaine/Prilocaine and other Chemicals

Minocycline hydrochloride (microspheres, 1 mg/cartridge) was obtained from OraPharma, Inc. (Langhome, PA). Lidocaine/prilocaine was obtained from Dentsply Pharmaceutical (York, PA). Chlorhexidine gluconate oral rinse (0.12%) was obtained from Patterson Dental (St. Paul, MN). Mitis salivarius agar, Todd Hewitt broth, and yeast extract were obtained from Becton, Dickinson and Company (Sparks, MD). Bacitracin (0.6 U/mg) was obtained from Acros Organics USA (Morris Plains, NJ) or from Sigma Chemical (St. Louis, MO).

Treatment of Transformants with Minocycline Hydrochloride, Lidocaine/ Prilocaine, or Chlorhexidine

Lux transformants UA 159 or ATCC 25175, or corresponding non-transformed *S. mutans* strains, were treated with minocycline hydrochloride (0 – 100 µg/ml) for up to 6 hours, and assayed every 30 minutes for bioluminescence using luminometry and for cell mass accumulation by measuring absorbance at 600 nm. Parallel cultures were also treated with minocycline hydrochloride and concurrent application using lidocaine/prilocaine (0 – 200 µg/ml), and also assayed every 30 minutes for bioluminescence and cell mass accumulation. In independent experiments, *lux* transformant UA 159 was treated with minocycline hydrochloride (0.1 µg/ml or 1.0 µg/ml) in the presence of absence of chlorhexidine (0.01%) for up to 5.5 hours, and assayed every 30 minutes for bioluminescence and cell mass accumulation.

Luminometry and Absorbance Assays and Culture Medium

Bioluminescence was measured as relative light units (RLUs) with the Turner Biosystems Veritas Luminometer. Absorbance at 600 nm wavelength was measured using a Novaspec II visible spectrophotometer. Streptococci were plated on mitis salivarius agar (MSA, Difco™; Becton, Dickinson and Company, Sparks, MD), which utilizes high saccharose and vital dyes (ie: crystal violet and bromophenol blue) as selective agents. MSA was supplemented with potassium tellurite (Difco™; Becton, Dickinson and Company, Sparks, MD); 1 ml of 1% aqueous potassium tellurite was added to 1 liter of MSA. To validate the sub-group of mutans streptococci, MSA including potassium tellurite, was supplemented with bacitracin (10 Units/ml).

Statistical Analysis

All bioluminescence determinations were conducted in quadruplicate. Descriptive statistics, including mean values and standard error of the mean for each data point, were conducted. Standard error bars, even those nearly indistinguishable from corresponding mean values, are displayed in graphs. In selected cases where multiple enumerations were conducted, as in the chlorhexidine experiments, we conducted pair-wise comparison using one-way between-subjects Analysis of Variance (ANOVA) modified for multiple comparisons with the use of the Bonferroni correction.

RESULTS

Validation of Streptococcus Mutans *Lux* Transformants

The two transformants used in these studies have been validated as *S. mutans* derivatives, consistent with the specific identification of *S. mutans* strains UA159 and ATCC 25175. This is based on selection and growth on mitis salivarius agar supplemented with bacitracin, in addition to an antibody test directed specifically against *S. mutans* cell wall proteins (Saliva Check Mutans test) and PCR experiments targeting sequences in the *S. mutans gtf* gene. Using the Saliva Check Mutans kit, positive immunoreactivity lines were formed using *S. mutans* strains UA159 and ATCC 25175, in addition to the two transformants, but not with *S. sobrinus* or *S. salivarius*. In addition, PCR using *S. mutans*-specific primers amplified the correct size fragment from the two transformants, and from stock cultures of *S. mutans* UA159 and ATCC 25175, but not from *S. sobrinus* or *S. salivarius* (unpublished observations). We conclude that both transformants are confirmed as *S. mutans* strains.

In addition, acidification reactions were conducted using a panel of metabolic substrates in the API 20 Strep kit (Table 1). Each ampule was inoculated with aliquots of *S. mutans* ATCC 25175 (two independent sources), UA159 or ATCC 35668, or the two transformants, or *S. sobrinus* or *S. salivarius*. All inocula were calibrated to the equivalent of 4 McFarland Units, as recommended by the manufacturer. As can be observed (Table 1), and as previously described [61-63], *S. mutans* and *S. sobrinus* can be distinguished by differential raffinose acidification (*S. mutans*: raffinose positive acidification; *S. sobrinus*: raffinose negative acidification). *S. mutans* strains UA159 and ATCC 25175 can be distinguished by differential sorbitol acidification (ATCC 25175: sorbitol positive acidification; UA159: sorbitol negative acidification). The combination of negative inulin acidification and positive raffinose acidification distinguish *S. salivarius* from *S. mutans* (either strain) or *S. sobrinus*. We therefore conclude that the two *S. mutans* transformants are consistent with the identification of derivatives of UA159 and ATCC 25175.

Table 1.

Bacterium	Sugars Metabolism									
	RIB	ARA	MAN	SOR	LAC	TRE	INU	RAF	AMD	GLYG
S. mutans, ATCC 25175, source A	-	-	+	+	+	+	+	+	-	-
S. mutans, ATCC 25175, source B	-	-	+	+	+	+	+	+	-	-
S. mutans, UA159	-	-	+	-	+	+	+	+	-	-
S. mutans, ATCC 35668	-	-	+	+	+	+	+	+	-	-
Lux Transformant A	-	-	+	-	+	+	+	+	-	-
Lux Transformant B	-	-	+	+	+	+	+	+	-	-
S. sobrinus	-	-	+	+	+	+	-	-	-	-
S. salivarius	-	-	+	-	+	+	-	+	-	-

The metabolic substrates include D-ribose, L-arabinose, D-mannitol, D-sorbitol, D-lactose, D-trehalose, inulin, D-raffinose, amidon, and glycogen. Manufacturer states that yellow color reactions are positive for acidification using varied substrates, and that orange/red colors are negative for acidification. *Lux* transformants A and B have been subsequently confirmed as derivatives of the UA159 and ATCC 25175 strains, respectively.

Growth Curve Analysis of UA159 Transformant Demonstrates Increase in Bioluminescence Activity, Reflective of Cell Mass Accumulation during Log Phase

Cultures of the UA159 transformant were inoculated for overnight incubation, and then re-initiated the following morning at reduced concentration in fresh medium to allow regenerated growth. Aliquots from the regenerated culture were measured for both absorbance (A=600 nm) and for bioluminescence (Figure 1, Panels A and B, respectively). We observe that bioluminescence increases as cell mass accumulates during logarithmic phase of growth, and as the culture enters stationary phase, bioluminescence drops, reflective of the decrease in the metabolic activity of the culture (Figure 1, Panel B). Similar results were also obtained using the ATCC 25175 transformant (unpublished observations).

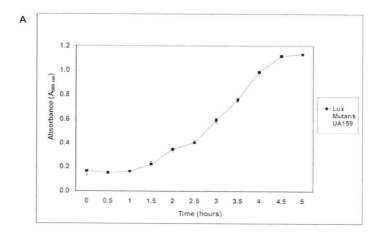

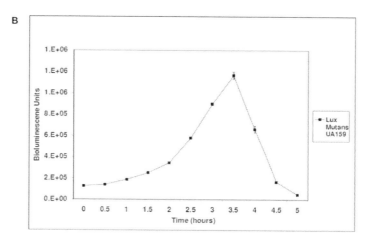

Figure 1. Panels A and B: Growth curve analysis of *lux* UA159 transformant examining absorbance and bioluminescence, respectively. Absorbances were measured at 600 nm. Note that measurements in Panels A and B were conducted with 4 replicate determinations, and that data points represent mean values. Standard error bars have been placed on each data point; in many cases, the standard error bars are indistinguishable from the data point itself.

S. *Mutans* UA159 Strain and S. *Mutans Lux* Transformants have Near-Equivalent Sensitivity to the Antibiotic Minocycline Hydrochloride

Cultures of non-transformed *S. mutans* UA159 were treated with varying doses of minocycline hydrochloride (0.01 – 100 µg/ml), and absorbance (A_{600} nm) was measured at specific time intervals (Figure 2, Panel A).

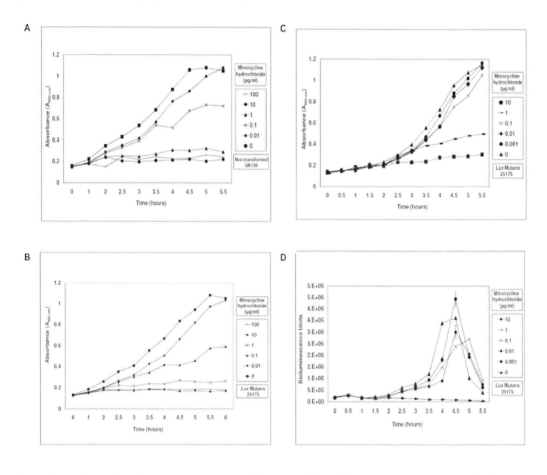

Figure 2. Panel A: Absorbance measurements of non-transformed *S. mutans* UA159 treated with varying doses of minocycline hydrochloride (0.01 – 100 µg/ml). Panel B: Absorbance measurements of *lux* ATCC 25175 transformant treated with varying doses of minocycline hydrochloride (0.1 – 100 µg/ml). Panel C and D: Matched experiment examining absorbance (Panel C) and bioluminescence (Panel D) measurements of *lux* ATCC 25175 transformant treated with intermediate range doses of minocycline hydrochloride (0.001 – 10 µg/ml). Absorbances were measured at 600 nm. Replicate determinations (n = 4) were conducted for all experiments displayed in Panel D. Standard error bars have been placed over all data points, with some standard error bars indistinguishable from the data point itself.

Non-treated cultures (0 µg/ml minocycline hydrochloride) served as controls for growth. Repeated experiments demonstrated that 1 µg/ml minocycline hydrochloride was the minimum effective dose for immediate and sustained reduction of accumulated cell mass as measured by absorbance (Figure 2, Panel A). Similar profiles were observed for both *S.*

mutans transformants, including the ATCC 25175 transformant (Figure 2, Panel B), which also demonstrated considerable inhibition of cell mass accumulation using 1 µg/ml minocycline hydrochloride. This was reproduced when using an intermediate range of minocycline hydrochloride (0.001–10 µg/ml; Figure 2, Panel C). When bioluminescence was simultaneously tracked in the ATCC 25175 transformant during the same matched experiment, we observe rapid and marked reduction of emitted light at the two highest minocycline hydrochloride doses (1 µg/ml and 10 µg/ml; line graphs are similar), with progressively less effect at the lower doses compared to the non-treated controls (Figure 2, Panel D). Interestingly, bioluminescence for the non-treated control peaked at approximately 4.5 hours and decreased with subsequent time points, indicative of the metabolic activity of the culture, which becomes slowed as the cultures become saturated and enter stationary phase (compare Panels C and D in Figure 2; also illustrated in Figure 1, Panels A and B).

When comparing bioluminescence values obtained at 4.5 hours, or the peak of metabolic activity, we find that the bioluminescence values for cultures treated with 1.0 or 10 µg/ml minocycline hydrochloride were statistically different from bioluminescence values for untreated cultures ($p=0.000058$ in both cases; p values have been factored with the Bonferroni correction for multiple comparisons). All other ATCC 25175 transformant cultures treated in this same experiment with sub-optimal doses of minocycline hydrochloride (0.001–0.1 µg/ml) also appeared to drop in bioluminescence activity at 4.5 hours or later, prior to saturation of growth (Figure 2, Panel D).

Lidocaine/Prilocaine has Antimicrobial Activity at Higher Concentrations in the UA159 Transformant and is not Contraindicative to the Antimicrobial Activity of Minocycline Hydrochloride

Cultures of the UA159 transformant were treated with varying doses of lidocaine/prilocaine (0 - 200 µg/ml) and absorbance was measured at specific time intervals (Figure 3, Panel A). The majority of doses of lidocaine/prilocaine (0.02–20 µg/ml) tested in this series had minimal effect on the growth of the UA159 transformant, with the exception of the highest dose (200 µg/ml), which resulted in immediate and sustained reduction of cell mass accumulation as measured by absorbance (Figure 3, Panel A).

We tested the hypothesis that lidocaine/prilocaine may have a contraindicative effect on the antimicrobial activity of hydrochloride by treating the UA159 transformant with combinations of minocycline hydrochloride (at 1 µg/ml) and varying doses of lidocaine/prilocaine (0–200 µg/ml), and determined that lidocaine/prilocaine has no contraindicative effects on the antimicrobial potency of minocycline hydrochloride (Figure 3, Panel B). In additional experiments, bioluminescence determinations (in relative light units or RLUs), which represent assessments of the metabolic activity of the cultures, were conducted with the UA159 transformant. Bioluminescence values in RLUs were depressed using the combination of minocycline hydrochloride at 1 µg/ml and all doses of lidocaine/prilocaine tested (compare Figure 3, Panel C to absorbance determinations in the absence of minocycline hydrochloride in Figure 3, Panel A).

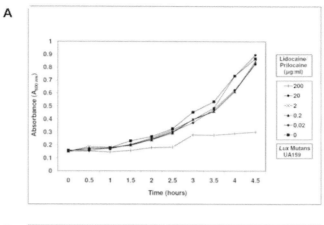

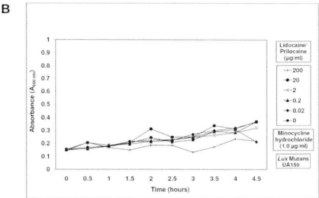

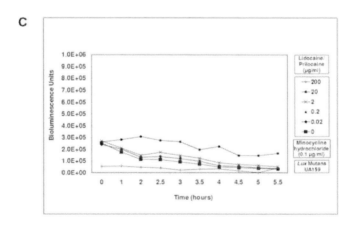

Figure 3. Panel A: Absorbance measurements of *lux* UA159 transformant treated with varying doses of lidocaine/prilocaine (0 – 200 μg/ml). Panels B and C: Matched experiment examining absorbance measurements (Panel B) and bioluminescence (Panel C) measurements of *lux* UA159 transformant treated with combination of Minocycline hydrochloride (1 μg/ml) and varying doses of lidocaine/prilocaine (0 – 200 μg/ml). Absorbances were measured at 600 nm. Replicate determinations (n = 4) were conducted for all experiments displayed in Panel C. Standard error bars have been placed over all data points, with some standard error bars indistinguishable from the data point itself.

Antimicrobial Activity of Lidocaine/Prilocaine is more Apparent when using Suboptimal Doses of Minocycline Hydrochloride

In order to more precisely test the sensitivity of the *lux* transformants to lidocaine/prilocaine, cultures of the ATCC 25175 transformant were treated with varied doses of lidocaine/prilocaine (0 – 100 µg/ml), combined with either near-optimal or suboptimal doses of minocycline hydrochloride (1 µg/ml and 0.1 µg/ml, respectively). In this experiment, we examined doses of lidocaine/prilocaine between 0-100 µg/ml, in the absence or presence of 1 µg/ml minocycline hydrochloride (Figure 4, Panels A and B, respectively). Consistent with the results of the UA159 transformant described above, we observe with the ATCC 25175 transformant, that lidocaine/prilocaine has weak antimicrobial activity when used alone at doses above 100 µg/ml (unpublished observations), and that no reductions in absorbance occurred using lidocaine/prilocaine at doses ≤ 100 µg/ml (Figure 4, Panel A). As described above in the case of the UA159 transformant, when lidocaine/prilocaine (25-100 µg/ml) is applied in conjunction with minocycline hydrochloride (1 µg/ml) in the ATCC 25175 transformant, we observe that lidocaine/prilocaine in this intermediate dose range does not have a contraindicative effect on the antimicrobial activity of minocycline hydrochloride, when minocycline hydrochloride is used at the near-optimal dose of 1 µg/ml (Figure 4, Panel B). Minocycline hydrochloride at that concentration will result in immediate and sustained reduction in absorbance. When minocycline hydrochloride is lowered to the suboptimal dose of 0.1 µg/ml, we observe that the combined effect of minocycline hydrochloride plus lidocaine/prilocaine at 100 µg/ml results in reductions in absorbance (Figure 4, Panel C). Other lower concentrations of lidocaine/prilocaine (< 100 µg/ml, when used with the suboptimal dose of minocycline hydrochloride (0.1 µg/ml) do not result in reductions in absorbance (Figure 4, Panel C). We conclude from these experiments that lidocaine/prilocaine at 100 µg/ml, when used in conjunction with suboptimal doses of minocycline hydrochloride, adds measureable bacteriostatic activity (Figure 4, Panel C).

Minocycline Hydrochloride and Antiseptic Chlorhexidine Display Additive Antimicrobial Activity in the UA159 Transformant

The UA159 transformant, when treated with chlorhexidine (0.01%) in conjunction with either high (1 µg/ml) or low (0.1 µg/ml) doses of minocycline hydrochloride, displayed reduced levels of cell mass accumulation, as measured by absorbance, that were additive when both antimicrobial agents were deployed (Figure 5, Panels A and B). When examining absorbance values at 5.5 hours, we find that the absorbance values of cultures treated with minocycline hydrochloride (1.0 µg/ml) plus chlorhexidine (0.01%) or minocycline hydrochloride (1.0 µg/ml) alone were statistically different from the absorbance values of untreated cultures ($p<10^{-6}$ in both cases with Bonferroni correction; Figure 5, Panel A). When comparing absorbance values at 5.5 hours for cultures treated with minocycline hydrochloride (1.0 µg/ml) with or without chlorhexidine (0.01%), we find that these values are nearly statistically distinct (p=0.059; Figure 5, Panel A). Similarly when examining data with minocycline hydrochloride at 0.1 µg/ml (Figure 5, Panel B), we observe statistical differences in absorbances between cultures treated with minocycline hydrochloride (0.1 µg/ml) plus chlorhexidine (0.01%) versus untreated cultures (p=0.00017 including Bonferroni correction), and cultures treated with minocycline hydrochloride (0.1 µg/ml) with or without chlorhexidine (0.01%) (p=0.0018 including Bonferroni correction).

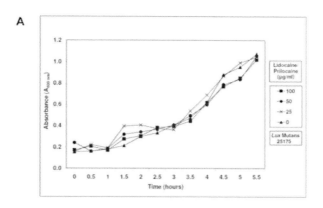

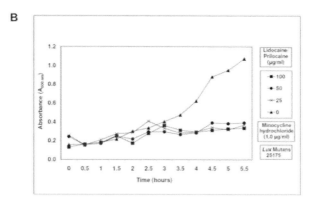

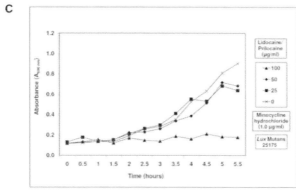

Figure 4. Panels A and B: Matched experiment examining the absorbance measurements of the *lux* ATCC 25175 transformant treated with varying doses of lidocaine/prilocaine (0 – 100 µg/ml), in the absence (Panel A) or presence (Panel B) of minocycline hydrochloride (1 µg/ml). Panel C: Absorbance measurements of the *lux* ATCC 25175 transformant treated with varying doses of lidocaine/prilocaine (0 – 100 µg/ml), in the presence of suboptimal doses of minocycline hydrochloride (0.1 µg/ml). Absorbances were measured at 600 nm.

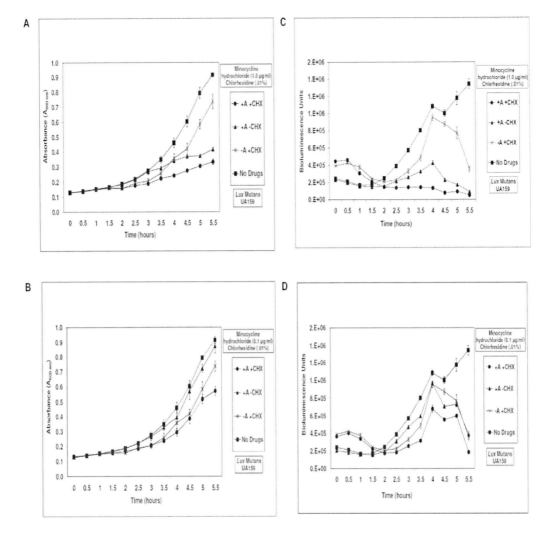

Figure 5. Panels A and C: Matched experiment examining absorbance (Panel A) and bioluminescence (Panel C) of the *lux* UA159 transformant treated with minocycline hydrochloride (1.0 μg/ml) or chlorhexidine alone or in combination. Panels B and D: Matched experiment examining absorbance (Panel A) and bioluminescence (Panel C) of the *lux* UA159 transformant treated with minocycline hydrochloride (0.1 μg/ml) or chlorhexidine alone or in combination. Absorbances were measured at 600 nm. Symbols A and CHX are reflective of Arestin and chlorhexidine.

Similar reductions in bioluminescence activity were also observed, with additive effects when both antimicrobial agents were deployed together (Figure 5, Panels C and D). When using bioluminescence values obtained at 4 hours for cultures treated with minocycline hydrochloride at 1.0 μg/ml (Figure 5, Panel C), and conducting multiple pair-wise comparisons, we find that all comparisons with the exception of the comparison between the untreated and chlorhexidine-treated cultures were statistically different with p values approaching zero ($p < 10^{-10}$ including Boneferroni correction). Similar statistically-significant differences were found with bioluminescence values obtained at 4 hours using the lower dose of minocycline hydrochloride (0.1 μg/ml; Figure 5, Panel D). In these comparisons, statistically-significant differences were found between untreated cultures and cultures treated with minocycline hydrochloride alone (0.1 μg/ml) or minocycline hydrochloride plus chlorhexidine (0.01%) ($p=0.012$ and $p<10^{-8}$, respectively including Bonferroni correction), between cultures treated with minocycline hydrochloride (0.1 μg/ml) alone or with chlorhexidine (0.01%) ($p=10^{-6}$ including Bonferroni correction) or between cultures treated with chlorhexidine (0.01%) alone or with minocycline hydrochloride (0.1 μg/ml) ($p=0.00018$ including Bonferroni correction).

DISCUSSION

The treatment of periodontal disease commonly involves mechanical and surgical interventions, such as scaling and root planing (SRP). SRP is now often augmented with adjunct antimicrobial therapies to treat supragingival and subgingival plaque, including the use of chlorhexidine [18,21,22]. More targeted antimicrobial adjunct therapies have recently emerged as additional tools for the treatment of subgingival plaque and periodontitis. These include the slow-release minocycline hydrochloride, which has shown some success when used in conjunction with standard SRP procedures [18,22].

Adverse drug interactions are a growing concern for all aspects of patient care, including periodontology. Pharmacodynamic drug interactions, including competition by enzyme inhibition and substrate bioavailability, may potentially antagonize the effectiveness of specific drugs [64,65]. We have sought to identify potential antagonistic or complementary effects of two commonly used products, one the anesthetic lidocaine/prilocaine, the other the antimicrobial agent chlorhexidine, on the bacteriostatic activity of the antibiotic minocycline hydrochloride, used as an adjunct therapy after scaling and root planing. Even though the application of minocycline hydrochloride and lidocaine/prilocaine are temporally distinct, these two agents are applied subgingivally in the same periodontal sulcus within a short time of each other, and interaction is plausible. The two antimicrobial agents chlorhexidine and minocycline hydrochloride are designed for use during the extended period of time following SRP.

There are known antagonistic interactions between bactericidal and bacteriostatic compounds [64,65]. Bactericidal antibiotics are dependent on active cell replication, and bacteriostatic antibiotics, when used in conjunction with bactericidal agents, will inhibit replication and diminish the effectiveness of the bactericidal agent. For example, there are well-documented instances where simultaneous administration of penicillin with either tetracycline or erythromycin is less effective than using penicillin alone [64,65].

The potential interactions between minocycline hydrochloride and lidocaine/prilocaine, and between minocycline hydrochloride and chlorhexidine, were determined using the *lux* biosensor system, where *lux* gene recombinants from *Photorhabdus luminescens* were transformed into the oral bacteria *Streptococcus mutans*. This system can serve as sensitive real-time biosensors in the determination of antimicrobial activity and can rapidly monitor inhibition of bacterial metabolism. The application of the *lux* biosensor system in this study represents its first use in examining drug interactions in dentistry.

Streptococci were selected as host strains for transformation using *lux* gene recombinants, because they are among the most common colonizers in plaque biofilm, which would be reforming in the period following SRP when minocycline hydrochloride is designed to be effective, and in fact may be beneficial in shifting the reforming biofilm away from periodontal pathogens [56]. Some streptococci species are initiators of biofilms, and are required for the colonization and expansion of subsequent periodontal biofilm [66-69]. Mutans streptococci, including *S. mutans*, have also recently been identified in the subgingival plaque of patients with periodontitis [56]. Streptococci were also selected because of the availability of known transformation protocols for these strains and ease of growth in culture, and because minocycline hydrochloride is a broad-spectrum antibiotic that inhibits common protein synthesis components found in both gram-positive streptococci and gram-negative periodontal bacteria [18-21].

Transformants that carry significant plasmid loads might be expected to have slowed growth kinetics because of the increased metabolic burden to replicate additional nucleic acids. Interestingly, this does not appear to be the case with the *lux* mutans transformants, where the saturating cell mass accumulation based on absorbance, and the duration of time necessary to obtain saturation, does not appear to be different from what occurs in nontransformed *S. mutans* (compare Figure 1, Panel C with Figure 2, Panel A).

The *lux A-E* operon reconstitutes an aldehyde-recycling pathway [60] and using bioluminescence can detect changes in metabolic activity before changes in cell mass occur. In this regard, we have determined that bioluminescence activity decreases as the culture enters stationary phase, reflective of the diminished metabolic activity of the culture at that stage, and occurs well in advance of the observed plateau in cell mass accumulation, which is an indirect measure of cell number (Figure 2, Panels C and D). Bioluminescence and the assessed metabolic activity of the culture approaches zero during prolonged periods of stationary phase (Figure 2, Panels C and D). Other similar systems using ATP-driven bioluminescence, also conducted in our laboratory [70], measures ATP content in bacterial cells using a luciferase-luciferin substrate, and like the *lux* biosensor system also demonstrates a dramatic decrease in metabolic activity during stationary phase of growth.

We have verified the two transformants used in this study as *S. mutans* derivatives, using the criteria of growth on MSA with bacitracin inhibitors, PCR using specific *S. mutans* primers and immunoreactivity using antibodies directed at unique *S. mutans* cell wall components. In spite of differences in utilization of metabolic substrates and acidification profiles (Table 1), both *S. mutans* transformants used in this study, *lux* UA159 and *lux* ATCC 25175, have near equivalent sensitivities to minocycline hydrochloride, where 1 μg/ml minocycline hydrochloride was noted to be the minimum effective dose for immediate and sustained reduction of accumulated cell mass as measured by absorbance (Figure 2). In addition, the influence of the *lux* recombinant plasmid in transformed cells on minocycline sensitivity is negligible, since both nontransformed and transformed mutans cells exhibit the same minimum effective dose of 1 μg/ml minocycline hydrochloride for sustained reduction of accumulated cell mass (compare Panel A versus Panel B of Figure 2). This reduction of accumulated cell mass is reproducible in an independently conducted experiment (Figure 2, Panel C) using an intermediate range of minocycline hydrochloride (0-10 μg/ml), where reduction in bioluminescence is also observed at the same dose of minocycline hydrochloride

(Figure 2, Panel D; 1 µg/ml and 10 µg/ml minocycline hydrochloride curves are merged as overlapping line graphs).

In additional experiments, we demonstrate that lidocaine/prilocaine has weak antimicrobial activity at the higher doses examined (200 µg/ml) in mutans transformants (Figure 3, Panel A). Minocycline hydrochloride at the optimal concentration of 1.0 µg/ml added to all doses of lidocaine/prilocaine resulted in the sustained reduction of the mutans transformant both in cell mass accumulation and bioluminescence (Figure 3, Panels B and C, respectively). Thus, in these instances, the addition of lidocaine/prilocaine does not have a contraindicative effect on the antimicrobial activity of minocycline hydrochloride. In some experiments, we used reduced amounts of minocycline hydrochloride (0.1 µg/ml), where the bacteriostatic activity of minocycline hydrochloride was purposefully weak, in order to confirm that the addition of lidocaine/prilocaine (at 200 µg/ml) had augmented antimicrobial activity. Interestingly, the dose of lidocaine/prilocaine used in the *lux* biosensor system (200 µg/ml) is much lower than the dose applied in the periodontal pocket (each cartridge contains 1.7 g of gel which contains 42.5 mg of lidocaine and 42.5 mg of prilocaine), where lidocaine/prilocaine is mixed with crevicular fluid and saliva, and one may presume that the effective dose of lidocaine/prilocaine in the periodontal pocket would be less than the applied dose.

The limited antimicrobial activity of lidocaine/prilocaine at the 100 µg/ml dose in the ATCC 25175 transformant (Figure 4, Panel C) has been found to be reproducible in additional experiments (unpublished observations). The ATCC 25175 transformant appears to retain similar sensitivity profiles for lidocaine/prilocaine when administered with the suboptimal dose of minocycline hydrochloride (0.1 µg/ml), but may be less sensitive than the UA159 transformant at the 100 µg/ml dose (unpublished observations). Thus again, lidocaine/prilocaine does not appear to be contraindicative to the bacteriostatic activity of minocycline hydrochloride, and may in fact augment the antimicrobial effect of suboptimal doses of minocycline hydrochloride in the *lux* biosensor system (Figure 4, Panel C).

The mechanism of the antimicrobial activity of lidocaine/prilocaine is unknown. The anesthetic composite of lidocaine and prilocaine has been found to retain antimicrobial properties in skin creams used to treat human skin flora [71,72]. Both lidocaine and prilocaine are sodium channel blockers [73], and voltage-gated sodium ion channels have been found in bacteria [74]. One potential mechanism of action may constitute blockade of ion flux and resultant dysregulation of osmolarity, ultimately resulting in slow disruption of the cell. Interestingly, chlorhexidine, another antimicrobial agent used in the treatment of supragingival and subgingival plaque, is a chemical antiseptic with both bactericidal and bacteriostatic properties that is believed to act through membrane disruption [75]. Like the combination of minocycline hydrochloride and lidocaine/prilocaine, the combination of the bacteriostatic antibiotic minocycline hydrochloride and the antiseptic chlorhexidine display additive antimicrobial effects in the *lux* biosensor system (Figure 5), and that the majority of pair-wise comparisons are statistically distinct. Statistically-significant differences were found 1) between untreated cultures and cultures treated with minocycline hydrochloride alone (0.1 µg/ml) or with minocycline hydrochloride plus chlorhexidine (0.01%) ($p=0.012$ and $p<10^{-8}$, respectively including Bonferroni correction), 2) between cultures treated with minocycline hydrochloride (0.1 µg/ml) alone or with chlorhexidine (0.01%) ($p=10^{-6}$ including Bonferroni correction) or 3) between cultures treated with chlorhexidine (0.01%) alone or with minocycline hydrochloride (0.1 µg/ml) (p=0.00018 including Bonferroni correction). Our results are consistent with other studies that indicate chlorhexidine may enhance the penetration and intracellular activity of antibiotics in bacterial cells [76,77]. This may have important implications for the periodontist when considering use of minocycline hydrochloride antibiotic as an adjunct therapy for SRP, followed by use of chlorhexidine for generalized control of supragingival plaque. Using the *lux* biosensor system, there appears to be no contraindicative effect when using minocycline hydrochloride and chlorhexidine in combination.

CONCLUSION

We have found that the *lux* biosensor system is an excellent monitor of the metabolic activity of the culture, and is especially useful when assessing single antimicrobial agents, or with combinations of multiple agents. We conclude that the anesthetic lidocaine/prilocaine, or the antiseptic chlorhexidine, does not interfere with the potent bacteriostatic activity of minocycline hydrochloride, and in fact has an additive antibacterial effect.

ACKNOWLEDGMENTS

The *lux* recombinant was a kind gift of Dr. Vyv Salisbury (Faculty of Applied Sciences, University of the West of England, Bristol, United Kingdom). We also thank Anna Nguyen (Integrative Biosciences, OHSU) for assistance in final development of the figures, and Dr. Michael Leo (Affiliate Assistant Professor, Integrative Biosciences, OHSU) for advice on statistical determinations. We also thank our OHSU colleagues, Drs. Don Adams and Marvin Levin, for their critical review of this work, and for Dr. Don Adams as the reviewer of this manuscript. Portions of this work were conducted by VTT and SN in fulfillment of the research component of the OHSU Periodontology graduate certification program. AR was supported by a special research fellowship award from Dean Clinton and the OHSU School of Dentistry. WSM was supported as a 2008 OCTRI Student Research Fellow from the Oregon Clinical and Translational Research Institute, OHSU. RS was the recipient of the 2008 OCMID Student Fellowship for Caries Microbiology Research. This research was supported by Dentsply Pharmaceutical, with funds for supplies provided to TM, and use of the luminometer was kindly provided by Oral Biotech. WC, TM and CM are supported by the OHSU School of Dentistry.

REVIEWED BY

Dr. Don Adams, Professor, Department of Periodontology, Oregon Health & Science University School of Dentistry, 611 SW Campus Drive, Portland, OR 97239.

REFERENCES

[1]   Armitage GC. *Clinical evaluation of periodontal diseases*. Periodontol 2000 1995;7:39-53.

[2]   Moore WEC, Moore LVH. *The bacteria of periodontal diseases*. Periodontol 2000 1994;5:66-77.

[3]   Consensus Report: *Periodontal diseases: pathogenesis and microbial factors*. Ann Periodontol 1996;1(1):926-932.

[4]   Socransky SS, Haffajee AD, Cugini MA, Smith C, Kent RL Jr. *Microbial complexes in subgingival plaque*. J Clin Periodontol 1998;25(2):134-144.

[5]   Costerton JW, Lewabdowski Z, DeBeer D, Caldwell D, Korber D, James G. *Biofilms, the customized microniche*. J Bacteriol 1994;176 (8):2137-2142.

[6]   Socransky SS, Haffajee AD. *Dental biofilms: difficult therapeutic targets*. Periodontal 2000 2002;28:12-55.

[7]   Cugini MA, Haffajee AD, Smith C, Kent RL Jr, Socransky SS. *The effect of scaling and root planing on the clinical and microbiological paramaters of periodontal diseases: 12 month results*. J Clin Periodontol 2000;27 (1):30-36.

[8]   Cobb CM. *Non-surgical pocket therapy: mechanical*. Ann Periodontol 1996;1:443-490.

[9]   Rabbani GM, Ash MM Jr, Caffesse RG. *The effectiveness of subgingival scaling and root planing in calculus removal*. J Periodontol 1981;52(3):119-23.

[10]   Adriaens PA, Adriaens LM. *Effects of nonsurgical periodontal therapy on hard and soft tissues*. Periodontol 2000 2004;36:121-145.

[11]   Clifford LR, Needleman IG, Chan YK. *Comparison of periodontal pocket penetration by conventional and microultrasonic inserts*. J Clin Periodontol 1999;26:124-130.

[12]   Caffesse RG, Sweeney PL, Smith BA. *Scaling and root planing with and without periodontal flap surgery*. J Clin Periodontol 1986;13:205-210.

[13]   Haffajee AD, Cugini MA, Dibart S, Smith C, Kent RL Jr, Socransky SS. *The effect of SRP on the clinical and microbiological parameters of periodontal diseases*. J Clin Periodontol 1997;24:324-334.

[14]   Adriaens PA, De Boever JA, Loesche WJ. *Bacterial invasion in root cementum and radicular dentin of periodontally diseased teeth in humans. A reservoir of periodontopathic bacteria*. J Periodontol 1988;59 (4):222-30.

[15]   Giuliana G, Ammatuna P, Pizzo G, Capone F, D'Angelo M. *Occurrence of invading bacteria in radicular dentin of periodontally diseased teeth: microbiological findings*. J Clin Periodontol 1997;24(7):478-85.

[16]   Williams RC, Paquette DW, Offenbacher S, Adams DF, Armitage GC, Bray K, Caton J, Cochran DL, Drisko CH, Fiorellini JP, Giannobile WV, Grossi S, Guerrero DM, Johnson GK, Lamster IB, Magnusson I, Oringer RJ, Persson GR, Van Dyke TE, Wolff LF, Santucci EA, Rodda BE, Lessem J. *Treatment of periodontitis by local administration of minocycline microspheres: a controlled trial*. J Periodontol 2001;72 (11):1535-1544.

[17]   Ah MK, Johnson GK, Kaldahl WB, Patil KD, Kalkwarf KL. *The effect of smoking on the response to periodontal therapy*. J Clin Periodontol 1994;21(2):91-97.

[18]   American Academy of Periodontology Research, Science and Therapy Committee. *Tobacco use and the periodontal patient*. J Periodontol 1999;70(11):1419-1427.

[19]   Fleischer HC, Mellonig JT, Brayer WK, Gray JL, Barnett JD. *Scaling and root planing efficacy in multirooted teeth.* J Periodontol 1989;60(7):402-409.

[20]   Slots J, Rams TE. *Antibiotics in periodontal therapy: advantages and disadvantages.* J Clin Periodontol 1990;17(7 Pt2):479-493.

[21]   Oringer RJ, Al-Shammari KF, Aldredge WA, Iacono VJ, Eber RM, Wang HL, Berwald B, Nejat R, Giannobile WV. *Effects of locally delivered minocycline microspheres on markers of bone resorption.* J Periodontol 2002;73:835-842.

[22]   Paquette DW. *Pocket depth reduction as an outcome measure of inflammation and soft tissue changes in periodontitis trials.* J Int Acad Periodontol 2005;7/4(Supplement): 147-156.

[23]   Paquette DW, Williams RC, Hanlon A, Lessem J. *Clinical relevance of adjunctive minocycline microspheres in patients with chronic periodontitis: secondary analysis of a phase 3 trial.* J Periodontol 2004;75:531-536.

[24]   Zambon JJ, Grossi SG, Machtei EE, Ho AW, Dunford R, Genco RJ. *Cigarette smoking increases the risk for subgingival infection with periodontal pathogens.* J Periodontol 1996;67:1050-1054.

[25]   Williams RC, Paquette DW, Offenbacher S, Adams DF, Armitage GC, Bray K, Caton J, Cochran DL, Drisko CH, Fiorellini JP, Giannobile WV, Grossi S, Guerrero DM, Johnson GK, Lamster IB, Magnusson I, Oringer RJ, Persson GR, Van Dyke TE, Wolff LF, Santucci EA, Rodda BE, Lessem J. *Treatment of periodontitis by local administration of minocycline microspheres: a controlled trial.* J Periodontol 2001;72 (11):1535-44.

[26]   Paquette DW, Ryan ME, Wilder RS. *Locally Delivered Antimicrobials: Clinical Evidence and Relevence.* J Dent Hyg 2008;82 Suppl 3:10-15.

[27]   Van Dyke TE, Offenbacher S, Braswell L, Lessem J. *Enhancing the value of scaling and root-planing: Arestin clinical trial results.* J Int Acad Periodontol 002;4(3):72-6.

[28]   Hellström MK, McClain PK, Schallhorn RG, Bellis L, Hanlon AL, Ramberg P. *Local minocycline as an adjunct to surgical therapy in moderate to severe, chronic periodontitis.* J Clin Periodontol 2008;35(6):525-31.

[29]   Salvi GE, Persson GR, Heitz-Mayfield LJ, Frei M, Lang NP. *Adjunctive local antibiotic therapy in the treatment of peri-implantitis II: clinical and radiographic outcomes.* Clin Oral Implants Res 2007;18(3):281-5.

[30]   Heitz-Mayfield LJ, Lang NP. *Antimicrobial treatment of peri-implant diseases.* Int J Oral Maxillofac Implants 2004;19 Suppl:128-39.

[31]   Renvert S, Lessem J, Lindahl C, Svensson M. *Treatment of incipient peri-implant infections using topical minocycline microspheres versus topical chlorhexidine gel as an adjunct to mechanical debridement.* J Int Acad Periodontol 2004;6(4 Suppl):154-9.

[32]   Hugo WB, Longworth AR. *Some aspects of the mode of action of chlorhexidine.* J Pharm Pharmacol 1964;16:655-662.

[33]   Lang NP, Brecx M. *Chlorhexidine digluconate. An agent for chemical plaque control and prevention of gingival inflammation.* J Periodontal Res 1986;21:74-89.

[34]   Greenstein G, Berman C, Jaffin R. *Chlorhexidine: An adjunct to periodontal therapy.* J Periodontal Res 1986;57:370-377.

[35]   Noiri Y, Okami Y, Narimatsu M, Takahashi Y, Kawahara T, Ebisu S. *Effects of chlorhexidine, minocycline, and metronidazole on Porphyromonas gingivalis strain 381 in biofilms.* J Periodontol 2003;74(11):1647-51.

[36] Bonesvoll P. *Oral pharmacology of chlorhexidine.* J Clin Periodontol 1977;4(5):49-65.

[37] Löe H, Schiott CR. *The effect of mouthrinses and topical application of chlorhexidine on the development of dental plaque and gingivitis in man.* J Periodontal Res 1970;5 (2):79-83.

[38] Armitage GC, Robertson PB. *The biology, prevention, diagnosis and treatment of periodontal diseases: scientific advances in the United States.* J Am Dent Assoc 2009;140 Suppl 1:36S-43S.

[39] Hallmon WW, Rees TD. *Local anti-infective therapy: mechanical and physical approaches. A systematic review.* Ann Periodontol 2003;8(1):99-114.

[40] Zanatta FB, Antoniazzi RP, Rösing CK. *The effect of 0.12% chlorhexidine gluconate rinsing on previously plaque-free and plaque-covered surfaces: a randomized, controlled clinical trial.* J Periodontol 2007;78(11):2127-34.

[41] Briner W, Grossman E, Buckner R, Rebitski G, Sox T, Setser R, Ebert M. *Assessment of susceptibility of plaque bacteria to chlorhexidine after six months oral use.* J Perodontal Res 1986;16:53-39.

[42] Flotra L, Gjermo P, Rolla G, Waerhaug J. *Side effects of chlorhexidine mouth washes.* Scand J Dent Res 1971;79:119–125.

[43] Loe H. *Does chlorhexidine have a place in the prophylaxis of dental disease?* J Periodont Res 1973; 8 (suppl 12):93.

[44] Löe H, Mandell M, Derry A, Schött CR. *The effect of mouthrinses and topical application of chlorhexidine on calculus formation in man.* J Periodontal Res 1971;6 (4):312-4.

[45] Cancro LP, Paulovich DB, Klein K, Picozzi A. *Effects of a chlorhexidine gluconate mouthrinse on dental plaque and calculus.* J Periodontol 1972;43(11):687-91.

[46] Sanz M, Vallcorba N, Fabregues S, Müller I, Herkströter F. *The effect of a dentifrice containing chlorhexidine and zinc on plaque, gingivitis, calculus and tooth staining.* J Clin Periodontol 1994;21(6):431-7.

[47] Lang NP, Mombelli A, Tonetti MS, Brägger U, Hämmerle CH. *Clinical trials on therapies for peri-implant infections.* Ann Periodontol 1997;2(1):343-56.

[48] Cannell JS. *The use of antimicrobials in the mouth.* J Int Med Res 1981;9(4):277-82.

[49] Ciancio S. *Expanded and future uses of mouthrinses.* J Am Dent Assoc 1994;125 Suppl 2:29S-32S.

[50] Sanz M, Newman MG, Anderson L, Matoska W, Otomo-Corgel J, Saltini C. *Clinical enhancement of post-periodontal surgical therapy by a 0.12% chlorhexidine gluconate mouthrinse.* J Periodontol 1989;60(10):570-6.

[51] Christensen, G. *Increasing the Quality and Predictability of Multiple Unit Impressions.* Dental Town Magazine July 2001, p.34.

[52] Soskolne WA, Chajek T, Flashner M, Landau I, Stabholtz A, Kolatch B, Lerner EI. *An in vivo study of the chlorhexidine release profile of the PerioChip in the gingival crevicular fluid, plasma and urine.* J Clin Periodontol 1998;25(12):1017-21.

[53] Stanley A, Wilson M, Newman HN. *The in vitro effects of chlorhexidine on subgingival plaque bacteria.* J Clin Periodontol 1989;16(4):259-64.

[54] Donaldson D, Gelskey SC, Landry RG, Matthews DC, Sandhu HS. *A placebo-controlled multi-centered evaluation of an anaesthetic gel (Lidocaine/prilocaine) for periodontal therapy.* J Clin Periodontol 2003;30:171-175.

[55] Jeffcoat MK, Geurs NC, Magnusson I, MacNeill SR, Mickels N, Robinson P, Salamati A, Yukna R. *Intrapocket anesthesia for scaling and root planing: Results of a double-blind multicenter trial using lidocaine-prilocaine dental gel.* J Periodontol 2001;72 (7):895-900.

[56] Teughels W, Newman MG, Coucke W, Haffajee AD, Van Der Mei HC, Haake SK, Schepers E, Cassiman JJ, Van Eldere J, van Steenberghe D, Quirynen M. *Guiding periodontal pocket recolonization: a proof of concept.* J Dent Res 2007;86(11):1078-1082.

[57] Van der Reijden WA, Dellemijn-Kippuw N, Stijne-van Nes AM, de Soet JJ, van Winkelhoff AJ. *Mutans streptococci in subgingival plaque of treated and untreated patients with periodontitis.* J Clin Periodontol 2001;28(7):686-691.

[58] Beard SJ, Salisbury V, Lewis RJ, Sharpe JA, MacGowan AP. *Expression of lux genes in a clinical isolate of Streptococcus pneumoniae: Using bioluminescence to monitor gemifloxacin activity.* Antimicrob Agents Chemother 2002;46(2):538-542.

[59] Gupta RK, Patterson SS, Ripp S, Simpson ML, Saylor GS. *Expression of the Photorhabdus luminescens lux genes (luxA, B, C, D, and E) in Saccharomyces cervisiae.* FEMS Yeast Research 2003;4(3):305-313.

[60] Welham PA, Stekel DJ. *Mathematical model of the lux luminescence system in the terrestrial bacterium Photorhabdus luminescens.* Mol Biosyst 2009;5(1):68-76.

[61] Shklair IL, Keene HJ. *A biochemical scheme for the separation of the five varieties of Streptococcus mutans.* Arch Oral Biol 1974;19(11):1079-1081.

[62] Gold OG, Jordan HV, Van Houte JV. *Identification of Streptococcus mutans colonies by mannitol-dependent tetrazolium reduction.* Arch Oral Biol 1974;19(3):271-272.

[63] Linke HAB. *New method for the isolation of Streptococcus mutans and its differentiation from other oral streptococci.* J Clin Microbiol 1977;5(6):604-609.

[64] Hersh EV, Moore PA. *Adverse drug interactions in dentistry.* Periodontol 2000 2008;46:109-142.

[65] Pelz K, Wiedmann-Al-Ahmad M, Bogdan C, Otten JE. *Analysis of antimicrobial activity of local anesthetics used for dental analgesia.* J Med Microbiol 2008;57 (Pt 1):88-94.

[66] Gibbons RJ. *Microbial ecology. Adherent interactions which may affect microbial ecology in the mouth.* J Dent Res 1984;63(3):378-385.

[67] Whittaker CJ, Klier CM, Kolenbrander PE. *Mechanisms of adhesion by oral bacteria.* Ann Rev Microbiol 1996;50:513-552.

[68] Jenkinson HF, Lamont RJ. *Streptococcal adhesion and colonization.* Crit Rev Oral Biol Med 1997;8(2):175-200.

[69] Lamont RJ, Hersey SG, Rosan B. *Characterization of the adherence of Poryphyrmonas gingivalis to oral streptocci.* Oral Microbiol Immunol 1993;7(4):193-197.

[70] Pellegrini P, Sauerwein R, Finlayson T, McLeod J, Covell DA Jr, Maier T, Machida CA. *Plaque retention by self-ligating vs elastomeric orthodontic brackets: Quantitative comparison of oral bacteria and detection with adenosine triphosphate-driven bioluminescence.* Am J Orthod Dentofacial Orthop 2009;135:426.e1-426.e9.

[71] Batai I, Bogar L, Juhasz V, Batai R, Kerenyi M. *A comparison of the antimicrobial property of lidocaine/prilocaine cream (EMLA) and an alcohol-based disinfectant on intact human skin flora.* Anesth Analg 2009;108(2):666-668.

[72] Kerenyi M, Batai R, Juhasz V, Batai I. *Lidocaine/prilocaine cream (EMLA) has an antibacterial effect in vitro.* J Hosp Infect 2004;56(1):75-76.

[73] Binshtok AM, Gerner P, Oh SB, Puopolo M, Suzuki S, Roberson DP, Herbert T, Wang CF, Kim D, Chung G, Mitani AA, Wang GK, Bean BP, Woolf CJ. *Coapplication of lidocaine and permanently charged sodium channel blocker QX-314 produces long-lasting nociceptive blockade in rodents.* Anesthesiol 2009;111(1):127-37.

[74] Koishi R, Xu H, Ren D, Navarro B, Spiller BW, Shi Q, Clapham DE. *A superfamily of voltage-gated ion channels in bacteria.* J Biol Chem 2004;279(10):9532-9538.

[75] Kuyyakanond T, Quesnel LB. *The mechanism of action of chlorhexidine.* FEMS Microbiol Lett 1992;79(1-3):211-215.

[76] Barnham M, Kerby J. *Antibacterial activity of combinations of chlorhexidine with neomycin and gentamycin.* J Hosp Infect 1980;1(1):77-81.

[77] Pons JL, Bonnaveiro N, Chevalier J, Cremieux A. *Evaluation of antimicrobial interactions between chlorhexidine, quaternary ammonium compounds, preservatives and excipients.* J Appl Bacteriol 1992;73(5):395-400.

In: Periodontitis Symptoms, Treatment and Prevention   ISBN: 978-1-61668-836-3
Editor: Rosemarie E. Walchuck, pp. 167-184   ©2010 Nova Science Publishers, Inc.

Chapter 6

THE ROLE OF THE T$_H$17 PATHWAY IN THE PROGRESSION OF PERIODONTAL DISEASE

Roger B. Johnson

Department of Periodontics and Preventive Sciences, University of Mississippi School
of Dentistry, Jackson, Mississippi, USA

CONCEPTS OF PERIODONTAL DISEASE PATHOGENESIS

Periodontitis is a chronic inflammatory disease which destroys the tooth-supporting tissues[1]. This disease is initiated by bacteria; in particular, faculative anaerobic Gram-negative microorganisms[2]. Several types of these pathogens initiate periodontal disease, and the host response determines the disease progression and ultimate tissue damage[3-4]. The early periodontal lesion (gingivitis) is characterized by the presence of large numbers of T cells and macrophages within the gingiva, while the presence of beta (B) and plasma cells characterize the advanced lesion[5]. These phenomena suggest that a shift in the type of host response occurs during the progression of periodontal disease[6]. However, there is little specific information available concerning the characteristics of this shift.

It is uncertain whether periodontal disease is a continuous process, or consists of episodes of exacerbation and remission[7-8]. It is generally accepted that periodontal health is a dynamic state where the activity of pro-inflammatory/antimicrobial cytokines and chemokines is balanced by anti-inflammatory cytokines and chemokines. When this balance is disrupted, severe inflammation and tissue destruction occur. Two models of the pathogenesis of periodontal disease have been proposed[9]. In the "linear model" of periodontal disease, specific bacteria initiate the disease. The inflammation is either resolved or progresses based on the host response to these bacteria[10]. The "circular model" contends that bacteria are required for both the initiation and progression of the disease. These bacteria constantly reshape the T-helper (T$_H$) cell response, which determines the ultimate fate of the infection. During the progression of the inflammation, alveolar bone resorption and soft tissue damage offer new niches for colonization of bacteria. These niches facilitate bacterial overgrowth, which reinforces this circular process and produces an ongoing vicious cycle.

In both models of pathogenesis of periodontal disease, innate and adaptive immune responses are featured. The initial response to bacterial infection is a local inflammatory reaction that activates the innate immune system[11-12]. In this response, neutrophils, macrophages and monocytes become activated by periodontal pathogens such as *Actinobacillus actinomycetemcomitans* and *Porphyromonas gingivalis*, and then produce a pattern of pro-inflammatory cytokines and chemokines[11-13]. Under normal circumstances, these innate immune cells are capable of preventing significant tissue invasion of the microbes. However, if these cells are unable to clear the infiltration of bacteria, the acquired immune responses become active. Cytokines produced by cells of the innate immune system are the first line of defense against pathogens. Their pattern recognition receptors, which are not specific for any particular epitope, allow them to respond to a wide variety of microbial invaders by producing cytokines that activate T and B cells of the adaptive immune system[14-16,17]. The failure to encapsulate this "inflammatory front" within gingival tissues results in the expansion of the inflammation adjacent to alveolar bone[12]. During the infectious process, inappropriate immune and inflammatory responses can reduce tissue damage or even undesired systemic reactions and outcomes[18-19].

PERIODONTOPATHOGENIC BACTERIA AND THE INNATE IMMUNE RESPONSE

A critical aspect of the host response is the detection of bacteria by Toll-like receptors (TLRs) on cells of the innate immune system. Activation of the innate immune response by the binding of various bacterial components to TLRs results in the production of cytokines and chemokines[20]. This process involves activation of the TLRs, which induces an intracellular signaling cascade that results in the activation of transcriptional factors and the production of various cytokines and chemokines[20].

The activation of TLR's depends on the type of microorganism and its specific component. For instance, *Porphyromonas gingivalis* fibriae promote monocyte or macrophage derived cytokine expression, such as IL-1-β, IL-8, or TNF-α[21,22-23], which are mediated through TLR2[24]. *P. gingivalis* type II fimA fimbriae are the predominant fimbrial phenotype associated with periodontal disease[25]. *P. gingivalis* lipopolysaccharide promotes the expression of a T_H2 pattern of proinflammatory cytokines and chemokines in monocytes/macrophages (which express IL-5, IL-10, and IL-13)[26,27] due to activation of a CD14/TLR-4 and/or a TRL-2 dependent pathway[28-30]. However, antigens to *P. gingivalis* produce IL-17[31].

THE T_H1/T_H2 PARADIGM

For almost two decades, the T_H1-T_H2 paradigm has prevailed in immunology[32]. Periodontopathogenic bacteria induce naïve CD4+ cells to differentiate into several lineages of T-helper (T_H) subsets with unique cytokine profiles and functions[5,33]. When a naïve CD4+ T cell is exposed to an antigen in the presence of IL-12, it is driven to develop into a T_H1 phenotype[34]. The T_H1 cell uniquely expresses the IL-12 receptor subunit IL-12Rβ2, which further commits the cell to proceed along this differentiation pathway. The process is dependent on the transcription factor STAT-4, which is activated by IL-12[35].

T_H1 cells activate macrophages, cytotoxic T cells and natural killer (NK) cells as well as driving anti-viral signals in target cells. T_H1 cells produce IFN-γ and lymphotoxin-α and are responsible for protection against intracellular pathogens such as viruses, mycobacteria and protozoa[36]. IFN-γ provides a positive feedback signal to reinforce T_H1 development by upregulating the IL-12 receptor. The key regulator of T_H1 lineage commitment is T-bet[37]. T-bet is upregulated in developing T_H1 cells[38], but not in T_H2 cells[39]. Thus, signals from T_H1 cytokines inhibit T_H2 and T_H17 differentiation.

Conversely, when a newly activated T_H cell is exposed to IL-4, differentiation to a T_H2 phenotype occurs[40]. This process is dependent on transcription factors STAT-6, GATA-3, and c-maf[41-43]. T_H2 cells produce IL-4, IL-5, IL-10, and IL-13[40]. IL-4 is the signature cytokine of the T_H2 population and promotes differentiation and expansion of this population. T_H2 cytokines are potent activators of B-cell IgE production, and eosinophil recruitment [40]. Thus, T_H2 cells mediate humoral responses and autoimmunity.

T cell subsets have distinct characteristics[44], which regulate their function in the immune response. Dysregulated T_H1 responses can promote tissue destruction and chronic inflammation, whereas dysregulated T_H2 responses can cause allergy and asthma [36, 45].

T-HELPER CELLS AND PERIODONTAL DISEASE

Lesions of advanced periodontitis are characterized by the presence of both T_H1 and T_H2 cytokines[46-48]. Several studies have reported that the expression of T_H1-type cytokines predominates over that of T_H2 cytokines within diseased periodontal tissue, indirectly suggesting T_H1 involvement in the inflammation[49-50]. There is likely an initial predominance of T_H1 cytokines followed by their decline and a rise in T_H2 cytokines at later stages of infection[11]. In this way, T_H2 cells have been associated with non-protective antibody responses and progressive periodontal lesions and T_H1 with stable lesions[51]. T_H1 cells are protective to the host through IL-12/IFN-γ-stimulated cell-mediated immunity[52-53] and by inhibition of osteoclastogenesis[54-55].

T cells play an important role in maintaining a balance between the host and the biofilm on the tooth and gingival surfaces[5, 56]. TLR4 agonists (*E.coli*) promote production of IL-12 and a T_H1 response in contrast to TLR2 agonists (bacterial lipopolysaccharides) which foster T_H2 responses[57].

Another method for control of T_H responses is by Treg cells, which are CD4+/CD25+ cells that antagonize T_H1 and T_H2 immune responses by secreting suppressive cytokines. Treg cells are formed in the presence of TGF-β and secrete IL-10 and additional TGF-β[58-59]. These cells are present in high amounts within tissues with periodontal disease[60-61].

T_H1 cells express the chemokines, CCR5 and CXCR3[62-66], while CCR3 is expressed by T_H2 cells[65-68]. Several recent studies suggest that a T-helper cell response in addition to the T_H-1 or T_H-2 immune response contributes to the pathogenesis of periodontal disease.

THE T$_H$17 IMMUNOLOGICAL RESPONSE: A NEW PARADIGM FOR PERIODONTAL INFLAMMATION

There is evidence that the initiation and progression of periodontal disease cannot be explained, in its entirety, by the T$_H$1/T$_H$2 paradigm. Recent studies describe a new pathway, which links gingival inflammation and bone resorption[69-70]. This pathway is the T$_H$17 immune response[45, 71]. T$_H$17 cells are an important early response to catastrophic injuries that require immediate neutrophil recruitment[72]. IL-17 plays a crucial role in innate immunity because its secretion triggers production of numerous chemokines, resulting in neutrophil and macrophage recruitment[73-77] and subsequent pathogen clearance[78-79].

Proinflammatory cytokines IL-17 and IL-17F have been reported to be expressed by T$_H$17 cells[80-82]. IL-17A and IL-17F induce the production of various proinflammatory cytokines such as TNF-α, IL-1-β, and IL-6, and CXC chemokines[82-83]. T$_H$17 cells also produce IL-21, IL-22, and IL-26[84]. T$_H$17 cells rapidly initiate an inflammatory response dominated by neutrophils, and when unregulated, have been reported to maintain chronic inflammation. These responses result in recruitment, activation, and migration of neutrophils to the sites of inflammation and infection[82]. In addition to cytokines and chemokines, T$_H$17 cells also induce secretion of matrix metalloproteinases[73, 76, 85], which destroy extracellular matrix. In addition to the proinflammatory effects, T$_H$17 cells stimulate osteoblasts to express RANKL, activating osteoclasts, resulting in loss of bone. In this way, T$_H$17 cells link gingival inflammation to alveolar bone resorption.

It has been long recognized that there are discrepancies with the T$_H$1-T$_H$2 model of periodontal inflammation[86]. The recent discovery of a new "T$_H$17" subset has resolved many of these controversies, but has also raised many new questions and research directions[87-89]. The protective role for IL-17 is consistent with the protective role played by T$_H$17 cells in infectious inflammatory diseases, compared to events in sterile inflammatory situations where IL-17 is tissue destructive[90]. T$_H$17 cells protect against extracellular bacteria and fungi, which are not dealt with by T$_H$1 mediated immunity[82].

The development of T$_H$17 cells is different from that of T$_H$1 and T$_H$2 cells. IFN-γ, IL-12, and IL-4, which are important for T$_H$1 and T$_H$2 differentiation, have been shown to be dispensable for T$_H$17 cell differentiation *in vitro* and *in vivo,* providing the first clue that T$_H$17 cells are an independent lineage from T$_H$1 or T$_H$2 cells[45, 73]. IL-6 and TGF-β initiate T$_H$17 differentiation[39, 91-92] and TNF-α and IL-1-β amplify T$_H$17 cell differentiation. IL-21 is not only expressed by T$_H$17 cells, but also controls the generation of T$_H$17 cells[93-95]. In addition, IL-21 can substitute for IL-6 in generation of T$_H$17 cells[93]. IL-23 synergizes with IL-6 to also induce T$_H$17 differentiation[96]. While IL-23 is not required for initial differentiation of T$_H$17 cells, it may play a role in the survival and expansion of the T$_H$17 cell population has been reported to promote T$_H$17 development/expansion in the presence of IL-6 and TGF-β[39, 97], which may be especially relevant to periodontal disease as IL-1-β concentrations are elevated within gingiva at sites of chronic periodontitis and within bone at sites of chronic periapical lesions[49, 69, 98-100]. For example, one study reports that IL-17 was 6.2 fold higher within gingiva obtained from sites of periodontitis patients than from healthy sites[101].

In addition, IL-18 synergizes with IL-23 in the induction of IL-17-producing CD4+ T cells [37]. IL-6 and IL-21 signal through STAT-3[102-103], which is essential for T$_H$17 differentiation. IL-21 also acts as a feedback factor to further reinforce T$_H$17 development. IL-27 inhibits T$_H$17 development[104] and IL-2/STAT-5 also limit this process [53, 73, 102].

IL-27 inhibits IL-17 production, suggesting that IL-27 may have an important role in switching the early pro-inflammatory effects of IL-17 toward a T$_H$1 response[105]. Both T$_H$1 and T$_H$2 subsets negatively regulate T$_H$17 differentiation[45, 73].

Following the discovery of the T$_H$17 subset, the role of T$_H$1 destructive inflammation has been questioned [90, 106]. T$_H$17 cytokines have been found in diseased gingiva[49, 69-70, 98]. In addition, IL-17 and IL-23 concentrations have been reported to be higher within gingiva adjacent to sites of clinical attachment loss[100,69, 107]. Thus, the inability to sustain a T$_H$1 response may lead to disease progression. PGE$_2$ inhibits IL-12p35, but enhances IL-23 expression and may contribute to T$_H$17 development[108]. IL-17 regulates COX-2 and PGE$_2$ production[109-110]. PGE$_2$ is strongly associated with periodontal tissue destruction[111-112].

IL-23 mediates autoimmunity, and may be a link between periodontal inflammation and autoimmune diseases[90, 113-114]. IL-23 is not the direct initiator of T$_H$17 production, but is an important factor for expanding and maintaining T$_H$17 cells[115,116].

Since molecules involved in the induction of T$_H$17 cells have been identified, they could be targets for prevention, or treatment, of chronic periodontal inflammation.

THE T$_H$17 PATHWAY AND ALVEOLAR BONE RESORPTION COINCIDENT TO PERIODONTAL DISEASE

Although a functional immune system is vital to protect against infectious diseases, dysfunctional immune responses may have deleterious effects on the host, which, in periodontal disease, is manifested in alveolar bone destruction and numerous systemic effects. Several studies have suggested that alveolar bone resorption coincident to periodontal disease was caused by the immune response, rather than directly by the infectious organism[4, 117]. Whether alveolar bone resorption will occur in response to gingival inflammation depends on two critical factors[12]. First, the concentration of proinflammatory mediators within the gingival tissue must be sufficient to activate pathways leading to bone resorption. Second, the inflammatory mediators must penetrate the gingival tissue to reach a critical distance from alveolar bone. There is increasing evidence that T$_H$17-type cytokines participate in the pathogenesis of periodontal disease, but whether their role is host-protective or host-destructive is uncertain, but is likely both roles[118-120].

During the pathogenesis of periodontitis, IL-17 appears within gingival tissues during the early stages of the inflammatory process, and begins to disappear from the gingiva at later stages of the inflammation[69, 49, 69, 98]. As these data were obtained from gingiva in a cross-sectional study, it was not certain whether this "removal" of IL-17 was a sign of impending resolution of the inflammation. A recent study of gingiva obtained from sites of severe clinical attachment loss indicated higher concentrations of IL-17, IL-23, IL-1-β, IL-6 and TNF-α within those tissues[70]. Thus, it seems that IL-17 could potentially be a factor for progression of periodontal disease from gingivitis to periodontitis when other related cytokine concentrations are also elevated.

Most of our knowledge about the relationship between IL-17 and bone resorption comes from studies of rheumatoid arthritis, a disease very similar to periodontal disease. IL-17, in conjunction with TNF-α, seems to be a primary factor in bone resorption at sites of inflammation at sites of rheumatoid arthritis[119-120]. IL-17 modulates the RANKL/OPG ratio: it increases RANKL (receptor activator of nuclear factor-kappa B ligand) expression and decreases osteoprotegerin (OPG) expression, resulting in enhanced formation of osteoclasts and bone resorption[121-122]. $T_H17$cells have been reported to also express higher levels of RANKL than T_H1 cells[106]. Similarly, IL-17 can induce osteoclast differentiation at other sites of inflammation, such as periodontal disease[12, 123].

In periodontal disease, there is an uncoupling of alveolar bone resorption from alveolar bone deposition, so that a net loss of alveolar bone occurs[124-125]. There is some evidence for IL-17 involvement in this destructive phase of periodontal disease[31,106].

During an inflammatory response involving bone, IL-17, IL-1-β, IL-6, and TNF-α, chemokines, and other mediators stimulate periosteal osteoblasts, enhancing their expression of RANKL on the osteoblast surface[122,125-127]. Bone resorption and deposition are regulated by the relative concentrations of RANKL, RANK (the RANKL receptor) and OPG on the surface of periosteal osteoblasts[126]. When RANKL expression is enhanced relative to OPG, RANKL is available to bind RANK on osteoclast precursors, enhancing the activation of osteoclast formation and bone resorption[126]. When OPG concentrations are high relative to RANKL expression, OPG binds RANKL, inhibiting it from binding to RANK[126]. Prevention of the binding of RANKL to RANK leads to reduced formation of osteoclasts and apoptosis of preexisting osteoclasts[126]. Relative decreases in OPG concentrations or increase in RANKL expression affect the RANKL/OPG ratio, which is indicative of the potential for bone resorption. The RANKL/OPG ratio is higher in individuals with periodontitis than in healthy persons[127-132]. An increased RANKL/OPG ratio may also be associated with the clinical severity of PD[131]. Thus, control of this ratio is likely to be crucial to control of alveolar bone loss coincident to periodontal disease and is likely regulated by the T_H17 immune pathway.

INDUCTION AND REGULATION OF THE T_H17 IMMUNE PATHWAY

A combination of TGF-β plus IL-6 has been reported to induce the differentiation of naïve T cells into T_H17 cells[39, 91-92]. T_H17 cells express a unique transcription factor, ROR-γt[133] which induces transcription of the IL-17 gene in naïve T-helper cells and is required for the development of IL-17 producing cells in the presence of IL-6 and TGF-β [134]. ROR-γt must act in cooperation with other transcription factors, including ROR-α, STAT3, IRF-4, and runt-related transcription factor (Runx1), for full commitment of precursors to the T_H17 lineage [96, 135-137]. Activation of ROR-γt also causes expression of the receptor for IL-23, indicating that IL-23 acts on T cells that are already committed to the T_H17 lineage. Exposure of developing T_H17 cells to IL-23 not only enhances their expression of IL-17 but also induces IL-22 and suppresses IL-10 and IFN-γ, which are not associated with the T_H17 phenotype[115]. Thus, IL-23 is essential for stabilizing the T_H17 phenotype.

IL-17 is neither a growth factor nor a differentiation factor for T_H17 cells and cannot amplify the T_H17 responses. However, IL-21, together with TGF-β, can amplify the T_H17 differentiation [93-95] and the expansion of the T_H17 cell population is defective in the absence of IL-21. TGF-β plus IL-21[138], TGF-β plus a combination of IL-6 and IL-23, or IL-6 plus IL-21[139] can induce the expression of ROR-c, the human counterpart of ROR-γt expressed in mice. Co-expression of the chemokine receptors CCR4 and CCR6[140] or expression of CCR2 in the absence of CCR5[141] also appears to define the T$_H$17 cells in humans. Inflamed tissues have large cells with a resemblance to plasma cells which produce IL17, suggesting that T$_H$17 cells acquire an activated phenotype at the tissue site[142].

The Treg cell population is driven to develop in opposition to T$_H$17, which is driven by TGF-β in the absence of STAT3. IL-2 is an important factor in expanding this lineage while simultaneously inhibiting T$_H$17 cell development[102]. There is a close relationship between Treg and T$_H$-17 cells, since TGF-β, which is required for the generation of Treg cells, is also necessary for the differentiation of T$_H$-17 cells[92] and the transcription factors required for the development of these two subsets might antagonize each other.

THE ROLE OF T$_H$17 CELLS IN OTHER DISEASES

Much of what we know about IL-17 in periodontal disease has been extrapolated from studies of other inflammatory diseases. Elevated IL-17 concentrations have been reported in individuals with a variety of autoimmune disease[143-144] and inflammatory bowel disease[145]. T$_H$17 cells can secrete IL-17 and IL-6 and TNF-α[146], and the presence of these cytokines has strong potential for initiating and intensifying systemic diseases. T$_H$17 cells have been shown to play important roles in many diseases ranging from inflammation and autoimmunity to infectious diseases and cancer[49, 98, 147-149]. IL-17 likely contributes to inflammatory pathologies such as atherosclerosis[150-151] and diabetes[152-154], which previously were attributed only to excessive levels of TNF-α and IL-6. For example, TNF-α and IL-6 are detectible in the sputum of COPD patients and are increased during exacerbations[155]. T$_H$17 cells attract numerous cells into inflamed tissues. These cells, acting in synergy with TNF-α and IL1-β, provides a potent inducer of CCL20, which is strongly chemotactic for lymphocytes. In this way, T$_H$17 cells are involved in psoriasis[156], multiple sclerosis[147], inflammatory bowel syndrome[145], and corticosteroid-resistant asthma[156-157].

Certain types of cancers use inflammatory mediators to induce angiogenesis and tissue remodeling[158]. Thus, IL-17 can promote tumor growth through the enhancement of angiogenesis-mediating factor production[159]. However, it has also been shown that IL-17 production can inhibit tumor cell growth due to the recruitment of CD8+ T lymphocytes with cytotoxic activity against the tumor[160].

Several studies have demonstrated a key role of IL-17 or IL-23 in the progression of arthritis[161-165]. Blockade of IL-17 after disease onset was able to prevent cartilage and bone destruction, leading to amelioration of the clinical symptoms of the disease[163]. Human IL-17 cells within the arthritic synovium expressed RANKL[106], which induces osteoclastogenesis[166]. Synovial fluids from human samples contained high levels of both CCL20 and IL-17, suggesting that both are required for disease progression[167-170]. IL-17 induced synovial fibroblasts to produce IL-6, IL-8, MMP-1, and MMP-3, contributing to the destruction of the joint[168]. In rheumatoid arthritis patients, the production of TNF, IL-1 and IL-17 by synovial cells is predictive of joint destruction[171].

Many reports have identified the presence of T$_H$-17 cytokines (IL-1-α, IL-1-β, IL-6, IL-17, IL-17F, and TNF-α) in psoriatic lesions[172-174]. A clinical trial using anti-IL-12/IL-23 p40 neutralizing antibodies has been conducted. Patients receiving the neutralizing antibodies had a significant improvement in psoriatic areas and disease index, demonstrating a crucial role for T_H-17 in the pathogenesis of that disease[175].

FUTURE QUESTIONS ABOUT THE T_H17 PATHWAY

Efforts are underway to test drugs that target the T_H17 pathway in humans[176-177]. Because periodontal disease cannot be characterized solely as a T_H1 or T_H2 response, discovery of the T_H17 cell subset may provide insight into the basis for this disease. Specific deletion of the T_H17 subset may be a more effective therapy than blocking IL-12, IL-17 or IL-23 alone. Specific deletion of the T_H17 cells would keep the IL-12/T_H1 immune pathway intact, which is an effective pathway for targeting many intracellular microbial infections and is important for the IFN-γ production that is required to resolve these infections.

Understanding the intricate interplay between cytokines and bone may allow for therapeutic intervention in diseases caused by an imbalance in bone remodeling. It seems that IL-17 blockade could be a treatment for periodontal disease; however, studies in rodents suggest that alveolar bone loss is exacerbated in animals infected with *P. gingivalis,* that were deficient in IL-17 receptors[178]. The amplification and propogation of the inflammatory response through gingival tissue is critical to the pathogenesis of periodontal disease. However, it is the spread of the response to the adjacent alveolar bone that drives the cellular machinery involved in bone loss. The RANKL-RANK-OPG axis is clearly involved in the regulation of bone metabolism in periodontitis and an increase in the relative expression of RANKL or a decrease in OPG can tip the balance in favor of alveolar bone loss. Interference with this axis may have a protective effect on alveolar bone loss. Thus, future therapeutic options are likely to have regulation of the RANK-RANKL-OPG axis as their goal.

LITERATURE CITED

[1]   Pihlstrom BL, Michalowicz BS, Johnson NW. *Periodontal diseases.* Lancet 2005; 366:1809-1820.

[2]   Socransky SS, Haffajee AD, Cugini MA, Smith C, Kent RL. *Microbial complexes in subgingival plaque.* J Clin Periodontol 1998; 25:134-144.

[3]   Bartova J, Kratka-Opatrina Z, Prochazkova J, et al. *Th1 and Th2 cytokine profile in patients with early onset periodontitis and their healthy siblings.* Mediators Inflamm 2000; 9:115-120.

[4]   Taubman MA, Valverde P, Han X, Kawai T. *Immune response: the key to bone resorption in periodontal disease.* J Periodontol 2005; 76(Suppl. 11):2033S-2041S.

[5]   Gemmell E, Yamazaki K, Seymour GJ. *The role of T cells in periodontal disease: homeostasis and autoimmunity.* Periodontol 2000 2007; 43:14-40.

[6]   Shapira L, van Dyke TE, Hart TC. *A localized absence of interleukin-4 triggers periodontal disease activity: a novel hyothesis.* Med Hypotheses 1992; 39:319-322.

[7]   Gilthorpe MS, Zamzuri AT, Griffiths GS, Maddick IH, Eaton KA, Johnson NW. *Unification of the "burst" and "linear" theories of periodontal disease progression: a multilevel manifestation of the same phenomenon.* J Dent Res 2003; 82:200-205.

[8]   Goodson JM, Tanner AC, Haffajee AD, Somberger GC, Socransky SS. *Patterns of progression and regression of advanced destructive periodontal disease.* J Clin Periodontol 1982; 9:472-481.

[9]   Gaffen SL, Hajishengallis G. *A new inflammatory cytokine on the block: re-thinking periodontal disease and the Th1/Th2 paradigm in the context of Th17 and IL-17.* J Dent Res 2008; 87:817-828.

[10] Salvi GE, Lang NP. *Host response modulation in the management of periodontal diseases.* J Clin Periodontol 2005; 32(Suppl. 6):108-129.

[11] Garlet GP, Cardoso CR, Silva TA, et al. *Cytokine pattern determines the progression of experimental periodontal disease induced by Actinobacillus actinomycetemcomitans through the modulation of MMPs, RANKL, and their physiological inhibitors.* Oral Microbiol Immunol 2006; 21:12-20.

[12] Graves DT, Cochran D. *The contribution of interleukin-1 and tumor necrosis factor to periodontal tissue destruction.* J Periodontol 2003; 74:391-401.

[13] Bachmann MF, Kopf M. *Balancing protective immunity and immunopathology.* Curr Opin Immunol 2002; 14:413-419.

[14] Ebersole JL, Taubman MA. T*he protective nature of host responses in periodontal diseases.* Periodontol 2000 1994; 5:112-141.

[15] Baker PJ. *The role of immune responses in bone loss during periodontal disease.* Microbes Infect 2000; 2:1181-1192.

[16] Zambon JJ. P*eriodontal diseases: microbial factors.* Ann Periodontol 1996; 1:879-925.

[17] Ebersole JL, Cappelli D, Holt SC. *Periodontal diseases: to protect or not to protect is the question?* Acta Odontol Scand 2001; 59:161-166.

[18] Hao L, Sasaki H, Stashenko P. *B-cell deficiency predisposes mice to disseminating anaerobic infections: protection by passive antibody transfer.* Infect Immun 2000; 68:5645-5651.

[19] Teng YT, Taylor GW, Scannapieco F, et al. *Periodontal health and systemic disorders.* J Can Dent Assoc 2002; 68:188-192.

[20] Mahanonda R, Pichyangkul S. *Toll-like receptors and their role in periodontal health and disease.* Periodontol 2000 2007; 43:41-55.

[21] Sandros J, Karlsson C, Lappin DF, Madianos PN, Kinane DF, Papapanou PN. *Cytokine responses of oral epithelial cells to Porphyromonas gingivalis infection.* J Dent Res 2000; 79:1808-1814.

[22] Steffen MJ, Holt SC, Ebersole JL. *Porphyromonas gingivalis induction of mediator and cytokine secretion by human gingival fibroblasts.* Oral Microbiol Immunol 2000; 15:172-180.

[23] Sugano N, Ikeda K, Oshikawa M, Sawamoto Y, Tanaka H, Ito K. *Differential cytokine induction by two types of Porphyromonas gingivalis.* Oral Microbiol Immunol 2004; 19:121-123.

[24] Hiramine H, Watanabe K, Hamada N, Umemoto T. *Porphyromonas gingivalis 67-kDa fimbriae induced cytokine production and ostoclast differentiation utilizing TLR2.* FEMS Microbiol Lett 2003; 229:49-55.

[25] Amano A, Nakagawa I, Okahashi N, Hamada N. *Variations of Porphyromonas gingivalis fimbriae in relation to microbial pathogenesis.* J Periodontal Res 2004; 39:136-142.

[26] Pulendran B, Kumar P, Cutler CW, Mohamadzadeh M, Van Dyke T, Banchereau J. *Lipopolysaccharides from distinct pathogens induce different classes of immune responses in vivo.* J Immunol 2001; 167:5067-5076.

[27] Zhou Q, Desta T, Fenton M, Graves DT, Amar S. *Cytokine profiling of macrophages exposed to Porphyromonas gingivalis, its lipopolysaccharide, or its FimA protein.* Infect Immun 2005; 73:935-943.

[28] Suthin K, Matsushita M, Machigashira M, et al. *Enhanced expression of vascular endothelial growth factor by periodontal pathogens in gingival fibroblasts.* J Periodontal Res 2003; 38:90-96.

[29] Tabeta K, Yamazaki K, Akashi S, et al. *Toll-like receptors confer responsiveness to lipopolysaccharide from Porphyromonas gingivalis in human gingival fibroblasts.* Infect Immun 2000; 68:3731-3735.

[30] Wang PL, Ohura K. *Porphyromonas gingivalis lipopolysaccharide signaling in gingival fibroblasts-CD14 and Toll-like receptors.* Crit Rev Oral Biol Med 2002; 13:132-142.

[31] Oda T, Yoshie H, Yamazaki K. *Porphyromonas gingivalis antigen preferentially stimulates T cells to express IL-17 but not receptor activator of NF-kappaB ligand in vitro.* Oral Microbiol Immunol 2003; 18:30-36.

[32] Dong C, Flavell RA. *Cell fate decision: T-helper 1 and 2 subsets in immune reponses.* Arthritis Res 2000; 2:179-188.

[33] Teng YT. *The role of acquired immunity and periodontal disease progression.*Crit Rev Oral Biol Med 2003; 14:237-252.

[34] Szabo SJ, Sullivan BM, Peng SL, Glimcher LH. *Molecular mechanisms regulating Th1 immune responses.* Annu Rev Immunol 2003; 21:713-758.

[35] Glimcher LH. *Trawling for treasure: tales of t-bet.* Nat Immunol 2007;8:448-450.

[36] Paul WE, Seder RA. *Lymphocyte responses and cytokines.* Cell 1994; 76:241-251.

[37] Mathur AN, Chang HC, Zisoulis DG, et al. *Stat 3 and Stat 4 direct development of IL-17 secreting Th cells.* J Immunol 2007; 178:4901-4907.

[38] Szabo SJ, Kim ST, Costa GL, Zhang X, Fathman CG, Glimcher LH. *A novel transcription factor, T-bet, directs Th1 lineage commitment.* Cell 2000; 100: 655-669.

[39] Veldhoen M, Hocking RJ, Atkins CJ, Locksley RM, Stockinger B. *TGFbeta in the context of an inflammatory cytokine milieu supports de novo differentiation of IL-17-producing T cells.* Immunity 2006; 24:179-189.

[40] Murphy KM, Reiner SL. *The lineage decisions of helper T cells.* Nat Rev Immunol 2002; 2:933-944.

[41] Yamashita M, Onodera A, Nakayama T. *Immune mechanisms of allergic airway disease: regulation by transcription factors.* Crit Rev Immunol 2007; 27:539-546.

[42] Ho IC, Hodge MR, Rooney JW, Glimcher LH. *The proto-oncogene c-maf is responsible for tissue -specific expression of interleukin-4.* Cell 1996; 85:973-983.

[43] Zheng W, Flavell RA. *The transcription factor GATA-3 is necessary and sufficient for Th2 cytokine gene expression in CD4 T cells.* Cell 1997; 89:587-596.

[44] Castellino F, Germain RN. *Cooperation between CD4+ and CD8+ T cells: when, where, and how.* Annu Rev Immunol 2006; 24:519-540.

[45] Harrington LE, Hatton RD, Mangan PR, et al. *Interleukin 17-producing CD4+ effector T cells develop via a lineage distinct from the T helper type 1 and 2 lineages.* Nat Immunol 2005; 6:1123-1132.

[46] Fujihashi K, Yamamoto M, Hiroi T, Bamberg TV, McGhee JR, Kiyono H. *Selected Th1 and Th2 cytokine mRNA expression by CD4(+) T cells isolated from inflamed human gingival tissues.* Clin Exp Immunol 1996; 103:422-428.

[47] Berglundh T, Liljenberg B, Lindhe J. *Some cytokine profiles of T-helper cells in lesions of advanced periodontitis.* J Clin Periodontol 2002; 29:705-709.

[48] Prabhu A, Michalowicz BS, Mathur A. *Detection of local and systemic cytokines in adult periodontitis.* J Periodontol 1996; 67:515-522.

[49] Takahashi K, Azuma T, Motohira H, Kinane DF, Kitetsu S. *The potential role of interleukin-17 in the immunopathology of periodontal disease.* J Clin Periodontol 2005; 32:369-374.

[50] Ukai T, Mori Y, Onoyama M, Hara Y. *Immunohistological study of interferon-gamma- and interleukin-4-bearing cells in human periodontitis gingiva.* Arch Oral Biol 2001; 46:901-908.

[51] Gemmell E, Yamazaki K, Seymour GJ. *Destructive periodontitis lesions are determined by the nature of the lymphocytic response.* Crit Rev Oral Biol Med 2002; 13:17-34.

[52] Alayan J, Gemmell E, Ford P, et al. *The role of cytokines in a Porphyromonas gingivalis-induced murine abscess model.* Oral Microbiol Immunol 2007; 22:304-312.

[53] Hajishengallis G, Shakhatreh MA, Wang M, Liang S. *Complement receptor 3 blockade promotes IL-12-mediated clearance of Porphyromonas gingivalis and negates its virulence in vivo.* J Immunol 2007; 179:2359-2367.

[54] Gowen M, Nedwin GE, Mundy GR. *Preferential inhibition of cytokine-stimulated bone resorption by recombinant interferon gamma.* J Bone Miner Res 1986; 1:469-474.

[55] Horwood NJ, Elliott J, Martin TJ, Gillespie MT. *IL-12 alone and in synergy with IL-18 inhibits osteoclast formation in vitro.* J Immunol 2001; 166:4915-4921.

[56] Iwasaki A, Medzhitov R. *Toll-like receptor control of the adaptive immune responses.* Nat Immunol 2004; 5:987-995.

[57] Re F, Strominger JL. *Toll-like receptor 2 (TLR2) and TLR4 differentially activate human dendritic cells.* J Biol Chem 2001; 276:37692-37699.

[58] Burns F, Marrack PC, Kappler JW, Janeway CA. *Functional heterogeneity among the T-derived lymphocytes of the mouse. IV. Nature of spontaneously induced suppressor cells.* J Immunol 1975; 114:1345-1347.

[59] Taams LS, Palmer DB, Akbar AN, Robinson DS, Brown Z, Hawrylowicz CM. *Regulatory T cells in human disease and their potential for therapeutic manipulation.* Immunology 2006; 118:1-9.

[60] Ito H, Honda T, Domon H, et al. *Gene expression analysis of the CD4+ T-cell clones derived from gingival tissues of periodontitis patients.* Oral Microbiol Immunol 2005; 20:382-386.

[61] Seymour GJ, Gemmell E. *Cytokines in periodontal disease: Where to from here?* Acta Odontol Scand 2001; 59:167-173.

[62] Kaplan G, Luster AD, Hancock G, Cohn ZA. *The expression of a gamma interferon-induced protein (IP-10) in delayed immune responses in human skin.* J Exp Med 1987; 166:1098-1108.

[63] Loetscher P, Uguccioni M, Bordoli L, et al. *CCR5 is characteristic of Th1 lymphocytes.* Nature 1998; 391:344-345.

[64]   Loetscher P, Pellegrino A, Gong JH, et al. *The ligands of CXC chemokine receptor 3, I-TAC,, Mig, and IP10, are natural antagonists for CCR3*. J Biol Chem 2001; 276:2986-2991.

[65]   Sallusto F, Lanzavecchia A, Mackay CR. *Chemokines and chemokine receptors in T-cell priming and Th1/Th2-mediated responses*. Immunol Today 1998; 19:568-574.

[66]   Sallusto F, Lenig D, Mackay CR, Lanzavecchia A. *Flexible programs of chemokine receptor expression on human polarized T helper 1 and 2 lymphocytes*. J Exp Med 1998; 187:875-883.

[67]   Bonecchi R, Bianchi G, Bordignon PP, et al. *Differential expression of chemokine receptors and chemotactic responsiveness of type 1 T helper cells (Th 1s) and Th2s*. J Exp Med 1998; 187:129-134.

[68]   Gu L, Tseng S, Horner RM, Tam C, Loda M, Rollins BJ. *Control of T_H2 polarization by the chemokine monocyte chemoattractant protein-1*. Nature 2000; 404:407-411.

[69]   Johnson RB, Wood N, Serio FG. *Interleukin-11 and IL-17 and the pathogenesis of periodontal disease*. J Periodontol 2004; 75:37-43.

[70]   Lester SR, Bain JL, Johnson RB, Serio FG. *Gingival concentrations of interleukin-23 and -17 at healthy sites and at sites of clinical attachment loss*. J Periodontol 2007; 78:1545-1550.

[71]   Harrington LE, Mangan PR, Weaver CT. *Expanding the effector CD4 T-cell repertoire: the Th17 lineage*. Curr Opin Immunol 2006; 18:349-356.

[72]   Miyamoto M, Prause O, Sjostrand M, Laan M, Lotvall J, Linden A. *Endogenous IL-17 as a mediator of neutrophil recruitment caused by endotoxin exposure in mouse airways*. J Immunol 2003; 170:4665-4672.

[73]   Park H, Li Z, Yang XO, et al. *A distinct lineage of CD4 T cells regulates tissue inflammation by producing interleukin 17*. Nat Immunol 2005; 6:1133-1141.

[74]   Ruddy MJ, Shen F, Smith JB, Sharma A, Gaffen SL. *Interleukin-17 regulates expression of the CXC chemokine LIX/CXCL5 in osteoblasts: Implications for inflammation and neutrophil recruitment*. J Leukoc Biol 2004; 76:135-144.

[75]   Shen F, Ruddy MJ, Plamondon P, Gaffen SL. *Cytokines link osteoblasts and inflammation: Microarray analysis of interleukin-17- and TNF-alpha-induced genes in bone cells*. J Leukoc Biol 2005; 77:388-399.

[76]   Yao Z, Fanslow WC, Seldin MF, et al. *Herpesvirus saimiri encodes a new cytokine, IL-17, which binds to a novel cytokine receptor*. Immunity 1995; 3:811-821.

[77]   Ye P, Rodriguez FH, Kanaly S, et al. *Requirement of interelukin 17 receptor signaling for lung CXC chemokine and granulocyte colony-stimulating factor expression, neutrophil recruitment, and host defense*. J Exp Med 2001; 194:519-527.

[78]   Stark MA, Huo Y, Burcin TL, Morris MA, Olson TS, Ley K. *Phagocytosis of apoptotic neutrophils regulates granulopoiesis via IL-23 and IL-17*. Immunity 2005; 22:285-294.

[79]   Cruz A, Khander SA, Torrado E, et al. *Cutting edge: IFN-{gamma} regulates the induction and expansion of IL-17 producing CD4 T cells during mycobacterial infection*. J Immunol 2006; 177:1416-1420.

[80]   Infante-Duarte C, Horton HF, Byrne MC, et al. *Microbial lipopeptides induce the production of IL-17 in Th cells*. J Immunol 2000; 165:6107-6115.

[81]   Aggarwal S, Ghilardi N, Xie MH, de Sauvage FJ, Gurney AL. *Interleukin-23 promotes distinct CD4 T cell activation state characterized by the production of interleukin-17*. J Biol Chem 2003; 278:1910-1914.

[82]   Kolls JK, Linden A. *Interelukin-17 family members and inflammation.* Immunity 2004; 21:467-476.

[83]   Ouyand W, Kolls JK, Zheng Y. *The biological functions of T helper 17 cell effector cytokines in inflammation.* Immunity 2008; 28:454-467.

[84]   Dong C. *TH17 cells in development: an updated view of their molecular identity and genetic programming.* Nat Rev Immunol 2008; 8:337-348.

[85]   Fossiez F, Djossou O, Chomarat P, et al. *T cell interleukin-17 induces stromal cells to produce proinflammatory and hematopoietic cytokines.* J Exp Med 1996; 183:2593-2603.

[86]   Gor DO, Rose NR, Greenspan NS. *TH-1-TH2: a procrustean paradigm.* Nat Immunol 2003; 4:503-505.

[87]   Weaver CT, Hatton RD, Mangan PR, Harrington LE. *IL-17 family cytokines and the expanding diversity of effector T cell lineages.* Annu Rev Immunol 2007; 25:821-852.

[88]   Steinman L. *A brief history of T(H)17, the first major revision in the T(H)1/T(H)2 hypothesis of T cell-mediated tissue damage.* Nat Med 2007; 13:139-145.

[89]   Weaver CT, Murphy KM. *T-cell subsets: the more the merrier.* Curr Biol 2007; 17:R61-R63.

[90]   Cua DJ, Sherlock J, Chen Y, et al. *Interleukin-23 rather than interleukin-12 is the critical cytokine for autoimmune inflammation of the brain.* Nature 2003; 421:744-748.

[91]   Mangan PR, Harrington LE, O'Quinn DB, et al. *Transforming growth factor-beta induces development of the T(H) 17 lineage.* Nature 2006;441:231-234.

[92]   Bettelli E, Carrier Y, Gao W, et al. *Reciprocal developmental pathways for the generation of pathogenic effector TH17 and regulatory T cells.* Nature 2006; 441:235-238.

[93]   Korn T, Bettelli E, Gao W, et al. *IL-21 initiates an alternative pathway to induce proinflammatory T(H) cells.* Nature 2007; 448:484-487.

[94]   Nurieva R, Yang XO, Martinez G, et al. *Essential autocrine regulation by IL-21 in the generation of inflammatory T cells.* Nature 2007; 448:480-483.

[95]   Zhou L, Ivanov IL, Spolski R, et al. *IL-6 programs T(H)-17 cell differentation by promoting sequential engagement of the IL-21 and IL-23 pathways.* Nat Immunol 2007; 8:967-974.

[96]   Yang XO, Papopoulos AD, Nurieva R, et al. *STAT3 regulates cytokine-mediated generation of inflammatory helper T cells.* J Biol Chem 2007; 282:9358-9363.

[97]   van Beelen AJ, Zelinkova Z, Taanman-Kueter EW, et al. *Stimulation of the intracellular bacterial sensor NOD2 programs dendritic cells to promote interleukin-17 production in human memory T cells.* Immunity 2007; 27:660-669.

[98]   Vernal R, Dutzan N, Chaparro A, Puente J, Antonieta Valenzuela M, Gamonal J. *Levels of interleukin-17 in gingival crevicular fluid and in supernatants of cellular cultures of gingival tissue from patients with chronic periodontitis.* J Clin Periodontol 2005; 32:383-389.

[99]   Colic M, Vasilijic S, Gazivoda D, Vucevic D, Marjanovic M, Lukic A. *Interleukin-17 plays a role in exacerbation of inflammation within chronic periapical lesions.* Eur J Oral Sci 2007; 115:315-320.

[100] Lester SR, Bain JL, Serio FG, Johnson RB. *Relationship between the gingival sulcus depth and interleukin-1 isoform concentrations within the adjacent gingival tissue.* J Periodontal Res 2009; 44:323-329.

[101] Beklen A, Ainola M, Hukkanen M, Gurgan C, Sorsa T, Konttinen YT. *MMPs, IL-1, and TNF are regulated by IL-17 in periodontitis.* J Dent Res 207; 86:347-351.

[102] Laurence A, Tato CM, Davidson TS, et al. *Interleukin-2 signaling via STAT5 constrains T helper 17 cell generation.* Immunity 2007; 26:371-381.

[103] Chen Z, Laurence A, Kanno Y, et al. *Selective regulatory function of Socs3 in the formation of IL-17-secreting T cells.* Proc Natl Acad Sci USA 2006;103:8137-8142.

[104] Stumhofer JS, Laurence A, Wilson EH, et al. *Interleukin 27 negatively regulates the development of interleukin 17-producing T helper cells during chronic inflammation of the central nervous system.* Nat Immunol 2006; 7:937-945.

[105] Tesmer LA, Lundy SK, Sarkar S, Fox DA. *Th17 cells in human disease.* Immunol Rev 2008; 223:87-113.

[106] Sato K, Suematsu A, Okamoto K, et al. *Th17 functions as an osteoclastogenic helper T cell subset that links T cell activation and bone destruction.* J Exp Med 2006; 203:2673-2682.

[107] Ohyama H, Kato-Kogoe N, Kuhara A, et al. *The involvement of IL-23 and the Th17 pathway in periodontitis.* J Dent Res 2009; 88:633-638.

[108] Sheibanie AF, Yen JH, Khayrullina T, et al. *The proinflammatory effect of prostaglandin E2 in experimental inflammatory bowel disease is mediated through the IL-23-->IL-17 axis.* J Immunol 2007; 178:8138-8147.

[109] Jovanic DV, Di Battista JA, Martel-Pelletier J, et al. *Modulation of TIMP-1 synthesis by antiinflammatory cytokines and prostaglandin E2 in interleukin 17 stimulated human monocytes/macrophages.* J Rheumatol 2001; 28:712-718.

[110] LeGrand A, Fermor B, Fink C, et al. *Interleukin-1, tumor necrosis factor alpha, and interleukin-17 synergistically up-regulate nitric oxide and prostaglandin E2 production in explants of human osteoarthritic knee menisci.* Arthritis Rheum 2001; 44:2078-2083.

[111] Roberts FA, Houston LS, Lukehart SA, Mancl LA, Persson GR, Page RC. *Periodontitis vaccine decreases local prostaglandin E2 levels in a primate model.* Infect Immun 2004; 72:1166-1168.

[112] Heasman PA, Benn DK, Kelly PJ, Seymour RA, Aitken D. *The use of topical flurbiprofen as an adjunct to non-surgical management of periodontal disease.* J Clin Periodontol 1993; 20:457-464.

[113] Yen D, Cheung J, Scheerens H, et al. *IL-23 is essential for T cell-mediated colitis and promotes inflammation via IL-17 and IL-6.* J Clin Invest 2006; 116:1310-1316.

[114] Hue S, Ahern P, Buonocore S, et al. *Interleukin-23 drives innate and T-cell-mediated intestinal inflammation.* J Exp Med 2006; 203:2473-2483.

[115] McGeachy MJ, Bak-Jensen KS, Chen Y, et al. *TGF-beta and IL-6 drive the production of IL-17 and IL-10 by T cells and restrain T(H)-17 cell-mediated pathology.* Nat Immunol 2007; 8:1390-1397.

[116] Gihilardi N, Ouyang W. *Targeting the development and effector functions of Th17 cells.* Semin Immunol 2007; 19:383-393.

[117] Baker PJ. *The role of immune responses in bone loss during periodontal disease.* Microbes Infect 2000; 2:1181-1192.

[118] Kramer JM, Gaffen S. *Interleukin-17: a new paradigm in inflammation, autoimmunity and therapy.* J Periodontol 2007; 78:1083-1093.

[119] Van Bezooijen RL, Farih-Sips HC, Papapoulos SE, Lowik CW. *Interleukin-17: a new bone acting cytkine in vitro.* J Bone Miner Res 1999; 14:1513-1521.

[120] Van Bezooijen RL, Papapoulos SE, Lowik CW. *Effect of interleukin-17 on nitric oxide production and osteoclastic bone resorption: Is there dependency on nuclear factor-kappaB and receptor activator of nuclear factor kappaB (RANK)/RANK ligand signaling?* Bone 2001; 28:378-386.

[121] Lubberts E, van den Bersselaar L, Oppers-Walgreen B, et al. *IL-17 promotes bone erosion in murine collagen-induced arthritis through loss of the receptor activator of NF-kappa B ligand/osteoprotegerin balance.* J Immunol 2003; 170:2655-2662.

[122] Nakashima T, Kobayashi Y, Yamasaki S, et al. *Protein expression and functional difference of membrane-bound and soluble receptor activator of NF-kappaB ligand: Modulation of the expression by osteotropic factors and cytokines.* Biochem Biophys Res Commun 2000; 275:768-775.

[123] Azuma M. *Fundamental mechanisms of host immune responses to infection.* J Periodontal Res 2006; 41:361-373.

[124] Graves D, Liu R, Alikhani M, Al-Mashat H, Trackman P. *Diabetes-enhanced inflammation and apoptosis-Impact on periodontal pathology.* J Dent Res 2006; 85:15-21.

[125] Lerner UH. *Inflammation-induced bone remodeling in periodontal disease and the influence of post-menopausal osteoporosis.* J Dent Res 2006; 85:596-607.

[126] Boyle WJ, Simonet WS, Lacey DL. *Osteoclast differentiation and activation.* Nature 2003; 423:337-342.

[127] Kawai T, Matsuyama T, Hosokawa Y, et al. *B and T lymphocytes are the primary source of RANKL in the bone resorptive lesion of periodontal disease.* Am J Pathol 2006; 169:987-998.

[128] Wara-aswapati N, Surarit R, Chayasadom A, Boch JA, Pitiphat W. *RANKL upregulation associated with periodontitis and Porphyromonas gingivalis.* J Periodontol 2007; 78:1062-1069.

[129] Crotti T, Smith MD, Hirsch R, et al. *Receptor activator NF kappaB ligand (RANKL) and osteoprotegerin (OPG) protein expression in periodontitis.* J Periodontal Res 2003; 38:380-387.

[130] Mogi M, Otogoto J, Ota N, Togari A. *Differential expression of RANKL and osteoprotegerin in gingival crevicular fluid of patients with periodontitis.* J Dent Res 2004; 83:166-169.

[131] Bostanci N, Ilgenli T, Emingil G, et al. *Gingival crevicular fluid levels of RANKL and OPG is periodontal diseases: implications of their relative ratio.* J Clin Periodontol 2007; 34:370-376.

[132] Lu HK, Chen YL, Chang HC, Li CL, Kuo MY. *Identification of the osteoprotegerin/receptor activator of nuclear factor-kappa B ligand system in gingival crevicular fluid and tissue of patients with chronic periodontitis.* J Periodontal Res 2006; 41:354-360.

[133] Ivanov II, McKenzie BS, Zhou L, et al. *The orphan nuclear receptor RORgammat directs the differentiation program of proinflammatory IL-17(+) T helper cells.* Cell 2006; 126:1121-1133.

[134] Zhou L, Lopes JE, Chong MM, et al. *TGF-beta-induced Foxp3 inhibits T(H)17 cell differentation by antagonizing RORgammat function.* Nature 2008; 453:236-240.

[135] Yang XO, Pappu BP, Nurieva R, et al. *T helper 17 lineage differentiation is programmed by orphan nuclear receptors RORalpha and RORgamma.* Immunity 2008; 28:29-39.

[136] Brustle A, Heink S, Huber M, et al. *The development of inflammatory T(H)-17 cells requires interferon-regulatory factor 4.* Nat Immunol 2007; 8:958-966.

[137] Zhang F, Meng G, Strober W. *Interactions among the transcription factors Runx1, RORgammat and Foxp3 regulate the differentiation of interleukin 17-producing T cells.* Nat Immunol 2008; 9:1297-1306.

[138] Yang L, Anderson DE, Baecher-Allan C, et al. *IL-21 and TGF-beta are required for differentiation of human T(H)17 cells.* Nature 2008; 454:350-352.

[139] Manel N, Unutmaz D, Littman DR. *The differentiation of human T(H)-17 cells requires transforming growth factor-beta and induction of the nuclear receptor RORgammat.* Nat Immunol 2008; 9:641-649.

[140] Acosta-Rodriguez EV, Rivino L, Geginat J, et al. *Surface phenotype and antigenic specificity of human interleukin 17-producing T helper memory cells.* Nat Immunol 2007; 8:639-646.

[141] Sato W, Aranami T, Yamamura T. *Cutting edge: human Th17 cells are identified as bearing CCR2+CCR5- phenotype.* J Immunol 2007; 178:7525-7529.

[142] Page G, Sattler A, Kersten S, Thiel A, Radbruch A, Miossec P. *Plasma cell-like morphology of Th1-cytokine-producing cells associated with the loss of CD3 expression.* Am J Pathol 2004; 164:409-417.

[143] Kotake S, Udagawa N, Takahashi N, et al. *IL-17 in synovial fluids from patients with rheumatoid arthritis is a potent stimulator of osteoclastogenesis.* J Clin Invest 1999; 103:1345-1352.

[144] Wong CK, Ho CY, Li EK, Lam CW. *Elevation of proinflammatory cytokine (IL-18, IL-17, IL-12) and Th2 cytokine (IL-4) concentrations in patients with systemic lupus erythematosis.* Lupus 2000; 9:589-593.

[145] Duerr RH, Taylor KD, Brant SR, et al. *A genome-wide association study identifies IL23R as an inflammatory bowel disease gene.* Science 2006; 314:1461-1463.

[146] Weaver CT, Harrington LE, Mangan PR, Gavrieli M, Murphy KM. *Th17: An effector CD4 T cell lineage with regulatory T cell ties.* Immunity 2006; 24:677-688.

[147] Matsuvicius D, Kivisakk P, He B, et al. *Interleukin-17 mRNA expression in blood and CSF mononuclear cells is augmented in multiple sclerosis.* Mult Scler 1999; 5:101-104.

[148] Teunissen MB, Koomen CW, de Waal Malefyt R, Wierenga EA, Bos JD. *Interleukin-17 and interferon-gamma synergize in the enhancement of proinflammatory cytokine production by human keratinocytes.* J Invest Dermatol 1998; 111:645-649.

[149] Zhang Z, Zhang M, Bindas J, Schwarzenberger P, Kolls JK. *Critical role of IL-17 receptor signaling in acute TNBS-induced colitis.* Inflamm Bowel Dis 2006; 12:382-388.

[150] Hashmi S, Zeng QT. *Role of interleukin-17 and interleukin-17-induced cytokines interleukin-6 and interleukin-8 in unstable coronary artery disease.* Coron Artery Dis 2006; 17:699-706.

[151] von der Thusen JH, Kuiper J, van Berkel TJ, Biessen EA. *Interleukins in atherosclerosis: Molecular pathways and therapeutic potential.* Pharmacol Rev 2003; 55:133-166.

[152] Miljkovic D, Cvetkovic I, Momcilovic M, Maksimovic-lvanic D, Stosic-Grujicic S, Trajkovic V. *Interleukin-17 stimulates inducible nitric oxide synthase-dependent toxicity in mouse beta cells.* Cell Mol Life Sci 2005; 62:2658-2668.

[153] Vukkadapu SS, Belli JM, Ishii K, et al. *Dynamic interaction between T cell-mediated beta-cell damage and beta-cell repair in the run up to autoimmune diabetes of the NOD mouse.* Physiol Genomics 2005; 21:201-211.

[154] Genco RJ. *A proposed model linking inflammation to obesity, diabetes and periodontal infections.* J Periodontol 2005; 76 (Suppl. 11):2075-2084.

[155] Chung KF. *Cytokines as targets in chronic obstructive pulmonary disease.* Curr Drug Targets 2006; 7:675-681.

[156] Krueger GG, Langley RG, Leonardi C, et al. *A human interleukin-12/23 monoclonal antibody for the treatment of psoriasis.* N Engl J Med 2007; 356:580-592.

[157] Barczyk A, Pierzchala W, Sozanska E. *Interleukin-17 in sputum correlates with airway hyperresponsiveness to methacholine.* Respir Med 2003; 97:726-733.

[158] Coussens LM, Werb Z. *Inflammation and cancer.* Nature 2002; 420:860-867.

[159] Numasaki M, Watanabe M, Suzuki T, et al. *IL-17 enhances the net angiogenic activity and in vivo growth of human non-small cell lung cancer in SCID mice through promoting CXCR-2-dependent angiogenesis.* J Immunol 2005; 175:6177-6189.

[160] Benchetrit F, Ciree A, Vives V, et al. *Interleukin-17 inhibits tumor cell growth by means of a T-cell-dependent mechanism.* Blood 2002; 99:2114-2121.

[161] Nakae S, Urakawa T, Yamamoto M, et al. *Suppression of immune-induction of collagen-induced arthritis in IL-17-deficient mice.* J Immunol 2003; 171:6173-6177.

[162] Nakae S, Saijo S, Horai R, et al. *IL-17 production from activated T cells is required for the spontaneous development of destructive arthritis in mice deficient in IL-1 receptor antagonist.* Proc Natl Acad Sci USA 2003; 100:5986-5990.

[163] Lubberts E, Koenders MI, Oppers-Walgreen B, et al. *Treatment with a neutralizing anti-murine interleukin-17 antibody after the onset of collagen-induced arthritis reduces joint inflammation, cartilage destruction, and bone erosion.* Arthritis Rheum 2004; 50:650-659.

[164] Ruddy MJ, Shen F, Smith JB, et al. *Interleukin-17 regulates expression of the CXC chemokine LIX/CXCL5 in osteoblasts: implications for inflammation and neutrophil recruitment.* J Leukoc Biol 2004;76:135-144.

[165] Murphy CA, Langrish CL, Chen Y, et al. *Divergent pro- and anti-inflammatory roles for IL-23 and IL-12 in joint autoimmune inflammation.* J Exp Med 2003; 198:1951-1957.

[166] Nakashima T, Takayanagi H. *The dynamic interplay between osteoclasts and the immune system.* Arch Biochem Biophys 2008; 473:166-171.

[167] Hirota K, Yoshitumi H, Hashimoto M, et al. *Preferential recruitment of CCR6-expressing Th17 cells to inflamed joints via CCL20 in rheumatoid arthritis and its animal model.* J Exp Med 2007; 204:2803-2812.

[168] Agarwal S, Misra R, Aggarwal A. *Interleukin 17 levels are increased in juvenile idiopathic arthritis synovial fluid and induce synovial fibroblasts to produce proinflammatory cytokines and matrix metalloproteinases.* J Rheumatol 2008;3 5:515-519.

[169] Nistala K, Moncrieffe H, Newton KR, Varsani H, Hunter P, Wedderburn LR. *Interleukin-17-producing T cells are enriched in the joints of children with arthritis, but*

have a reciprocal relationship to regulatory T cell numbers. Arthritis Rheum 2008; 58:875-887.

[170] Kohno M, Tsutsumi A, Matsui H, et al. *Interleukin-17 gene expression in patients with rheumatoid arthritis.* Mod Rheumatol 2008; 18:15-22.

[171] Kirkham BW, Lassere MN, Edmonds JP, et al. *Synovial membrane cytokine expression is predictive of joint damage progression in rheumatoid arthritis: a two-year prospective study (the DAMAGE study cohort).* Arthritis Rheum 2006; 54:1122-1131.

[172] Piskin G, Sylva-Steenland RM, Bos JD, *Teunissen MB. In vitro and in situ expression of IL-23 by keratinocytes in healthy skin and psoriasis lesions: enhanced expression in psoriatic skin.* J Immunol 2006; 176:1908-1915.

[173] Lee E, Trepicchio WL, Oestreicher JL, et al. *Increased expression of interleukin 23 p19 and p40 in lesional skin of patients with psoriasis vulgaris.* J Exp Med 2004; 199:125-130.

[174] Wolk K, Witte E, Wallace E, et al. *IL-22 regulates the expression of genes responsible for antimicrobial defense, cellular differentaion, and mobility in keratinocyes: a potential role in psoriasis.* Eur J Immunol 2006; 36:1309-1323.

[175] Schmechel S, Konrad A, Diegelmann J, et al. *Linking genetic susceptibility to Crohn's disease with TH17 cell function: IL-22 serum levels are increased in Crohn's disease and correlate with disease activity and IL23R genotype status.* Inflamm Bowel Dis 2008; 14:204-212.

[176] Kikly K, Liu L, Na S, Sedgwick JD. *The IL-23/Th(17) axis: therapeutic targets for autoimmune inflammation.* Curr Opin Immunol 2006; 18:670-675.

[177] McInnes IB, Schett G. *Cytokines in the pathogenesis of rheumatoid arthritis.* Nat Rev Immunol 2007; 7:429-442.

[178] Yu JJ, Ruddy MJ, Wong G, et al. *An essential role for IL-17 in preventing pathogen-initiated bone destruction: recruitment of neutrophils to inflamed bone requires IL-17 receptor-dependent signals.* Blood 2007; 109:3794-3802.

In: Periodontitis Symptoms, Treatment and Prevention   ISBN: 978-1-61668-836-3
Editor: Rosemarie E. Walchuck, pp. 185-195   ©2010 Nova Science Publishers, Inc.

Chapter 7

NATURAL AVOCADO SUGARS INDUCE SECRETION OF ß-DEFENSIN-2 BY EPITHELIAL CELLS: EFFECTS ON *PORPHYROMONAS GINGIVALIS*

Martine Bonnaure-Mallet[*1,3], *Fatiha Chandad*[1,4], *Astrid Rouillon*[1^],
Zohreh Tamanai-Shacoori[1^], *Vincent Meuric*[1,3], *Patrice Gracieux*[1],
Caroline Baudouin[2], *Stéphanie Brédif*[2], *and Philippe Msika*[2]

Equipe de Microbiologie, UPRES-EA 1254, Rennes 1, Université Européenne
de Bretagne, 2 avenue du Professeur Léon Bernard, 35043 Rennes, France[1]
Laboratoires Expanscience, R&D Center, rue des 4 filles, 28230 Epernon, France[2]
CHU Rennes, Pôle Microbiologie et Pôle Odontologie[3]
Groupe de recherche en Écologie Buccale, Faculté de Médecine Dentaire,
Université Laval, Québec, Canada[4]

ABSTRACT

Oral epithelia represent the first physical and chemical barrier against bacterial invasion and colonization of the underlying tissues. This protection results from the production of epithelial innate immune responses, including the secretion of cationic antimicrobial peptides with a large spectrum of activity against pathogenic microorganisms. Among these antimicrobial cationic peptides, ß-defensin 2 (hBD-2) is expressed in the gingival epithelia upon stimulation by microorganisms or inflammatory mediators such as interleukin-1β or tumour necrosis factor-α. The aim of the present study was to investigate the effect of AV119, a patented blend of two sugars from avocado, on the induction of hBD-2 in two epithelial cell lines and a primo-culture of gingival epithelial cells. Culture supernatant from epithelial cells treated with AV119 was also evaluated for its antimicrobial activity against the periodontopathogen *Porphyromonas gingivalis*. Cell ELISA assays revealed that AV119 induces the

---

*Corresponding author: Martine Bonnaure-Mallet, Equipe de Microbiologie, UPRES-EA 1254, Université de Rennes 1, 2 avenue du Professeur Léon Bernard, 35043 Rennes, France, Tel.: (33) 2 23 23 43 58, Fax: (33) 2 23 23 49 13, E-mail: martine.bonnaure@univ-rennes1.fr
^Authors contributed equally to this work.

production of hBD-2 by all the epithelial cells tested. Minimal Inhibition Concentration assay also showed that the culture supernatant of epithelial cells treated with AV119 possesses antibacterial activity. In conclusion, our data revealed that AV119 component, through hBD2 induction and antibacterial activity, could be considered for potential use in the control of oral mucosal infections and reduction of microbial tissue invasion during periodontitis.

Keywords: ß-defensin, natural avocado sugars, epithelial cells, *Porphyromonas gingivalis*

INTRODUCTION

Periodontitis, the result of bacterial infection of the gingival sulcus, is the most common infectious disease in humans [1]. This infectious disorder is caused by a subset of periodontal Gram-negative anaerobic bacteria where the major pathogen is *Porphyromonas gingivalis* [2]. These microorganisms lead to the destruction of periodontal tissues, including both connective tissue and the alveolar bone surrounding the teeth. Oral epithelial cells, which are directly invaded by periodontal bacteria, act as mechanical and immunological barriers by producing cytokines and metalloproteinases that regulate the host defense against periodontal microorganisms. Antimicrobial proteins and peptides constitute a diverse class of host-defense molecules that act early in protection against invasion and infection by microorganisms [3]. Two main antimicrobial peptide families are defensins and cathelicidins [4]. Defensins are small cationic peptides with a vast spectrum of antimicrobial activity [1, 5-7]. Actually, there are 6 different α-defensins, including 4 peptides (HNP-1 to HNP-4) in neutrophils and 2 peptides (HD5 and HD6), and six β-defensins (hBDs) (hBD-1–6) expressed in numerous epithelial cell surfaces [8, 9]. Only the first three hBDs (hBD-1–3) have been characterized in some details [10]. hBD-1 is constitutively expressed by various tissues and may be modulated by inflammation [11]. hBD-2 and hBD-3 are expressed by the epithelial cells upon stimulation with proinflammatory cytokines such as interleukin (IL)-1β, tumor necrosis factor (TNF)-α, interferon (IFN)-γ and by microorganisms [6]. These peptides are regarded as primary effector molecules in defense against invading microorganisms [12]. Human hBD-1, hBD-2 and hBD-3 are expressed by epithelia of the gingival tissues [13] and hBDs may play a role in the control of the many commensal and putative periodontopathogenic bacteria.

hBD-2, a cysteine-rich, cationic, low-molecular-weight antimicrobial peptide, was first discovered in psoriatic lesions and was thought to be involved in cutaneous defense and inflammation. hBD-2 exhibits strong antimicrobial activity against *Escherichia coli*, *Pseudomonas aeruginosa* and *Staphylococcus aureus* [14, 15]. Yin and Dale [16] have shown that both commensal bacteria and hBD2 activate protective responses of oral epithelial cells and play an important role in immune modulation in the oral cavity.Until now, bacteria did not show any resistance to antimicrobial peptides. Therefore, antimicrobial peptides become valuable antibiotic compounds and natural products that promote the increase of the secretion of antimicrobial peptides are of great interest.

The aim of the present study was to investigate the effect of natural sugars AV119, extracted from the avocado fruit (*Persea gratissima*), on the induction of production of hBD2 in and on antibacterial activity of their culture supernatant against the major periodontal pathogen *Porphyromonas gingivalis*.

MATERIAL AND METHODS

AV119 Extraction Process

AV119 is a patented extract from the avocado fruit (*Persea gratissima*) (Patent N° 0607651 FRANCE 08/31/2006 and EP2007/059136 08/31/2007) (Laboratoires EXPANSCIENCE). AV119 was prepared from sliced and dried avocado fruit. After elimination of fats, the dry matter was ground and extracted in a water-alcoholic solution. The insoluble material was eliminated by filtration and the final product was obtained by concentrating the solution to obtain 5% of active substance. The final solution was mainly composed of two rare sugars, D-mannoheptulose and perseitol, which together represent 80% of the dry matter.

Bacterial Strain and Growth Conditions

P. gingivalis ATCC 33277 was maintained on Colombia agar plates and grown in Brain Heart Infusion (BHI) broth (AES CHEMUNEX, France) supplemented with hemin (5 µg/ml) (Sigma, France), vitamin K1 (1 µg/ml) (Sigma, France) and yeast extract (0.5%) (AES CHEMUNEX, France). The bacterial cultures were incubated overnight at 37°C in an anaerobic chamber (80% N_2, 10% H_2, 10% CO_2).

Epithelial Cells

Two cell lines, KB cells (ATCC CCL-17), and Ca9-22 cells (TKG 0485, Japanese Cancer Research Resources Bank) and primary human gingival epithelial (HGE) cells were used in this study. The cell lines and HGE cells were grown in RPMI 1640 medium with Glutamax™ (Invitrogen, France), supplemented with 10% fetal calf serum, 100 IU/ml penicillin and 100 µg/ml streptomycin. Cells were maintained in a humidified incubator at 37°C under 5% CO_2 atmosphere.

MTT Assay for Cell Viability

Cell viability was estimated by the MTT assay, which is based on the cleavage of a tetrazolium salt by mitochondrial dehydrogenases in viable cells [17]. Epithelial cells were seeded in a 96 well plate at 1×10^5 cells/ml. Twenty-four hours after plating, cells were treated with two concentrations of AV119 (0.01% and 0.03%) and incubated for additional 24 h at 37°C. Twenty microlitres of sterile filtered (3-(4,5-dimethylthiazol-2-yl)-2,5-diphenyl tetrazolium bromide) (MTT, Sigma, France) stock solution in phosphate buffered saline (PBS) pH 7.4 (5 mg/ml) were added to each well reaching a final concentration of 0.5 mg MTT/ml. After 4 hs, culture supernatants were removed by aspiration, the insoluble formazan crystals were dissolved in 200 µl/well dimethylsulfoxide (Sigma, France) and the optical density (OD) measured spectrophotometrically using an ELISA microplate reader at a wavelength of 570 nm. The OD_{570nm} of the formazan formed in the control cells was taken as 100% viability. Assays were performed in triplicate and repeated three times.

Cell ELISA Assay for hBD-2 Production

hBD2 production was measured following a modification of the protocol described by Arunachalam *et al.* [18]. Briefly, epithelial cells were seeded into 96-well culture plates at a density of 3×10^4 cells/well. After 24 h incubation, cell monolayers were treated with AV119 (0.01%, 0.03%) or 200 ng/ml TNFα (T0157 Sigma, France) and incubated for additional 48 h at 37°C under 5% CO_2 atmosphere. Untreated cells were used as control for the basal production of hBD2. The cell monolayers were then washed twice with PBS and fixed with 4% formaldehyde (Sigma, France) for 15 min. Primary Goat polyclonal antibody against hBD-2 (0.5 µg/ml) (Ab9871, Abcam, France) was applied for 1 h at room temperature. After three washes, the plates were treated with rabbit horseradish peroxidase-conjugated secondary antibody (Abcam, France, 1:1000 dilution) for 1 h at room temperature. After washing, the tetramethylbenzidine (TMB™)-substrate (Sigma, France) was added for 15 min and the OD was measured at 450 nm using an ELISA microplate reader. Results were expressed as OD_{450nm} percentage of the control cells. Assays were performed in triplicate and repeated five times.

Effect of AV119 on P. Gingivalis Viability and Growth

To determine the effect of AV119 on *P. gingivalis* viability and growth, serial dilutions of AV119 (ranging from 0.03 µg/ml to 20 µg/ml), hBD-2 peptide (ranging from 2.5 µg/ml to 25 µg/ml) and metronidazole (ranging from 0.03 µg/ml to 2 µg /ml) (Sigma, France) were prepared in BHI culture medium. *P. gingivalis* suspensions 10^5 to 10^6 CFU/ml were incubated with or without various concentrations of AV119, hBD2 or metronidazole for 5 days at 37°C under anaerobic conditions. Antibacterial activities were assessed by $OD_{660 nm}$ measurement. Bacterial susceptibility to the various compounds was expressed as minimal inhibitory concentration (MIC) values. Each assay was performed three times in duplicate.

Antibacterial Activity of Epithelial Cell Culture Supernatants

The antibacterial activity of epithelial cell culture supernatants, harvested from cells treated with AV119, was determined against *P. gingivalis*. Briefly, epithelial cells were seeded into 96-well plates for 24 h at 37°C in a 5% CO_2 atmosphere to allow cells to adhere. The culture medium was replaced with antibiotic-free RPMI medium supplemented with

0.01% or 0.03 % of AV119 or TNFα (20 ng/ml). After 48 h, the cell supernatants of two wells (400 µl) were harvested and tested for antimicrobial activity against equal volume of *P. gingivalis* suspension (~ 5 x 10^3 CFU/ml). After 5 h of incubation in an anaerobic atmosphere, bacterial growth was determined by plate counting method. A negative control consisted of bacteria treated with culture supernatant from untreated epithelial cells (RPMI 1640 medium without AV119).

Statistical Analysis

All the experiments were performed at least three times for each assay conducted in duplicate or triplicate. Results are expressed as means ± SDs. Statistical analyses of all data between the treated and untreated cells were performed by the Student t test. A *p* value <0.05 was considered statistically significant.

RESULTS

Effect of AV119 on Cell Viability

To assess the effect of AV119 on epithelial cell viability, dose-response curves were generated using data from the MTT assay. Treatment of cells with AV119 for 24 h did not affect the cell viability of HGE cells (Fig. 1). However, treatment of KB and Ca9-22 cells with 0.03% of AV119 resulted in slight but negligible decrease (7%, *p* <0.001) of cell viability compared to untreated cells (Fig. 1). For the following experiments, both 0,01 and 0,03 % of AV119 were tested.

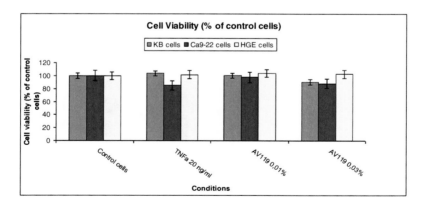

Figure 1. Cell viability of KB, Ca9-22 and human gingival epithelial cells (HGE) treated for 24 hours with 2 concentrations of AV119. The cell viability was determined by an MTT assay as described in Materials and Methods. The absorbance was measured with an enzyme-linked immunosorbent assay reader at a wavelength of 570 nm. Each assay was performed in triplicate, and the data are presented as percent cell viability in terms of control (untreated cells). Data shown are the mean ± SD of three independent experiments, and the values marked with asterisks (*) are significantly different from the control (p <0.05).

Natural Avocado Sugars Induce hBD-2 Production in Epithelial Cells

The production of the antimicrobial peptide hBD-2 by KB, Ca9-22 and HGE cells was determined by a cellular ELISA assay after treatment of cells with AV119 (0.01%, 0.03%) or TNF-α (20 ng/ml). ELISA results revealed that AV119 and TNF-α (positive control for hBD2 induction), dose dependently increased the production of hBD-2 in the three epithelial cell types. In particular, 0.03% AV119 increased significantly hBD-2 production in KB cells (+4 X, $p < 0.05$) as well as in Ca9-22 and HGE cells (+3 X, $p < 0.05$) compared to untreated cells (Fig. 2A, B and C).

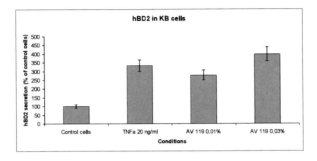

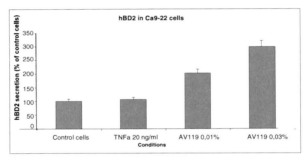

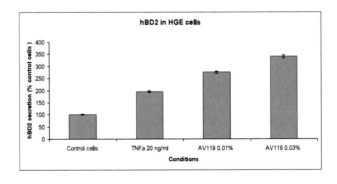

Figure 2. hBD-2 secretion by epithelial cells. The production of hBD-2 was assessed by cell ELISA assay. KB cells (A), Ca9-22 (B) and HGE (C) were treated with TNF-α **920 ng/mL)** or AV119 (0,01% or 0,03%). Induced hBD-2 production was compared to hBD-2 in untreated (control) cells. The data are presented OD_{450nm} percent in terms of control untreated cells. The percentages indicate hBD-2 production as measured in three independent experiments. Data shown are the mean ± SD of three independent experiments. The significant differences in hBD-2 production were determined by the Student's t-test. (*p < 0.05).

Effect of Natural Avocado Sugars on P. Gingivalis Growth

The antibacterial activities of various concentrations of AV119, hBD-2 and metronidazole against *P. gingivalis* were examined by MIC determination. AV119 showed no significant effects on *P. gingivalis* viability or growth at the concentrations tested (0.01% and 0.03%), indicating that AV119 has no inherent antibacterial activity. In contrast, hBD-2 and metronidazole MIC values for *P. gingivalis* were respectively ≤ 2.5 µg/ml and 0.122 µg/ml.

Antibacterial Activity of Epithelial Cell Culture Supernatants

The antimicrobial effect of the supernatants of AV119-treated KB and Ca9-22 cells was measured by plate counting. Plate counts from the supernatants of KB cells treated with AV119 and TNFα revealed higher antimicrobial effect on *P. gingivalis* ($2 \times 10^2 \pm 0.02$ and $1.9 \times 10^2 \pm 0.10$ respectively) compared to untreated KB control cells. A lower antimicrobial activity was observed with supernatants of Ca9-22 cells treated with AV119 and TNFα reduction ($3.00 \times 10^2 \pm 0.20$ and $4.10 \times 10^2 \pm 0.1$ respectively) (Table 1). The positive control with the antibiotic metronidazole showed the most efficient antimicrobial activity.

Table 1. Antimicrobial activity against P. gingivalis in the supernatant of KB cells treated with AV119.

Cellular supernatant	Number of culturable bacteria (UFC ml^{-1})
Untreated KB cells	$5.8 \times 10^2 \pm 0.05$
KB cells treated with TNF☐(20 ng/ml)	$1.9 \times 10^2 \pm 0.10$
KB cells treated with AV119 0.03%	$2.00 \times 10^2 \pm 0.02$
Untreated Ca-22 cells	$4.47 \times 10^2 \pm 0.37$
Ca9-22 cells treated with TNF☐(20 ng/ml)	$4.10 \times 10^2 \pm 0.1$
Ca9-22 cells treated with AV119 0.03%	$3.00 \times 10^2 \pm 0.20$
Media	Number of culturable bacteria (UFC ml^{-1})
BHI + Metronidazole (0.12 µg/ml)	3×10

DISCUSSION

Detection and elimination of periodontal pathogens by gingival epithelial cells is a crucial step in the maintenance of the homeostasis of oral health. Constitutive or induced expression of antimicrobial peptides provides a first line of defense against colonization by pathogens [19]. These cationic peptides are important in protection against invading microorganisms by modulating the innate immune response [10]. Among the antimicrobial peptides, numerous studies have focused on the expression of ß-defensins in gingival epithelial cells [20, 21] suggesting a role of these peptides in the oral mucosal immunity. hBD-2 has been shown to be expressed in all tissue samples and to play a role in the initial mucosal defense system. In most epithelia, it has been reported that hBD2 is present only in inflamed tissue [22]. In the oral cavity, clinically healthy gingival tissue is permanently stressed by microorganisms. In order to maintain a balanced equilibrium between epithelial tissues and the bacterial invasion, cells increase their basal production of antimicrobial peptides including hBD2. Hence, hBD2 is potent therapeutic agent in oral diseases. Its antimicrobial activity could be useful in the prevention and treatment of periodontal diseases.

Identification of natural products, endowed with active properties that can increase the secretion of hBD2 is of high importance in oral health care. In the present study, we investigated the effect of two concentrations of natural sugars derived from avocado fruit (AV119) on the secretion of the antimicrobial peptide hBD-2 by 2 epithelial cell lines and by primary culture of HGE cells. We showed that AV119 increases the secretion of hBD2 by the all tested epithelial cells. The effect of AV119 on the signaling pathways involved in hBD2 secretion is still uncharacterized. However, the signaling pathways involved in hBD-2 induction in response to commensal and pathogenic bacteria [23] have been partially characterized. It has been stated that JNK and p38 pathways were involved in the induction of hBD2 and that hBD-2 induction, in both oral and skin keratinocytes, was blocked by inhibitors of NF-kappaB [23]. In addition, Krisanaprakornkit et al. [24] have demonstrated that phorbol ester induces hBD-2 via the p44/42 extracellular signal-regulated kinase pathway. The upregulation of hBD-2 secretion in cells treated with AV119 could be related to a potential effect of avocado sugars on these pathways. A recent study, using skin keratinocytes examined the intracellular signaling pathways and the nuclear responses that contribute to HBD-2 gene expression upon treatment with AV119 [25]. The reported data suggest that the activation of protein tyrosine kinases and protein kinase C could be involved and could lead to hBD-2 gene activation. These signaling pathways were obtained in a skin keratinocyte model and should be investigated in a gingival model.

The antibacterial activity of culture supernatants obtained from AV119 treated cells was also investigated against the major etiologic agent of periodontitis, *P. gingivalis*. Results of the MIC assays did not reveal any antibacterial effect of AV119 on *P. gingivalis*. Similar results have been obtained when AV119 was tested against *Staphylococcys aureus*, *Pseudomonas aeruginosa* or *Streptococcus pyogenes* [26]. These results exclude the direct antimicrobial effect of AV119 but not that of the culture supernatant of AV119 treated epithelial cells. Indeed, an antimicrobial effect on *P. gingivalis* was observed when KB and Ca9-22 cells were treated with 0.03 % AV119. These results are in agreement with those of Joly et al. [27], who demonstrated that hBD-2 possesses antimicrobial activity against Gram-negative bacteria. Nevertheless, these series of experiments do not exclude the fact that other antimicrobial peptides could be secreted by epithelial cells following AV119 treatment. The antibacterial effect of hBD1, hBD3, cathelicidin LL37 and other cytokines against *P. gingivalis* was not observed in similar conditions [28].

In conclusion, these results show that it is possible to stimulate antimicrobial peptides secretion with natural sugars AV119, and this could help in the maintenance of a healthy mucosal surface by preparing epithelial cells to subsequent exposure to oral pathogens. Avocado natural sugars are potential agents for use in managing gingival and periodontal diseases.

ACKNOWLEDGMENTS

We are grateful to Céline Allaire for editorial assistance. The manuscript was edited by San Francisco Edit. This work was supported by Fondation Langlois, Conseil Régional de Bretagne.

CONFLICT OF INTEREST STATEMENT

No conflict of interest.

REFERENCES

[1]   Offenbacher, S; Salvi, GE; Beck, JD; Williams, RC. *The design and implementation of trials of host modulation agents.* Ann Periodontol 1997;2 (1):199-212.

[2]   Holt, SC; Ebersole, JL. *Porphyromonas gingivalis, Treponema denticola, and Tannerella forsythia: the "red complex", a prototype polybacterial pathogenic consortium in periodontitis.* Periodontol 2000 2005;38 (72-122.

[3]   Gorr, SU. *Antimicrobial peptides of the oral cavity.* Periodontol 2000 2009;51(152-80.

[4]   Ganz, T. *Defensins: antimicrobial peptides of innate immunity.* Nat Rev Immunol 2003;3 (9):710-20.

[5]   Abiko, Y; Saitoh, M. S*alivary defensins and their importance in oral health and disease.* Curr Pharm Des 2007a;13 (30):3065-72.

[6]   Abiko, Y; Saitoh, M; Nishimura, M; Yamazaki, M; Sawamura, D; Kaku, T. *Role of beta-defensins in oral epithelial health and disease.* Med Mol Morphol 2007b;40 (4):179-84.

[7]   Taylor, K; McCullough, B; Clarke, DJ; Langley, RJ; Pechenick, T; Hill, A; Campopiano, DJ; Barran, PE; Dorin, JR; Govan, JR. *Covalent dimer species of beta-defensin Defr1 display potent antimicrobial activity against multidrug-resistant bacterial pathogens.* Antimicrob Agents Chemother 2007;51 (5):1719-24.

[8]   Droin, N; Hendra, JB; Ducoroy, P; Solary, E. *Human defensins as cancer biomarkers and antitumour molecules.* J Proteomics 2009;72 (6):918-27.

[9]   Vordenbaumen, S; Pilic, D; Otte, JM; Schmitz, F; Schmidt-Choudhury, A. *Defensins are differentially expressed with respect to the anatomic region in the upper gastrointestinal tract of children.* J Pediatr Gastroenterol Nutr 2009; 49(1):139-42.

[10] Finlay, BB; Hancock, RE. *Can innate immunity be enhanced to treat microbial infections?* Nat Rev Microbiol 2004;2(6):497-504.

[11] Dunsche, A; Acil, Y; Dommisch, H; Siebert, R; Schroder, JM; Jepsen, S. *The novel human beta-defensin-3 is widely expressed in oral tissues.* Eur J Oral Sci 2002;110 (2):121-4.

[12] Wehkamp, J; Schauber, J; Stange, EF. *Defensins and cathelicidins in gastrointestinal infections.* Curr Opin Gastroenterol 2007;23 (1):32-8.

[13] Schutte, BC; Mitros, JP; Bartlett, JA; Walters, JD; Jia, HP; Welsh, MJ; Casavant, TL; McCray, PB, Jr. *Discovery of five conserved beta -defensin gene clusters using a computational search strategy.* Proc Natl Acad Sci U S A 2002; 99(4):2129-33.

[14] Harder, J; Bartels, J; Christophers, E; Schroder, JM. *A peptide antibiotic from human skin.* Nature 1997; 387(6636):861.

[15] Scott, MG; Hancock, RE. *Cationic antimicrobial peptides and their multifunctional role in the immune system.* Crit Rev Immunol 2000;20 (5):407-31.

[16] Yin, L; Dale, BA. *Activation of protective responses in oral epithelial cells by Fusobacterium nucleatum and human beta-defensin-2.* J Med Microbiol 2007;56 (Pt 7):976-87.

[17] Hansen, MB; Nielsen, SE; Berg, K. *Re-examination and further development of a precise and rapid dye method for measuring cell growth/cell kill.* J Immunol Methods 1989;119 (2):203-10.

[18] Arunachalam, B; Talwar, GP; Raghupathy, R. *A simplified cellular ELISA (CELISA) for the detection of antibodies reacting with cell-surface antigens.* J Immunol Methods 1990;135 (1-2):181-9.

[19] Yang, D; Biragyn, A; Kwak, LW; Oppenheim, JJ. *Mammalian defensins in immunity: more than just microbicidal.* Trends Immunol 2002;23 (6):291-6.

[20] Dale, BA; Kimball, JR; Krisanaprakornkit, S; Roberts, F; Robinovitch, M; O'Neal, R; Valore, EV; Ganz, T; Anderson, GM; Weinberg, A. *Localized antimicrobial peptide expression in human gingiva.* J Periodontal Res 2001a;36 (5):285-94.

[21] Dale, BA; Krisanaprakornkit, S. *Defensin antimicrobial peptides in the oral cavity.* J Oral Pathol Med 2001b;30 (6):321-7.

[22] Liu, L; Wang, L; Jia, HP; Zhao, C; Heng, HH; Schutte, BC; McCray, PB, Jr.; Ganz, T. *Structure and mapping of the human beta-defensin HBD-2 gene and its expression at sites of inflammation.* Gene 1998;222 (2):237-44.

[23] Chung, WO; Hansen, SR; Rao, D; Dale, BA. *Protease-activated receptor signaling increases epithelial antimicrobial peptide expression.* J Immunol 2004a;173 (8):5165-70.

[24] Krisanaprakornkit, S; Kimball, JR; Dale, BA. *Regulation of human beta-defensin-2 in gingival epithelial cells: the involvement of mitogen-activated protein kinase pathways, but not the NF-kappaB transcription factor family.* J Immunol 2002;168 (1):316-24.

[25] Paoletti, I; Buommino, E; Tudisco, L; Baudouin, C; Msika, P; Tufano, MA; Baroni, A; Donnarumma, G. *Patented natural avocado sugars modulate the HBD-2 expression in human keratinocytes through the involvement of protein kinase C and protein tyrosine kinases.* Arch Dermatol Res 2009;

[26] Donnarumma, G; Buommino, E; Baroni, A; Auricchio, L; De Filippis, A; Cozza, V; Msika, P; Piccardi, N; Tufano, MA. *Effects of AV119, a natural sugar from avocado, on Malassezia furfur invasiveness and on the expression of HBD-2 and cytokines in human keratinocytes.* Exp Dermatol 2007;16 (11):912-9.

[27] Joly, S; Maze, C; McCray, PB, Jr.; Guthmiller, JM. *Human beta-defensins 2 and 3 demonstrate strain-selective activity against oral microorganisms.* J Clin Microbiol 2004;42 (3):1024-9.

[28] Ji, S; Kim, Y; Min, BM; Han, SH; Choi, Y. *Innate immune responses of gingival epithelial cells to nonperiodontopathic and periodontopathic bacteria.* J Periodontal Res 2007;42 (6):503-10.

In: Periodontitis Symptoms, Treatment and Prevention ISBN: 978-1-61668-836-3
Editor: Rosemarie E. Walchuck, pp. 197-208 ©2010 Nova Science Publishers, Inc.

Chapter 8

PERIODONTITIS AS A TRIGGER FOR CUTANEOUS DISORDER, CHEILITIS GRANULOMATOSA; REVIEW OF THE JAPANESE LITERATURE

Kazuyoshi Fukai[*]

Department of Dermatology, Osaka City University Graduate School of Medicine, Osaka, Japan

COMMENTARY

It is evident that periodontitis is the cause at least in part of the cases of cheilitis granulomatosa. Considering that periodontitis is extremely common, it is paradoxical that cheilitis granulomatosa is relatively rare, although mild cases might well be overlooked. Since most of the bacterial species found in periodontitis are not virulent by themselves, the notion of 'endogenous infection' might be reconsidered for the pathogenesis of cheilitis granulomatosa. Since only a small fraction of bacteria (~1%) can be cultured by conventional culture system, it should be necessary to employ PCR-based molecular approaches for identifying bacteria in diseases of unknown etiology. In the future, development of DNA-array system for identifying bacteria (or organisms) might be a promising approach for identifying the bacteria.

ABSTRACT

Cheilitis granulomatosa is characterized by the non-inflammatory swelling of the lips, and is considered as the incomplete expression of the Melkersson-Rosenthal syndrome, which consists of the triad of recurrent orofacial swelling, relapsing facial paralysis, and fissuring of the tongue. Rapid improvement after the treatment of

---

[*] Correspondence: Kazuyoshi Fukai, MD, Department of Dermatology, Osaka City University Graduate School of Medicine, 1-4-3 Asahimachi Abenoku, Osaka 545-8585, JAPAN, TEL +81-6-6645-3826, FAX +81-6-6645-3828, E-mail fukai@msic.med.osaka-cu.ac.jp

periodontitis was first reported in 1961 by Kawamura et al in Japan, and 46 such cases have been reported since then in the Japanese literature. We experienced a typical case of cheilitis granulomatosa. The swollen lip showed marked improvement following the treatment of apical periodontitis. A 57-year-old woman presented with a swelling of the lower lip for the period of two months. Skin biopsy of the lip disclosed non-caseous giant cell granuloma. Neither facial nerve palsy nor fissuring of the tongue was present, excluding the diagnosis of Melkersson-Rosenthal syndrome. Patch testing for metal allergy was negative for all dental metallic ions, except for only mild irritation reaction for Zinc ion. The patient was first treated with topical corticosteroid ointment and oral tranilast, which inhibits the release of chemical mediators from leukocytes, for 4 months. Although the treatment was ineffective, rapid and remarkable improvement of the swelling was noted soon after the treatment of apical periodontitis. Thus, it is highly likely that the periodontitis was the cause of cheilitis granulomatosa in this case. In this article, we review such 46 cases in the Japanese literature.

INTRODUCTION

The Melkersson-Rosenthal syndrome is characterized by the triad of recurrent orofacial swelling, relapsing facial paralysis, and fissuring of the tongue. The complete form with simultaneous occurrence of the above three symptoms is rare, and the most observed feature is the swelling of the orofacial region [1]. The incomplete expression of Melkerson-Rosenthal syndrome was first reported by Miescher in 1945 as cheilitis granulomatosa, for the localized, episodic non-inflammatory swelling of the lips [2].

The etiology and pathogenesis of cheilitis granulomatosa is still unknown. Genetic factors, infectious agents, allergies, and vasomotor disturbances have been postulated, but there have been no clear evidence for any of these [3-6].

The importance of dental infection as the cause for Melkersson-Rosenthal syndrome/cheilitis granulomatosa was first described by Rintala et al in 1973 in the English literature [7]. Worsaae et al then reported in 1982 that elimination of such foci is associated with regression or disappearance of orofacial swelling in 11 out of 16 patients [3].

REVIEW OF THE JAPANESE LITERATURE

In the Japanese literature, the association of cheilitis granulomatosa and the periodontitis was described much earlier. In 1961, Kawamura et al [8] described a 39-year-old male patient with cheilitis granulomatosa successfully treated along with the management of the chronic apical periodontitis, and concluded that the association of the periodontitis and cheilitis granulomatosa. At first, the patient was treated by the 'old-fashioned' irradiation therapy with Cobalt 60 (200 Roentogen), but the swelling of the lower lip was unchanged. Then the patient was administered by vitamin D and INAH. During the drug therapy, the patient complained of the teeth pain when biting. The removal of the teeth with apical lesions resulted in marked reduction of the swelling of the lip within a few days. The second case in Japan was reported by Baba et al in 1964 [9]. A 39-year-old man presented with swollen lower lip. Four days after the teeth with apical lesions were removed, the swelling of the lip markedly improved. In 1968, Dr. Katsusuke Yokoyama at the University of Tokyo reported an extensive study regarding cheilitis granulomatosa [10]. He experienced 17 cases and was able to evaluate 16 cases. One was lost to follow-up just after the initial examination. All of the 16 cases had periodontitis and the treatment of the dental lesions resulted in the reduction of the swelling of the lips (Table 1). Since then, the association of the periodontitis and cheilitis granulomatosa is well-recognized in Japan, and 46 such cases were reported. As noted in the Table 1, treatments which were not effective for the management of cheilitis granulomatosa include anti-histamines, tranilast (mast-cell membrane stabilizer inhibiting the release of histamine), and oral antibiotics. These treatments were also effective when administered along with the treatment of periodontitis. Therefore, these treatments are not effective alone and the management of the periodontitis is essential for controlling cheilitis granulomatosa. Administration of corticosteroid is very effective even without the treatment of periodontitis. Corticosteroid may be carefully considered against the possible systemic side-effect. Minor plastic surgery has been performed in some recalcitrant cases, particularly for long standing lesions. If the lesion is old and the granulomas might be hard and solid, plastic surgery might be an option of the treatments. Some of the Japanese dermatologists stress the importance of metal allergy as the cause for the development of cheilitis granulomatosa. Positive patch testing for dental metal ions and the removal of those metals resulted in improvement of cheilitis granulomatosa. Some of these anectodal case reports must be carefully reevaluated, since it is also possible that the removal of the metals might have resulted in the improvement of associated periodontitis itself.

TYPICAL CASE REPORT OF THE ASSOCIATION

Here is a summary of a typical case of cheilitis granulomatosa with marked improvement after the treatment of apical periodontitis, which had been already published by Kawakami et al [28].

A 57-year-old woman presented with asymptomatic swelling of the lower lip for the period of two months. The treatment with topical corticosteroid ointment and oral tranilast showed no improvement during the preceding one-month period. On examination, diffuse swelling and erythema of the lower lip was noted. Facial nerve palsy or fissuring of the tongue was not observed, excluding the diagnosis of Melkersson-Rosenthal syndrome. The results of laboratory tests, including hematological and biochemical investigations, liver and adrenal function tests, immunoglobulin levels, and serum angiotensin converting enzyme measurement, were within normal range. Cutaneous patch testing with a metal allergy series revealed only mild irritation to Zinc ion. Strong positive patch testing suggests the presence of allergic reaction toward metal ion(s). Some of the previous studies had reported the presence of the positive patch test and the removal of the metal crowns resulted in the improvement of the swelling of the lips of cheilitis granulomatosa. In this case, however, the test was negative. Histological examination of biopsy specimens from the lower lip revealed noncaseating epithelioid cell granulomas with inflammatory cell infiltrates, which is in agreement with the histology of the typical cheilitis granulomatosa. These clinical and histopathological findings led to the diagnosis of cheilitis granulomatosa. We asked her if she had seen a dentist. Although she had been seeing a dentist for ten years, obviously no treatment had been administered for possible periodontitis. We advised her to see another dentist, who found infections in the roots of the right upper 5th and 7th, right lower 6th, and left lower 7th molar teeth. In spite that the treatment of the swollen lip with topical corticosteroid and oral tranilast had been ineffective, one month after treatment of two lesions of apical periodontitis (right upper 5th and right upper 7th lesions), remarkable improvement of the swelling was noted, despite lack of treatment of the two lower lesions. Four months after the start of dental treatment, when treatment of the upper lesions had been completed, the swelling of the lower lip disappeared, although treatment of the lower two lesions was still ongoing. This patient had four foci of periodontitis, and treatment of the upper two lesions resulted in rapid improvement of cheilitis granulomatosa. The presence of apical periodontitis was clearly revealed on X-ray films. It is likely that the swelling of the lip in the present case was due to the apical periodontitis in either or both of the upper teeth.

BACTERIAL SPECIES OF PERIODONTITIS

A variety of bacterial species have been isolated from the periodontitis lesions: *Peptostreptococcus spp.*, *Eubacterium spp.*, and *Streptococcus spp.*. Less commonly, *Enterococcus spp.*, *Propionibacterium spp.*, and *Prevotella spp.* are observed in foci of periodontitis [31]. Recently, *Propionibacterium acnes* has been a focus of attention as a cause for sarcoidosis [32]. By quantitative PCR analysis, significantly higher copy numbers of *P. acnes* are reported to be found in the lymph nodes of patients with sarcoidosis [33]. *P. acnes* can produce components with strong chemoattractivity. In addition, *P. acnes* can activate the complement system by both the classical and alternative pathways. It is also evident that *P. acnes* induces pro-inflammatory cytokines, such as IL-1β, IL-1α, IL-8, and TNF-α [34]. Therefore, *P. acnes* might be a strong candidate as a causative agent for cheilitis granulomatosa.

In addition, the periodontopathic bacteria can give rise to virulence factors such as leukotoxins, cytolethal distending toxin, lipopolysaccharide, and proteases [35]. Cardiovascular diseases (atherosclerosis, heart attack, and stroke), complications of pregnancy (spontaneous preterm birth), and diabetes mellitus have been suggested to be associated with periodontitis [36]. Some of the above virulence factors and as yet unknown virulence factors may contribute to the production of cytokines and/or inflammatory mediators for these systemic disorders as well as cheilitis granulomatosa/Melkersson-Rosenthal syndrome.

Although periodontitis is caused by multiple bacteria, it is most likely that the interaction between the bacteria and host contributes the inflammation of periodontitis.

Table 1. The list of cheilitis granulomatosa patients improved after the treatment of periodontitis. In the column of the treatment, NA denotes 'not available'.

patient No.	Investigator	age	sex	duration	other treatment(s) along with the treatment of periodontitis	non-effective treatment	dental lesion(s)	reference
1	Kawamura	39	M	2M	isoniazide	radiation with cobalt60,	chronic apical 'lesion'	8
2	Baba	39	M	1Y	oral corticosteroid (3mg of metazolone)	NA	apical 'lesion'	9
3	Yokoyama	62	M	6M	NA	NA	chronic apical periodontitis	10
4	Yokoyama	50	M	6M	NA	NA	chronic apical abscess chronic apical	10
5	Yokoyama	33	F	1M	NA	NA	periodontitis, chronic apical abscess	10
6	Yokoyama	57	M	3Y	oral antibiotics	NA	chronic apical periodontitis chronic apical	10
7	Yokoyama	48	F	1Y	oral antibiotics, and corticosteroid	NA	periodontitis, chronic apical abscess	10
8	Yokoyama	36	M	3Y	NA	NA	chronic apical periodontitis chronic apical	10
9	Yokoyama	51	M	15Y	oral antibiotics	NA	periodontitis, chronic marginal periodontitis	10
10	Yokoyama	56	F	2Y	oral antibiotics	NA	chronic marginal periodontitis	10
11	Yokoyama	58	F	3Y	NA	NA	chronic marginal periodontitis	10

Table 1 (Continued).

12	Yokoyama	20	M	8M	antibiotics	NA	chronic marginal periodontitis	10
13	Yokoyama	29	F	5Y	NA	NA	chronic marginal periodontitis	10
14	Yokoyama	37	F	2Y	NA	NA	chronic apical periodontitis	10
15	Yokoyama	34	F	3M	NA	NA	chronic apical periodontitis	10
16	Yokoyama	47	M	2Y	NA	NA	chronic apical abscess	10
17	Yokoyama	23	M	3M	oral antibiotics	NA	chronic apical granuloma	10
18	Yokoyama	40	F	2Y	NA	NA	chronic apical periodontitis	10
19	Oogase	29	M	6M	oral antibiotics	ABPC	chronic periodontitis	11
20	Yurashige	53	F	5Y	NA	NA	suprodontis	12
21	Inamura	50	F	5M	NA	NA	chronic apical and marginal periodontitis	13
22	Inamura	60	M	2M	NA	NA	periodontitis	13
23	Inamura	54	F	8M	oral antibiotics	NA	periodontitis	13
24	Yano	51	F	1Y	NA	oral antibiotics	chronic periodontitis	14
25	Kounoe	38	M	2Y	oral corticosteroid	NA	periodontitis	15
26	Kondo	53	M	1Y	repeated injection of 4mg of triamcinolone acetonide		chronic marginal periodontitis	16
27	Ezura	61	M	1Y	NA	NA	chronic marginal periodontitis	17
28	Takeshita	39	M	4M	oral antibiotics	NA	periodontitis	18
29	Hattori	31	M	2Y	NA	NA	chronic apical periodontitis	19

Table 1 (Continued).

No.	Author	Age	Sex	Duration	Treatment	Drug	Diagnosis	Ref.
30	Yokoya	25	M	1Y	oral anti-histamine	NA	apical 'lesion'	20
31	Yokoya	47	M	5Y	oral corticosteroid	NA	chronic periodontitis	20
32	Yokoya	30	M	7M	oral anti-histamine	NA	chronic apical periodontitis	20
33	Yokoya	30	M	5M	oral corticosteroid	NA	chronic marginal periodontitis	20
34	Yokoya	19	F	1W	NA	NA	chronic apical periodontitis	20
35	Yoshida	53	M	1Y	NA	200mg of minocycline hydrochloride, and 300mg of tranilast	chronic apical periodontitis	21
36	Hasegawa	50	M	9M	tranilast	NA	chronic apical periodontitis	22
37	Hasegawa	45	F	1M	NA	tranilast	removal of the dental metal that contains Zn^{++} which showed positive patch testing	22
38	Tatsumi	45	F	8M	NA	NA	chronic periodontitis	23
39	Tsukamoto	34	M	5M	NA	tranilast	apical cyst	24
40	Tsukamoto	47	M	6M	NA	NA	apical granuloma	24
41	Tadokoro	24	F	6M	NA	NA	suprodontis	25
42	Sato	50	F	1M	NA	NA	apical 'lesion'	26

Table 1 (Continued).

43	Hattori	51	F	6M	NA	10mg of oral predonizolone, 120mg of fexofenadine hydrochloride, and other anti-histamines	chronic apical periodontitis	27
44	Kawakami	57	F	2M	NA	oral tranilast and topical corticosteroid ointment	chronic apical periodontitis	28
45	Kawa	6	M	4M	injection of corticosteroid, tranilast	NA	chronic apical periodontsis	29
46	Izumiyama	47	F	10M	NA	NA	apical periodontitis	30

THE NOTION OF ENDOGENOUS INFECTION

Koch's postulate for exogenous infection has long been the 'Gold-standard' for identifying the cause of a particular infectious disease. However, it has become increasingly clear that many disease-causing bacteria are difficult to culture and do not meet Koch's postulate, for examples, *Helicobacter pylori* in gastritis, *Campylobacter jejuni* in Guillain-Barre syndrome, *Chlamydia pneumoniae* in arteriosclerosis, *Propionibacterium acnes* in sarcoidosis, and *Bartonella henselae* in bacillary angiomatosis. Since 99% of bacteria cannot be cultured by conventional culture system [37], it should be necessary to employ PCR-based molecular approaches for identifying bacteria in diseases of unknown etiology. In the future, development of DNA-array system for identifying bacteria (or organisms) might be a promising approach for identifying the causes.

Escherlish, who discovered *E. coli*, might have been aware of or predicted this situation. He introduced the concept of 'endogenous infection' to describe and focus upon the pathologies due to normal flora. Endogenous infection is distinct from opportunistic infection in that the host is not immunologically compromised. Endogenous infection has been defined by Nakatani as follows: 1) the disease is caused by one of the normal host flora; 2) certain species of bacteria proliferate abnormally within the flora or expand in ectopic locations; 3) the disease is caused by non-virulent bacteria; 4) no latent period exists; 5) the disease is not contagious; 6) obtaining immunity to block recurrence is difficult; and 7) preceding precipitating factors exist along with the bacteria themselves [38].

Since most of the bacterial species found in periodontitis are not virulent by themselves, the notion of 'endogenous infection' might be reconsidered for the pathogenesis of cheilitis granulomatosa.

SARCOIDOSIS VS CHEILITIS GRANULOMATOSA

Generally, the formation of granuloma is the pathological process against bacterial agents. Macrophages are trying to eat bacteria but the process is not sufficient to kill those agents. Since *Propionibacterium acnes* has become a promising causative agent for developing sarcoidosis, the bacteria might also be a candidate pathogen for cheilitis granulomatosa. Sarcoidosis is a systemic disorder affecting lung, heart, skin, lymph nodes, and so on. On the other hand, cheilitis granulomatosa is limited to the orofacial swelling, adjacent to the dental lesion(s). In many cases, the treatment of the dental lesion(s) rapidly results in the improvement of the swelling in cheilitis granulomatosa, whereas in sarcoidosis no such foci have been reported.

CONCLUSION

Thus, it is evident that periodontitis is the cause at least in part of the cases of cheilitis granulomatosa. Considering that periodontitis is extremely common, it is paradoxical that cheilitis granulomatosa is relatively rare, although mild cases might well be overlooked. From

46 Japanese reported cases, no particular associated diseases, such as diabetes mellitus, allergic disorders, liver diseases or others, were noted. What is the missing piece linking between the two conditions, periodontitis and cheilitis granulomatosa? Are there any specific genetic background? Specific bacterial species? Special cytokines or virulence factors? Allergic host reaction? Molecular approaches should be tried to analyze the enigmatic disorder.

REFERENCES

[1]   Rogers RS III. (1996) *Melkersson-Rosenthal syndrome and orofacial granulomatosis.* Dermatol Clin 14: 371-379

[2]   Miescher G. (1945) *Uber essentielle granulomatose Makrocheilie (cheilititis granulomatosa).* Dermatologica 91: 57-85

[3]   Worsaae N, Christensen KC, Schiedt M, Reibel J. (1982) *Melkersson-Rosenthal syndrome and cheilitis granulomatosa. A clinicopathologic study of thirty-three patients with special reference to their oral lesions.* Oral Surg 54:404-413

[4]   Smeets E, Fryns JP, van den Berghe H. (1994) *Melkersson-Rosenthal syndrome and de novo autosomal t(9; 21) translocation.* Clin Genet 45:323-324

[5]   Morales C, Penarrocha M, Bagan JV, Burches Pelaes A. (1995) *Immunological study of Merkersson-Rosenthal syndrome. Lack of response to food additive challenge.* Clin Exp Allgergy 25:260-264

[6]   Hornstein OP. (1973) *Melkersson-Rosenthal syndrome: A neuro-muco-cutaneous disease of complex origin.* Curr Probl Dermatol 5:117-156

[7]   Rintala A, Alhopuro S, Ritsila V, Saksela E. (1973) *Cheilitis granulomatosa: The Melkerson-Rosenthal syndrome.* Scand J Plast Resonctr Surg 7:130-7

[8]   Kawamura M, Sato H, Raina AM. (1961) *A case of cheilitis granulomatosa.* Journal of the Japanese Stomatological Society. 7:2-4 (in Japanese)

[9]   Baba K, Aoki H, Saito M. (1964) *A case of cheilitis granulomatosa.* Journal of the Japanese Stomatological Society 10:75-7 (in Japanese)

[10]   Yokoyama K. (1968) *A clinical study of cheilitis granulomatosa.* Journal of the Japanese Stomatological Society 17:17-54 (in Japanese)

[11]   Oogase H, Hasegawa K, Matsumura T, Miyachi T, Kawakatsu K. (1976) *A case of cheilitis granulomatosa.* The Journal of Osaka University Dental Society 21:264-8 (in Japanese)

[12]   Kurashige T, Noguchi T. (1978) *Two cases of cheilitis granulomatosa.* Rinsho Derma (Tokyo) 20:1013-8 (in Japanese)

[13]   Inamura T, Kanai M, Seto K, Sugawara N. (1981) *Three cases of cheilitis granulomatosa.* Journal of the Japanese Stomatological Society 27:181-6 (in Japanese)

[14]   Yano K, Yokoyama N, Katagiri S. (1984) *A curative case of cheilitis granulomatosa.* The Journal of the Tokyo Dental College Society 84:359-64 (in Japanese)

[15]   Kounoe N, Kiyono K, Ohta S, Kurokawa H, Kajiyama M. (1984) *Cheilitis granulomatosa-report of a case.* The Journal of Kyushu Dental Society 38:737-42 (in Japanese)

[16] Kondo S, Aso K, Yasukawa K. (1988) *A case of cheilitis granulomatosa.* Japanese Journal of Clinical Dermatology 42:111-6 (in Japanese)

[17] Ezura A, Kitano Y, Kawasaki K. (1994*) A successful endodontic treatment for a case of cheilitis granulomatosa-suspected of focal dental infection from periapical lesions.* The Japanese Journal of Conservative Dentistry. 37:1915-20 (in Japanese)

[18] Takeshita T, Koga T, Yashima Y. (1995) *Case report: Cheilitis granulomatosa with periodontitis.* J Dermatol 22:804-6

[19] Hattori K, Mihara M, Tanio K. (1997) *A case of cheilitis granulomatosa successfully cured after treatment of apical periodontitis.* Rinsho Derma (Tokyo) 39:1540-1 (in Japanese)

[20] Yokoya S, Kinoshita Y, Kuzuhara T, Honma Y, Otsuka T, Ozono S. (1998) *Cheilitis granulomatosa-report of 5 cases.* Journal of the Japanese Stomatological Society. 47:56-60 (in Japanese)

[21] Yoshida M, Onishi Y, Tajima S, Ishibashi A. (1999) *A case of cheilitis granulomatosa subsided after the removal of dental metal and the treatment of apical lesions.* Rinsho Derma (Tokyo) 41:1300-1 (in Japanese)

[22] Hasegawa J, Horiuchi N. (2001) *A case of Melkersson-Rosenthal syndrome and a case of cheilitis granulomatosa subsided after dental treatment.* Rinsho Derma (Tokyo) 43:153-6 (in Japanese)

[23] Tatsumi H, Kometani H, Tsuji I, Mikayama S, Ohnishi A, Hojou H. (2002) *A case of cheilitis granulomatosa recovered with dental treatment.* Japanese Journal of Oral Diagnosis/Oral Medicine. 15:342-6 (in Japanese)

[24] Tsukamoto K, Nagata A, Misawa T, Kasai H, Yoshie H. (2003) *Two cases of cheilitis granulomatosa improved after the treatment of apical lesions.* Rinsho Derma (Tokyo) 45:709-12 (in Japanese)

[25] Tadokoro T, Osawa K, Muso Y, Ito H, Itami S, Yoshikawa K. (2003) *Melkersson-Rosenthal syndrome aused by saprodontia: a case report.* J Dermatol 30:679-82

[26] Sato T, Makino S, Kitagawa E, Hayashi N, Muranishi K, Fukazawa T. (2004) *A case of cheilitis granulomatosa.* The Journal of Hokkaido Dental Association 59:155-7 (in Japanese)

[27] Hattori T, Tamura A, Ishikawa O. (2004) *A case of cheilitis granulomatosa improved by the removal of dental metal crowns and root canal treatment.* Japanese Journal of Clinical Dermatology. 58:946-8 (in Japanese)

[28] Kawakami T, Fukai K, Sowa J, Ishii M, Teramae H, Kanazawa K. (2008) Case of cheilitis granulomatosa associated with apical periodontitis. J Dermatol 35:115-9

[29] Kawa R, Kambe Y, Obi Y, Ikeda K, Kusama M, Idemitsu T. (2008) *A case of cheilitis granulomatosa in a child.* Journal of Japanese Society for Oral Mucous Membrane. 14:46-50 (in Japanese)

[30] Izumiyama Y, Yura S, Kato T. (2008) *A case off cheilitis granulomatosa successfully treated by surgical removal of infectious dental focuses.* Hospital Dentistry and Oral-Mixillofacial Surgery. 20:153-4 (in Japanese)

[31] Yoshida M, Fukushima H, Yamamoto K, Ogawa K, Toda T. (1987) *Correlation between clinical symptoms and microorganisms isolated from root canals of teeth with periapical pathosis.* J Endod 13:24-28

[32] Moller DR, Chen ES. (2002) *What causes sarcoidosis?* Curr Opin Pulm Med 8: 429-434

[33] Eishi Y, Suga M, Ishige I, Kobayashi D, Yamada T. Takemura T, Takizawa T. Koike M et al. (2002) *Quantitative analysis of mycobacterial and propionibacterial DNA in lymh nodes of Japanese and European patients with sarcoidosis.* J Clin Microbiol 40: 198-204

[34] Perry AL, Lambert PA. (2006) *Under the microscope: Propionibacterium acnes.* Lett Appl Microbiol 42: 185-188

[35] Nishihara T, Koseki T. (2004) *Micobial etiology of periodontitis.* Periodontology 2000, 36:14-26.

[36] Moutsopoulos NM, Madianos PN. (2006) *Low-grade inflammation in chronic infectious diseases: paradigm of periodontal infections.* Ann N Y Acad Sci 1088: 251-264

[37] Relman DA. (1999) *The search for unrecognized pathogens.* Science 284: 1308-1310

[38] Nakatani R. (1971) *The role of the normal flora, particulary within the intestine.* Kansensho 1:2-8 (in Japanese)

In: Periodontitis Symptoms, Treatment and Prevention   ISBN: 978-1-61668-836-3
Editor: Rosemarie E. Walchuck, pp. 209-219   ©2010 Nova Science Publishers, Inc.

Chapter 9

GENETIC POLYMORPHISMS AND PERIODONTITIS

L. Chai, E. F. Corbet and W.K. Leung[*]
The University of Hong Kong, Hong Kong SAR, China

ABSTRACT

Periodontitis is a complex disease which is associated with multiple factors, including host immune responses, and genetic, behavioral and environmental factors. It is generally accepted that genetic polymorphisms can modulate host immune responses to bacterial challenge, hence influencing subjects' susceptibility to periodontitis. Genetic association with periodontal disease experience has been a subject of interest for more than a decade. With the completion of Human Genome Project, genetic association studies emerged in many fields of research including research into periodontitis, one of the most common human diseases. This chapter summarizes past and current research approaches with respect to periodontal disease experience and genetic polymorphisms, and suggests anticipated directions of future studies.

HISTORY OF RESEARCH ON GENETIC POLYMORPHISMS AND PERIODONTITIS

Early Days

Back in the 1970s, researchers had already realized that inheritance could possibly be involved in pathogenesis of what was then termed early onset or juvenile periodontitis. Evidence came from studies on families, from studying syndrome-associated juvenile periodontitis and also from research involving animal models. Some researchers considered juvenile periodontitis as possibly an X-linked disease with a decreased penetration dominant trait but a relatively consistent gene expressivity (Melnick et al., 1976; Marazita et al., 1994),

---

[*] Correspondence: W. Keung Leung, Periodontology, Faculty of Dentistry, The University of Hong Kong, Hong Kong SAR, China. Tel: +852-2959-0417, Fax: +852-2858-7874, E-mail: ewkleung@hkucc.hku.hk

whereas others suggested it was an autosomal recessive disease (Saxen, 1980; Saxen and Nevanlinna, 1984; Long et al., 1987). Although the inheritance pattern was unclear at that stage, the concept of heredity as one of the etiologic factors in this form of periodontitis was recognized. A common consensus was reached that genetic factors play a role in determining early onset periodontal disease susceptibility by modulating host immune responses rather than by causing the disease directly. Along with juvenile periodontitis, studies on twins also provided solid evidence of genetic predisposition on pathogenesis of adult chronic periodontitis. Michalowicz and colleagues reported clinical, radiographic, and bacteriologic findings in reared-together and reared-apart adult twins, including 21 pairs of reared-apart monozygous twins, 17 pairs of reared-apart dizygous twins, 83 pairs of reared-together monozygous twins and 43 pairs of reared-together dizygous twins. They concluded that about 50% of population variance in both severity and distribution of chronic periodontitis was influenced by genetic factors (Michalowicz et al., 1991). Another large study of twins confirmed these earlier findings and extended these by reporting that the concordance rates for chronic periodontitis were higher for monozygous twins (0.38) than dizygous twins (0.16), noting in addition, that the mean difference in age at diagnosis for concordant pairs was less for monozygous twins (0.94 years) than for dizygous twins (5.38 years) (Corey et al., 1993). Thus genetic predisposition and risk for periodontitis was confirmed, however any particular gene or genotype association with periodontitis remained unclear due to limited genotyping technology available at that time.

Association Study Era

In 1997, Kornman and co-workers reported a possible genetic basis for different levels of host immune responses in adult periodontal disease, which was considered as a major advance in genetic studies in Periodontology (Kornman et al., 1997). They found that a specific genotype of polymorphic interleukin-1 (IL-1) cluster to be associated with severity of periodontitis. Their study showed a strong and clear association between IL-1 cluster genotype and periodontitis. IL-1 and other pro-inflammatory cytokines and inflammatory mediators, such as tumor necrosis factor and prostaglandin E2, have been found that can be stably induced to be secreted under the influence of lipopolysaccharide (LPS) a product of the plaque biofilm. The 1997 study of Kornman and co-workers provided genotype evidence of these phenotypic traits. A simple test performed on a drop of peripheral blood was developed to screen IL-1 cluster genotype for determining periodontitis susceptibility in patients (Kornman et al., 1997). It was hoped that such a test could become a routine in screening periodontitis patients for high susceptibility to the disease, hence allowing recognition of those with high susceptibility to severe periodontal destruction so that special active and supportive periodontal care could be delivered for those at greater susceptibility. However, after diverse data from different populations emerging from differently designed studies were published, hope in the promise of periodontitis susceptibility testing was dampened, and it came to be realized that genetic study in Periodontology was still in its infancy. After 1997, genetic association studies became one of the 'hot spots' in periodontal research in the following years. The number of such studies on different candidate genes, most of which related to cytokines and inflammatory mediators, in different populations investigating associations with different types of periodontitis, was large. The results were diverse, even opposite to each other in some studies. The main problems of genetic studies in this association studies era will be discussed in following sections. Restriction fragment length polymorphisms polymerase chain reaction (RFLP-PCR) was the main method for genotyping in that era. Along with the burst of genetic association studies, some attention was devoted to the incorporation of genetic variance as a risk factor in periodontitis risk assessment. Page and Kornman put genetic risk factors into their working hypothesis of periodontitis pathogenesis, in which genetic variance can modulate host immune responses to bacterial challenge hence influencing the inflammatory and tissue events in response to the bacterial challenge resulting in the clinical manifestations of disease (Page and Kornman, 1997).

Post Human Genome Project Era

In 2003, a milestone in genetic research history, even human history, was established with the completion of the human genome project (HGP). Without question the HGP has provided detailed knowledge of the human genome, and such knowledge it is expected will revolutionize the traditional ways to diagnose, treat and prevent many diseases. Some genetic tests based on the results of the HGP have been starting to benefit clinical practice, for example screening subjects with high risk for breast cancer. However, completion of the HGP does not mean that associated variance with most diseases will be established soon. One reason is that many diseases, such as diabetes and periodontitis, are complex diseases, in other words, these are multi-factorial diseases which are likely associated with the effects of multiple, not single, genes in combination with lifestyle and environmental factors. Therefore, new strategies other than direct association studies and new technologies other than or in addition to direct PCR need to be developed. Recent emergence of genotyping and sequencing technologies such as SEQUNOM MassARRAY system, Illumina GoldenGate system and gene chips have made large-scale population and genome-wide investigation possible. Research on diabetes recently commenced employing different combined strategies other than direct association studies (Sladek et al., 2007; Nejentsev et al., 2009). It is coming to be realized that not only DNA sequence variance can affect gene expression and phenotype, and are heritable at the same time, other changes such as DNA methylation and chromatin remodeling can affect gene expression and also last for generations, which is called epigenetics. The association between epigenetic change and pathogenesis of disease is drawing more and more attention in recent years. Although there is the potential for dramatic progress in genetic studies using approaches mentioned above, most genetic studies in Periodontology seem to have remained as traditional association studies. There are only limited number of studies that have utilized advanced genotyping or statistical methods in searching disease associated single nucleotide polymorphisms (SNPs) (Chai et al., 2010a & 2010b). Periodontal researchers are encouraged to incorporate the use of recently developed technologies and concepts in searching for genetic variance in periodontal disease susceptibility, so that they can provide more reliable data from different populations and help in fostering greater understanding of genetic roles in the pathogenesis of periodontitis.

STRATEGIES FOR GENETIC ASSOCIATION STUDIES

Before the completion of the Human Genome Project and the emergence of dense genetic maps, investigators used linkage studies and positional cloning to identify DNA mutations that caused rare disorders, such as cystic fibrosis (Riordan et al. 1989; Rommens et al. 1989) and Huntington's disease (Gusella et al., 1983; THsDCR Group, 1993). However such approaches were unsuccessful when attempting to identify loci that contribute to complex diseases. In 1996, Risch and Merikangas suggested that for complex human diseases association study could be more powerful than linkage study in identifying the elusive susceptibility loci that geneticists seek (Risch and Merikangas, 1996). Furthermore, the common variant/common disease (CV/CD) hypothesis suggested that common DNA variation, as opposed to rare mutations, could be responsible for a proportion of common diseases (Lander, 1996; Collins et al., 1997; Chakravarti, 1999). Though that hypothesis remains controversial, resources for association studies, such as dense genetic maps of SNPs across the human genome, were channeled to enable investigators to identify disease-causing loci that could potentially have a major impact on public health (Collins et al., 2003). Nowadays association studies have become the focus of most study designs for identifying loci involved in complex diseases, such as cardiovascular diseases, diabetes, cancer and also periodontal diseases.

Direct Association Study

There are two approaches for studying candidate genes: direct and indirect. Direct association study means the putative causative SNP is genotyped directly. Although the direct approach using non-synonymous SNPs has proven successful (Cohen et al., 2004), it is facing some challenges. The major challenge is envisaging or determining *a priori* which SNPs are likely to be causative or to predict the phenotype of interest. However, our current knowledge about the pathogenesis of most complex diseases and related SNP functions is so small that the selection of the candidate SNPs has turned out to be tough in most situations.

Indirect Association Study

The indirect approach, on the other hand, is much more like a linkage study in that the study design assays many, presumably, neutral markers and makes no assumption on the location of the causative gene or locus (Crawford et al., 2005). The indirect approach is most often a case-control study drawn from the general population, using a measure of allelic association or site correlation, known as linkage disequilibrium (LD), to detect historical recombination. However, this strategy also has some problems. Sample selection looses statistical power, particularly for rare alleles, haplotypes at multiple loci cannot be resolved, precluding some powerful mapping strategies, and finally clinical samples are less readily stratified by phenotypic differences and environmental factors, yet such analyses may be critical to understanding disease susceptibility (Kruglyak and Nickerson, 2001).

Genome-Wide Association Studies and Other Combined Strategies

Genome-wide association study (GWAS) is one strategy based on the CD/CV hypothesis. This approach utilizes current high-throughput, array-based technologies to investigate DNA throughout the genome (Khor and Goh, 2010). Most GWAS arrays are for investigation of SNPs. Current arrays with 500,000 to 1 million SNPs have provided reasonable representation (>80% in Caucasians) of the common variants across the genome. GWAS is an unbiased approach since it makes no prior assumptions about the biological process or the mode of inheritance of the trait. The whole genome is scanned for association, which enables the discovery of genetic variants in genomic regions that would not have been suspected based on current knowledge. A good GWAS requires accurate phenotyping to reduce trait heterogeneity, a substantial sample size, a reliable genotyping platform, and the proper statistical strategies for handling large amounts of data and performing complex data analysis on large volumes of data, as well.

Another current strategy is the resequencing of extremes. This strategy is based on an opposite hypothesis, that is a common disease/rare variant (CD/RV) hypothesis in which common disease is considered to be due to the aggregate contribution of multiple different rare variants rather than being due to common variants (Sandhu et al., 2008). In this strategy, individuals at both extremes of the phenotypes are selected for further sequencing, which entails detailed examination of their DNA. It was not until recently, following the development of high throughput sequencing platforms, that resequencing could be carried out in large populations. Unlike GWAS, resequencing requires a selection of candidate genes or candidate regions for sequencing, and this selection is usually based on previous knowledge of the disease pathogenesis. Therefore this approach is unlikely to find out novel causal gene(s) or novel pathways for any disease under investigation. However, it can detect some rare variants other than common SNPs which cannot be detected through GWAS due to their low frequencies.

With respect to periodontitis, limited resources and heterogeneity of the disease manifestations usually prevent large-scale GWAS being conducted. On the other hand, our current limited understanding of the molecular pathogenesis of periodontitis also makes it tricky for periodontal researchers to select proper candidate genes or regions for resequencing. Nejentsev and colleagues targeted resequenced regions selected from results of GWAS and found out that a new variant may be protective in diabetes (Nejentsev et al., 2009). Such a combined strategy of resequencing on the basis of GWAS results may enlighten the pathogenesis of or susceptibility for, periodontitis and the outcomes to its treatment.

CURRENT UNDERSTANDING OF GENETIC POLYMORPHISMS AND PERIODONTITIS

Summary of Meta-Analyses and Systematic Reviews

In the past decade, much research into genetic polymorphism in periodontitis has been performed. The focus mostly has been directed to genetic association with infection processes and aspects of immunoregulation, such as cytokines, cell-surface receptors, chemokines, enzymes and other biologics that are related to antigen recognition. The results have been diverse, even studies on the same locus or same gene having shown opposite results sometimes, therefore it is difficult to draw a general conclusion without systemic review or meta-analysis of available appropriately designed and well conducted studies. Several systemic reviews or meta-analyses have been performed and published in recent years and an overview of these should hopefully consolidate some general ideas of the current status of the study of genetic polymorphism in Periodontology.

Cytokine gene polymorphisms have been the most extensively investigated genetic polymorphisms in Periodontology, due to the importance of cytokines in the pathogenesis of periodontitis. The number of such studies makes it possible to use meta-analysis or systemic review to establish a gross view of current understanding derived from genetic studies on cytokine polymorphisms in relation to clinical expressions and behaviour of periodontitis. In 2007, a systemic review on the association between composite IL-1 genotype (IL-1A-889 and IL-1B+3954) and periodontitis progression and treatment outcomes was published (Huynh-Ba et al., 2007). The systematic review screened 122 possible studies and finally included 11 longitudinal studies that reached the requirements for study design and conduct. Possibly due to the small number of studies included, no association between IL-1 composite genotype and periodontitis progression or treatment outcomes was confirmed in this systemic review. The authors also suggested a more cautious interpretation of the results obtained by using commercially available test kits. A meta-analysis which retrieved 53 studies, covering 4178 cases and 4590 controls (Nikolopoulos et al., 2008), analyzed the most investigated cytokine polymorphisms in periodontitis including IL-1A-889, IL-1A+4845, IL-1B-511, IL-1B+3954, IL-6-174 and additionally TNFA-308. A significant association of IL-1A-889 and IL-1B+3954 with chronic periodontitis was reported, with a weak association between IL-1B-511 and chronic periodontitis being noted. However there was great heterogeneity between different study populations, therefore the conclusions of this meta-analysis need cautious interpretation in certain populations. For example, IL-1 composite genotype has very low frequency in Han Chinese (Armitage et al., 2000), which makes the significant association of little importance when explaining pathogenesis of periodontitis in 19% of the world's 2009 population.

Another meta-analysis performed was on human leukocyte antigen polymorphism in both chronic and aggressive periodontitis among Caucasians (Stein et al., 2008). The authors selected 12 suitable studies from 174 publications and found HLA-A9 and HLA-B15 to be significantly associated with aggressive periodontitis, while HLA-A2 and HLA-B5 were suggested to be potential protective factors against aggressive periodontitis among Caucasians. There are currently no other systematic reviews or meta-analyses on other genetic polymorphisms and periodontitis, probably because of the limited number of suitable studies for inclusion.

PROBLEMS OF CURRENT GENETIC STUDIES AND PROSPECT

From the overview of the systematic reviews and meta-analyses, it is not difficult to realize that although the number of genetic studies in Periodontology is large, only a small proportion have been of a high standard which can provide complete data necessary for meta-analysis. The main problems are to do with ethnic heterogeneity, clinical classification and diagnosis of periodontal conditions, choice of controls, size of study groups, and data presentation and handling.

Ethnic Heterogeneity

There is a clear understanding that in the presence of large biological and environmental variability, genetic effects can differ across different populations, or even among generations within the same population (Ioannidis et al., 1998). Frequencies of the genetic marker of interest may also show large heterogeneity between races (Thomas and Witte, 2002). Variations in genotype frequencies across diverse populations may affect the number of individuals at increased risk for a disease, and population substructure imbalances may create spurious differences in genotype frequencies of the compared groups in gene-disease association studies (Kornman et al., 1997; Meisel et al., 2003; Scapoli et al., 2005). The current research-based understandings are derived from different populations and ethnic backgrounds, therefore it is not surprising, from the different results presented, that the current knowledge is not robust. This should warn periodontal researchers to try to ensure reasonable homogeneity of any selected study population, and also to be cautious when trying to replicate the same study of a certain gene marker in a different population. One example of this limited approach are studies conducted on Caucasian populations which suggested the IL-1 cluster composite genotype may associate with the severity of periodontitis (Kornman et al., 1997), however, the prevalence of such composite genotype is very low in those of Chinese heritage (Armitage et al., 2000), suggesting it plays a limited role in the pathogenesis of the periodontitis in Chinese.

Clinical Classification

Classifying periodontal diseases has been a longstanding dilemma largely influenced by paradigms that reflect the understanding of the nature of periodontal diseases during a given historical period (Armitage, 2002). Microbial plaque deposition, smoking, systemic diseases and other environmental factors influence the clinical expression of the periodontal disease condition, and its response to treatment, dramatically. In addition, it is probable that aggressive and chronic periodontitis share a common pathogenic pathway, therefore the periodontist is challenged regarding into which classification a patient would properly fall. Different classification criteria chosen by different studies can also result in different and sometimes conflicting findings.

Choice of Controls

Though control selection is well known to be very important in any genetic association study, it appears there is no clear definition of appropriate controls for a case-control study in periodontitis. Many of the reported association studies showed diverse criteria for control selection. Hence it is not necessarily easy to compare results from different research reports on a certain gene polymorphism given a wide diversity in the controls against which the genetic features of the diseased subjects were compared.

Size of Study Groups

One major concern related to genotype studies is the sample size of the groups of study subjects. Size of the study group clearly contributes to differences in statistical power of the study in its ability to interpret the results, especially in a complex disease like periodontitis. The results of small studies might differ significantly from the results of larger studies, but large studies with thousands of participants might not be easily performed (Ioannidis et al., 1998 & 2001). Experience from other clinical domains suggests that small studies may mistakenly yield more favorable outcomes than larger studies. The sample sizes in genetic association studies in relation to periodontitis have varied from around 50 (Caffesse et al., 2002) to more than 1000 (Meisel et al., 2003), thus making it difficult to combine relevant study results to draw a general view as to the interpretation of the results.

Data Presentation

Expressing differences in results in terms of p-values only is extremely popular in genetic association studies on periodontitis. However, the overuse and misuse of the venerable p-value has been criticized (Visintainer and Tejani, 1998; Sterne and Smith, 2001). It has been suggested that the data should be presented and evaluated not only by p-value but by confidence interval (CI), relative risk (RR) or odds ratio (OR) because these can provide more useful information than those which just use statistics applicable to hypothesis testing. Moreover, most of the current available periodontal data from existing studies do not have quality control measures, e.g. Hardy-Weinberg Equilibrium (HWE) testing, and genotyping success rates have been rarely presented calling for great caution in the interpretation of results.

PROSPECTS

Proper experimental design, including sensible control selection protocols, appropriate sample size calculations, quality control measures, and careful data analysis approaches are necessary before commencing periodontal genetic polymorphism studies, and failure to pay attention to these considerations would limit advances in our current understanding. Periodontal researchers are also encouraged to use combined strategies in genetic investigations of periodontal disease and to utilize newly developed technologies for investigating possible associated SNPs. Periodontitis is a multi-factorial, multi-gene involved disease, thus it is also important that suitable statistical strategies are employed allowing environmental factors which are relevant to genetic predisposition and gene-gene interaction to be taken into account. It is very likely that there is still a journey of discovery to be taken in relation to the understanding of genetic polymorphisms and periodontitis.

REFERENCES

Armitage, G.C. (2002). Classifying periodontal diseases--a long-standing dilemma. *Periodontol* 2000 *30*, 9-23.

Armitage, G.C., Wu, Y., Wang, H.Y., Sorrell, J., di Giovine, F.S., and Duff, G.W. (2000). Low prevalence of a periodontitis-associated interleukin-1 composite genotype in individuals of Chinese heritage. *J Periodontol 71*, 164-171.

Caffesse, R.G., De LaRosa, M.R., De LaRosa, M.G., and Mota, L.F. (2002). Prevalence of interleukin 1 periodontal genotype in a Hispanic dental population. *Quintessence Int 33*, 190-194.

Chai, L., Song, Y.Q., Zee, K.Y., and Leung, W.K. (2010a). Single nucleotide polymorphisms of complement component 5 and periodontitis. *J Periodontal Res 44*: doi: 10.1111/j.1600-0765.2009.01234.x.

Chai, L., Song, Y.Q., Zee, K.Y., and Leung, W.K. (2010b). SNPs of Fc-gamma receptor genes and chronic periodontitis. *J Dent Res* In press.

Chakravarti, A. (1999). Population genetics--making sense out of sequence. *Nat Genet 21*, 56-60.

Cohen, J.C., Kiss, R.S., Pertsemlidis, A., Marcel, Y.L., McPherson, R., and Hobbs, H.H. (2004). Multiple rare alleles contribute to low plasma levels of HDL cholesterol. *Science 305*, 869-872.

Collins, F.S., Green, E.D., Guttmacher, A.E., and Guyer, M.S. (2003). A vision for the future of genomics research. *Nature 422*, 835-847.

Collins, F.S., Guyer, M.S., and Charkravarti, A. (1997). Variations on a theme: cataloging human DNA sequence variation. *Science 278*, 1580-1581.

Corey, L.A., Nance, W.E., Hofstede, P., and Schenkein, H.A. (1993). Self-reported periodontal disease in a Virginia twin population. *J Periodontol 64*, 1205-1208.

Crawford, D.C., Akey, D.T., and Nickerson, D.A. (2005). The patterns of natural variation in human genes. *Annu Rev Genomics Hum Genet 6*, 287-312.

Gusella, J.F., Wexler, N.S., Conneally, P.M., Naylor, S.L., Anderson, M.A., Tanzi, R.E., Watkins, P.C., Ottina, K., Wallace, M.R., Sakaguchi, A.Y., *et al.* (1983). A polymorphic DNA marker genetically linked to Huntington's disease. *Nature 306*, 234-238.

Huynh-Ba, G., Lang, N.P., Tonetti, M.S., and Salvi, G.E. (2007). The association of the composite IL-1 genotype with periodontitis progression and/or treatment outcomes: a systematic review. *J Clin Periodontol 34*, 305-317.

Ioannidis, J.P., Cappelleri, J.C., and Lau, J. (1998). Issues in comparisons between meta-analyses and large trials. *JAMA 279*, 1089-1093.

Ioannidis, J.P., Ntzani, E.E., Trikalinos, T.A., and Contopoulos-Ioannidis, D.G. (2001). Replication validity of genetic association studies. *Nat Genet 29*, 306-309.

Khor, C.C., and Goh, D.L. (2010). Strategies for identifying the genetic basis of dyslipidemia: genome-wide association studies vs. the resequencing of extremes. *Curr Opin Lipidol* doi:10.1097/MOL.0b013e328336eae9.

Kornman, K.S., Crane, A., Wang, H.Y., di Giovine, F.S., Newman, M.G., Pirk, F.W., Wilson, T.G., Jr., Higginbottom, F.L., and Duff, G.W. (1997). The interleukin-1 genotype as a severity factor in adult periodontal disease. *J Clin Periodontol 24*, 72-77.

Kruglyak, L., and Nickerson, D.A. (2001). Variation is the spice of life. *Nat Genet 27*, 234-236.

Lander, E.S. (1996). The new genomics: global views of biology. *Science 274*, 536-539.

Long, J.C., Nance, W.E., Waring, P., Burmeister, J.A., and Ranney, R.R. (1987). Early onset periodontitis: a comparison and evaluation of two proposed modes of inheritance. *Genet Epidemiol 4*, 13-24.

Marazita, M.L., Burmeister, J.A., Gunsolley, J.C., Koertge, T.E., Lake, K., and Schenkein, H.A. (1994). Evidence for autosomal dominant inheritance and race-specific heterogeneity in early-onset periodontitis. *J Periodontol 65*, 623-630.

Meisel, P., Siegemund, A., Grimm, R., Herrmann, F.H., John, U., Schwahn, C., and Kocher, T. (2003). The interleukin-1 polymorphism, smoking, and the risk of periodontal disease in the population-based SHIP study. *J Dent Res 82*, 189-193.

Melnick, M., Shields, E.D., and Bixler, D. (1976). Periodontosis: a phenotypic and genetic analysis. *Oral Surg Oral Med Oral Pathol 42*, 32-41.

Michalowicz, B.S., Aeppli, D., Virag, J.G., Klump, D.G., Hinrichs, J.E., Segal, N.L., Bouchard, T.J., Jr., and Pihlstrom, B.L. (1991). Periodontal findings in adult twins. *J Periodontol 62*, 293-299.

Nejentsev, S., Walker, N., Riches, D., Egholm, M., and Todd, J.A. (2009). Rare variants of IFIH1, a gene implicated in antiviral responses, protect against type 1 diabetes. *Science 324*, 387-389.

Nikolopoulos, G.K., Dimou, N.L., Hamodrakas, S.J., and Bagos, P.G. (2008). Cytokine gene polymorphisms in periodontal disease: a meta-analysis of 53 studies including 4178 cases and 4590 controls. *J Clin Periodontol 35*, 754-767.

Page, R.C., and Kornman, K.S. (1997). The pathogenesis of human periodontitis: an introduction. *Periodontol* 2000 *14*, 9-11.

Riordan, J.R., Rommens, J.M., Kerem, B., Alon, N., Rozmahel, R., Grzelczak, Z., Zielenski, J., Lok, S., Plavsic, N., Chou, J.L., *et al.* (1989). Identification of the cystic fibrosis gene: cloning and characterization of complementary DNA. *Science 245*, 1066-1073.

Risch, N., and Merikangas, K. (1996). The future of genetic studies of complex human diseases. *Science 273*, 1516-1517.

Rommens, J.M., Iannuzzi, M.C., Kerem, B., Drumm, M.L., Melmer, G., Dean, M., Rozmahel, R., Cole, J.L., Kennedy, D., Hidaka, N., *et al.* (1989). Identification of the cystic fibrosis gene: chromosome walking and jumping. *Science 245*, 1059-1065.

Sandhu, M.S., Waterworth, D.M., Debenham, S.L., Wheeler, E., Papadakis, K., Zhao, J.H., Song, K., Yuan, X., Johnson, T., Ashford, S., *et al.* (2008). LDL-cholesterol concentrations: a genome-wide association study. *Lancet 371*, 483-491.

Saxen, L. (1980). Heredity of juvenile periodontitis. *J Clin Periodontol 7*, 276-288.

Saxen, L., and Nevanlinna, H.R. (1984). Autosomal recessive inheritance of juvenile periodontitis: test of a hypothesis. *Clin Genet 25*, 332-335.

Scapoli, C., Trombelli, L., Mamolini, E., and Collins, A. (2005). Linkage disequilibrium analysis of case-control data: an application to generalized aggressive periodontitis. *Genes Immun 6*, 44-52.

Sladek, R., Rocheleau, G., Rung, J., Dina, C., Shen, L., Serre, D., Boutin, P., Vincent, D., Belisle, A., Hadjadj, S., *et al.* (2007). A genome-wide association study identifies novel risk loci for type 2 diabetes. *Nature 445*, 881-885.

Stein, J.M., Machulla, H.K., Smeets, R., Lampert, F., and Reichert, S. (2008). Human leukocyte antigen polymorphism in chronic and aggressive periodontitis among Caucasians: a meta-analysis. *J Clin Periodontol 35*, 183-192.

Sterne, J.A., and Smith, D.G. (2001). Sifting the evidence-what's wrong with significance tests? *BMJ 322*, 226-231.

Thomas, D.C., and Witte, J.S. (2002). Point: population stratification: a problem for case-control studies of candidate-gene associations? *Cancer Epidemiol Biomarkers* Prev *11*, 505-512.

THsDCR Group (1993). A novel gene containing a trinucleotide repeat that is expanded and unstable on Huntington's disease chromosomes. *Cell 72*, 971-983.

Visintainer, P.F., and Tejani, N. (1998). Understanding and using confidence intervals in clinical research. *J Matern Fetal Med 7*, 201-206.

In: Periodontitis Symptoms, Treatment and Prevention   ISBN: 978-1-61668-836-3
Editor: Rosemarie E. Walchuck, pp. 221-238   ©2010 Nova Science Publishers, Inc.

Chapter 10

IMMUNE RESPONSES TO HEAT SHOCK PROTEINS IN CHRONIC PERIODONTITIS AND CORONARY HEART DISEASE

A. Hasan, D. Sadoh and M. Foo

Department of Periodontology, King's College London Dental, Institute at Guy's, King's College and St. Thomas', Hospitals, London, UK

ABSTRACT

Coronary heart disease (CHD) shares a number of features with chronic periodontitis (CP) including risk factors such as smoking and diabetes; an aetiopathogenesis implicating a number of microbial species, as well as chronic inflammation. However, the link between these two conditions remains unclear. The prevalence of CHD increases with age and is higher in males than females. CP is a chronic inflammatory condition which destroys the supporting tissues of teeth and also increases in prevalence with age. Immune responses against heat shock proteins (HSP) can be cross-reactive among bacterial and human antigens. There is evidence that microbial HSP65 and human HSP60 is involved in periodontal disease and CHD and may therefore provide a mechanistic link between CP and CHD. The aim of this study is to investigate immune responses to the human HSP60 and microbial HSP65 in patients with CP and CHD and relate these to the level of inflammation. We collected serum samples from 100 male subjects divided into 4 groups, each matched for age: (a) Healthy control group with minimal gingivitis, (b) CP, (c) CHD with gingivitis (d) CHD with CP. ELISA was used to determine the levels of serum anti-HSP and C-reactive protein (CRP) in the 4 groups. Peripheral blood mononuclear cells were also isolated from these 4 groups and stimulated with HSPs. Significant lymphoproliferation was seen in CHD with or without CP when stimulated with human HSP60. CRP and serum anti-human HSP60 IgG were elevated in the patients groups compared to the healthy control group, but not serum anti-microbial HSP 65 IgG,. In view of the potential confounding effects of smoking in CP and CHD, a group of current smokers (n=24) were also recruited to investigate whether smoking affects HSP immune responses.There was no significant difference in HSP-induced lymphoproliferation between smokers and non-smokers in any of the four groups. There was a significant correlation between CRP and lymphoproliferative responses to Human HSP60.

This study shows that serum anti-human HSP60 IgG and serum CRP are raised in CHD with or without CP. In CHD with or without CP, serum CRP levels correlated significantly with human HSP60-induced lymphoproliferation, but not with anti-HSP antibody levels.

INTRODUCTION

Cardiovascular disease arising as a result of atherosclerosis is a major cause of death in western societies and has been associated with periodontal disease (Beck et al 1996, DeStefano et al 1993). Both atherosclerosis and chronic periodontitis share risk factors, most relevantly smoking, and this has led some groups to conclude that shared risk factors are acting as confounders and that there is no link between the two conditions (Hujoel et al 2001); however further evidence for an association continue to appear in the literature (Desvarieux et al 2005).

The periodontium in the diseased state is a complex polymicrobial niche (Lang et al 1998). Over 300 species of bacteria have been isolated and characterised from plaque deposits (Moore & Moore 1994). In 1mg of dental plaque, more than 10^8 bacteria are present (Lang et al 1998). In a neglected dentition, common oral hygiene procedures may result in bacteraemias with consequent systemic inflammation (Carroll & Sebor 1980, Silver et al. 1977).

Chronic periodontitis (CP) is an inflammatory disease characterised by connective tissue destruction and bone resorption. The aetiology of CP is associated with a number of bacteria, autoimmunity or microbial cross-reactivity (Listgarten et al 2003). There is evidence from cross-sectional studies implicating *Porphyromonas gingivalis, Tannerella forsythia* as well as other microbial species including Gram-negative and Gram-positive bacteria, some of which are unculturable (Kumar et al 2003). These findings support the hypothesis that the aetiology of CP is polymicrobial. Serum concentration of CRP, a marker of systemic inflammation, is raised in patients with chronic periodontitis (Amar et al 2003, Buhlin et al 2003}.

HSPs are the most highly conserved group of proteins known in phylogeny with respect to biochemical function, mode of regulation and structure (Ellis 1995, Jindal et al 1989, Thole et al 1988). They are expressed in all eukaryotic and prokaryotic cells including Gram-positive and Gram-negative bacteria (Ellis 1995). The high degree of homology between microbial and human HSPs has led to the hypothesis that tissue damage can occur as a result of cross-reactivity between bacterial and human HSPs. Humoral and T cell response to HSPs have been demonstrated in CP (Hasan et al 2005, Buhlin et al 2003, Tabeta et al 2000, Lopatin et al 1999, Schett et al 1997a, Ando et al 1995).

Chronic infection may also play a role in coronary heart disease (CHD) (Danesh et al 1997, Zhu et al 2000, Saikku et al 1988). As well as DNA from *Chlamydia pneumoniae,* studies have also demonstrated the presence of DNA from periodontotopathic organisms such as *Porphyromonas gingivalis, Tannerella forsythia,* and *Actinobacillus actinomycetemcomitans* in atheromatous plaques (Ford et al 2005, Haraszthy et al 2000). Furthermore, antibodies to periodontal pathogens are associated with CHD (Pussinen et al 2003).

Animal models provide evidence for shared pathogenic mechanisms between atherosclerosis and periodontitis. When apolipoprotein-E-deficient (-/-) mice are immunized with a major periodontopathogen, *Porphyromonas gingivalis,* thereby increasing the burden of pathogen, atherogenesis was enhanced (Ford et al 2007). Host HSP could be detected in atherosclerotic lesions and lesion progression correlated with anti-GroEL antibody levels suggesting that molecular mimicry between GroEL and host HSP60 is involved (Ford et al 2007).

Many studies have focused on identifying a single pathogen, however it has been postulated that the risk factor is the cumulative pathogen burden rather than mono-infections (Epstein 2002). Given the wide range of microbial species implicated in both conditions, a role for HSPs seems probable and in CHD has been suggested by a number of findings: autoantibodies to microbial HSP65 have been shown to mediate macrophage lysis (Schett et al 1997b) and endothelial cytotoxicity (Schett et al 1995) and mucosal administration of microbial HSP65 reduced the presence of atherosclerosis and inflammation in the aortic arch of LDL receptor deficient mice (Maron et al 2002).

The objectives of this investigation are to determine whether serum anti HSP60/65 IgG and IgA are associated with chronic periodontitis and/or CHD in male Caucasian patients and to determine if inflammation, as reflected by CRP levels, correlates with these immune responses.

MATERIAL AND METHODS

Subjects

Patients with CP and CHD were recruited from the department of Periodontology at Guy's, King's and St Thomas's Institute and the Coronary Care Unit St Thomas's Hospital (Table 1). All subjects were male caucasians, aged between 35 and 69 years of age and had at least 15 standing teeth. CHD patients with angiographic evidence of atherosclerosis but no history of myocardial infarction or previous heart bypass operation were recruited. A small number of smokers were also recruited and matched in age and condition to the 4 groups (Table 2). Subjects were excluded from the study if they had systemic disease including diabetes mellitus, recurrent aphthous stomatitis and autoimmune disease, a history of malignancies, previous treatment for periodontitis, or a history of antibiotic therapy within the past six months prior to recruitment .

Subjects were allocated into:

1) Healthy control with minimal gingivitis group
2) Chronic periodontitis only group (CP)
3) CHD group with minimal gingivitis(CHD-G)
4) CHD group with Chronic Periodontitis (CHD-CP).

In each subject, probing depths and recession of all teeth (rounded down to the nearest millimetre) were determined using a William's probe. Recession was measured as the distance from the cemento-enamel junction to the gingival margin. Measurements were rounded down to the nearest mm from 6 sites: mesio-buccal, mid-buccal, disto-buccal, mesiolingual, mid-lingual and disto-lingual, probing attachment loss was then calculated as the sum of probing pocket depth and recession.

Table 1. Clinical data and optical densities at 1:100 for serum IgA antibodies to human HSP60 and microbial HSP65 of patients showing median (interquartile range).

Group & Number of patients	Healthy controls n=25	CP n=25	CHD-G n=25	CHD-CP n=25
Age (years) ANOVA p=0.239	48.0 (44-58)	49.0 (43-53)	52.0 (48-56)	54.0 (50-55)
Probing attachment level (mm)	0.9 (0.8-1.0)	3.2 (2.8-4.2)	1.0 (0.8-1.2)	3.2 (2.4-4.8)
Anti-microbial HSP65 IgA ANOVA p=0.362	0.38 (0.28-0.54)	0.33 (0.24-0.66)	0.30 (0.24-0.41)	0.47 (0.27-0.75)
Anti-human HSP60 IgA ANOVA p=0.559	0.62 (0.41-1.07)	0.58 (0.43-0.84)	0.50 (0.36-0.76)	0.53 (0.37-0.94)

Table 2. Clinical data from smokers in each of the 4 groups. showing median (interquartile range).

Present Smokers	Healthy controls n=6	CP n=6	CHD-G n=6	CHD-CP n=6
Age (yrs) ANOVA P=0.331	47 (43-57)	48 (44-51)	50 (47-52)	53 (47-51)
Probing attachment level (mm) p=0.3	0.8 (0.7-1.0)	3.0 (2.7-4.1)	0.9 (0.7-1.1)	3.0 (2.2-4.3)

Periodontitis was defined as probing attachment loss ≥4mm in at least 4 teeth and healthy control group as probing attachment loss < 2mm in all teeth. Probing attachment loss was calculated as the sum of the probing depth and recession. Ethical committee approval was obtained (code no 98/12/04) and subject consent obtained. 50ml of venous blood were withdrawn from each subject before periodontal probing or angiography.

HSP

Recombinant HSP65 derived from *Mycobacterium bovis* was prepared at the National Institute of Public Health and Environmental Protection, Bilthoven, the Netherlands and used at a predetermined optimal concentration of 10μg/ml. Human HSP60 was purchased from Stressgen (Victoria, Canada). The two HSPs were detoxified using Detoxi-gel columns (Pierce, Oxford, UK) and the endotoxin level was determined by Limulus Amoebocyte Lysate assay (Sigma-Aldrich, Poole, Dorset, UK). The concentration of endotoxin was <0·007 U/μg or 7 pg endotoxin/μg for both HSPs.

Serum ELISA Measurements

Antibodies to the HSP (human HSP60 and microbial HSP65) were detected by enzyme-linked immunosorbent assay. 96-well flat-bottomed polystyrene microtitre plates were coated (Immulon 4 HBX USA) with HSP60 (Stressgen, Victoria, Canada) or microbial HSP65 diluted (1μg/ml) with phosphate buffered saline (PBS, pH 7.4) and left overnight at room temperature. HSPs were detoxified using Detoxigel columns (Pierce, Oxford, UK) and the endotoxin level was determined by Limulus Amoebocyte Lysate assay Sigma-Aldrich, Poole, Dorset, UK). Uncoated sites were then blocked with 0.5% wt/vol BSA (Sigma-Aldrich Irvine U.K.) in PBS (200μl/well) for 60 minutes at room temperature. In addition, human sero-negative and sero-positive samples were identified by running the whole series of patient serum samples and obtaining the most positive and negative samples as positive and negative controls respectively. Serum from rabbits previously immunised with microbial HSP65 and human HSP60 (kindly provided by Dr L Bergmeier and Dr A Hasan, KCL Dental Institute, London) was also used as positive control. Serum samples obtained from patients including positive and negative controls were then diluted as follows in PBS containing 0.5% BSA and 0.05% tween 20; 2 fold dilution of serum at 1:100 for anti-human HSP60 IgG, anti-microbial HSP 65 IgG and anti-HSP60 IgA, 2 fold dilution of serum at 1:50 for anti-microbial HSP65 IgA. 100μl of each diluted sample or positive/negative control were then added in duplicates to each well and serially diluted to 1:6400, except for anti-microbial HSP65 IgA which had a final dilution of 1:3200.

Plates were then incubated at room temperature for 2 hours and washed 4 times with PBS containing 0.05% Tween 20. Secondary antibody goat anti-human IgG, or IgA Fc specific, alkaline phosphatase conjugates (Sigma-aldrich, U.K.) were diluted in diluent buffer to an optimal concentration. 100μl were then added to each well and incubated at room temperature for 2 hours. Anti-human IgG alkaline phosphatase conjugate was used at 1:2000. Anti-human IgA alkaline phosphatase conjugate was used at 1:1000 for detection of serum anti-human HSP60 IgA and at 1:500 for the detection of serum anti- microbial HSP65 IgA. Plates were then washed 4 times with wash buffer and were developed with para-nitrophenylphosphate in diethanolamine buffer (pH 9.8) at room temperature. The absorbance was determined using a microplate reader (Anthos 2001, Anthos labtec instruments U.K.) for IgG, and (Opsys MR DYNEX technologies) for IgA at 405nm with wavelength correction at 620nm. Inter-assay variation was monitored using a standard positive serum in each assay (Direskeneli et al 1996). The variation of the titre of this positive serum was within one dilution step.

Separation of Cells

Peripheral blood mononuclear cells (PBMC) were separated from blood by density gradient centrifugation and cultured as described previously (Pervin et al 1993). Briefly, 10^5 cells were cultured in RPMI with or without antigens, including ovalbumin (Sigma, Poole, UK) as an unrelated protein control, in quadruplicate in 96-well round-bottomed plates for 6 days. Cells were cultured in RPMI-1640 and 10% autologous serum for 1 h at 37 °C in 5% CO^2. In the final 6 h of culture the cells were pulsed with [3H]-thymidine (0·5 µCi or 18·5 mBq per well; Amersham International, Amersham, UK). The results were assessed by calculating the stimulation index (SI), which is the ratio of antigen-stimulated to antigen-unstimulated cultures (Pervin et al 1993).

Detection of C-reactive Protein by ELISA

50µL of pre-diluted standard and blank were added to a 96 well plate precoated with anti-serum CRP IgG (Kalon Biological Ltd). Serum samples were diluted 1:1000 with assay diluent (Kalon Biological Ltd) and dispensed in duplicates to designated wells in CRP precoated plates. The Plate was then incubated at room temperature for 60 minutes. Plates were washed 4 times with wash buffer (Kalon Biological Ltd). 100µL of CRP tracer (affinity purified sheep anti-CRP labelled with alkaline phosphatase, Kalon Biological Ltd U.K) were then dispensed to each well and incubated uncovered for 30 minutes at room temperature. Plates were washed again 4 times with washing buffer (Kalon Biological Ltd, U.K).

100µl of substrate solution (4-nitrophenylphosphate in substrate buffer Kalon Biological Ltd) were then dispensed to each well and incubated at room temperature for 30 minutes. The reaction was stopped with 100µl of (120g/L) sodium hydroxide. Optical densities were read at 405nm with micoplate reader (Anthos 2001, Anthos labtec instruments U.K.). A standard curve was constructed with standard points and curve fitted with four parameter logistic curve fitting software. Test serum values were then read off the standard curve.

Statistical Method

Kruskal-Wallis ANOVA test was used to assess differences between the groups. ELISA for serum anti-HSP IgG or IgA was analysed by using data consisting of optical density readings for the performed test. The mean optical density was then analysed at 1:100. The significance level was set at $p<0.05$. Post-ANOVA pair wise comparisons between the healthy with CP group; healthy with CHD-G group CP, and with CHD-CP group was carried out using the Mann-Whitney U test, using the Bonferroni correction test to set the significance level at $p<0.02$. Inter-relationships between serum anti-HSP60 IgG and serum CRP levels were tested using Spearman ranked correlation coefficients (r_s). Non-parametric data is displayed in graphs as median (1st and 3rd quartile, minimum, maximum).

RESULTS

Clinical Data

We recruited 120 patients (non-smokers) divided into 4 groups, The median (interquartile range) age of the subjects in the control group was 48 (44-58) years, in the CP group 49 (43-53) years, in the CHD-G group 52 (48-56) and in the CHD-CP group 54 (50-55) and there was no statistically significant difference between the groups, (ANOVA p=0.239, Table 1). In order to investigate the effect of smoking on lymphoproliferative responses, we recruited a small number of current smokers (Table 2). The current smokers were matched for age, gender, and disease status with non-smokers from the 4 groups. There were no significant differences in the age and periodontal status of non-smokers in each of the 4 groups when compared with smokers in the 4 groups (p>0.05).

For the non-smokers, the median (interquartile range) probing attachment level in the control group was 0.9 (0.8-1.0) mm, in the CP group 3.2 (2.8-4.2) mm, in the CHD-G group 1.0 (0.8-1.2) mm and in the CHD-CP group 3.2 (2.4-4.8) mm (Table 1). In view of the confounding effect of smoking in studies associating periodontitis to cardiovascular disease, the data from smokers and non-smokers have been kept separate in all figures and tables.

IgA Antibodies to Microbial HSP65 and Human HSP60

The OD at 1:100 dilution of serum for anti-microbial HSP65 IgA was 0.38 (0.28-0.54) in the control group, 0.33 (0.24-0.66) in the CP group, 0.30 (0.24-0.41) in the CHD-G group and 0.47 (0.27-0.75) in the CHD-CP group, and was not significant ANOVA, p=0.362 (Table 1). Similarly, there was no difference in serum anti-human HSP60 IgA in the 4 groups (Table 1). The median (interquartile range) OD at 1:100 dilution of serum was 0.62 (0.41-1.07) in the control group, 0.58 (0.43-0.84) in the CP group, 0.50 (0.36-0.76) in the CHD-G group, and 0.53 (0.37-0.94), or in the CHD-CP group ANOVA (p=0.559) (Table 1).

IgG Antibodies to Microbial HSP65 and Human HSP60

The median (interquartile range) optical density at 1:100 dilution of serum for anti-microbial HSP65 IgG was 0.34 (0.17-0.63) in the control group, 0.46(0.25-0.85) in the CP group, 0.35 (0.23-0.71) in the CHD-G group and 0.59 (0.2-0.94) in the CHD-CP group (Figure 1). There was no significant difference amongst the 4 groups in serum anti-HSP65 IgG titres by ANOVA (p=0.661).

Serum levels of anti-microbial HSP65 IgG were significantly associated with serum levels of anti-human HSP60 IgG in only 2 groups: the CP group (r_s= 0.538, p= 0.005) and the CHD-G group (r_s =0.524, p=0.007) (Table 3). No statistically significant relationship was revealed between serum anti-microbial HSP 65 IgG and serum anti-human HSP60 IgG in the control group (r_s=0.005, p=0.983) and the CHD-CP group (r_s=0.255, p=0.219) (Table 3).

Lymphoproliferative Responses to Human HSP60 in Smokers and Non-smokers

The results of the lymphoproliferative assays are expressed as stimulation indices (the ratio of antigen-stimulated to unstimulated cultures). An analysis of smokers and non-smokers in each group yielded no significant differences in lymphoproliferative responses between any of the four groups (figure 3). All patient groups responded significantly to human HSP60, in contrast to the healthy controls which yielded a median (interquartile range) stimulation index of 2.0 (0.45) (p<0.001). Smoking does not appear to influence HSP60-induced proliferation in CP or CHD. In all groups of non-smokers except the controls, HSP proliferative responses correlated with CRP levels (p<0.02).

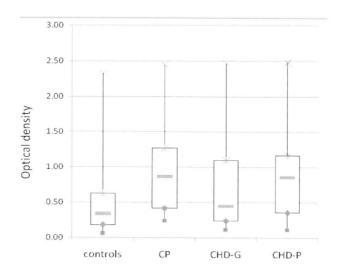

Figure 1. Boxplots showing median, interquartile range, minimum and maximum OD for serum anti-microbial HSP65 IgG in 4 groups of patients The median (interquartile range) OD of 1:100 dilution of serum for anti-human HSP60 IgG was 0.26 (0.17-0.34) in the control group, 0.87 (0.42-1.27) in the CP group, 0.33 (0.24-1.1) in the CHD-G group and 0.86 (0.36-1.17) in the CHD-CP group and this was statistically significant by ANOVA (p<0.001) (figure 2). Post-ANOVA analysis revealed a significant difference between the controls and the CP group (p<0.001). There was also a significant difference between the control and the CHD-G group (p=0.019), but no significant difference between the chronic periodontitis and the CHD-CP group (p=0.907).

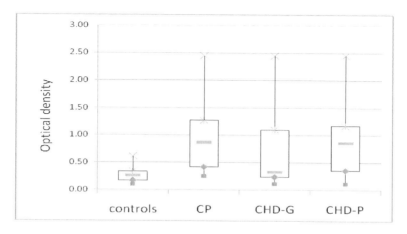

Figure 2. Boxplots showing median, interquartile range, minimum and maximum OD for serum anti-human HSP60 IgG in 4 groups of patients

Table 3. Correlation between serum anti-human HSP60 IgG and serum CRP levels to serum anti-microbial HSP 65 IgG

		anti-microbial HSP65 IgG	CRP
Control	r_s	0.005	0.115
n=25	p	0.983	0.583
CP	r_s	#0.538	-0.194
n=25	p	*0.005	0.352
CHD-G	r_s	#0.524	-0.099
n=25	p	*0.007	0.637
CHD-CP	r_s	0.255	#0.417
n=25	p	0.219	*0.038

significant correlation coefficient (r_s) * Significant p value

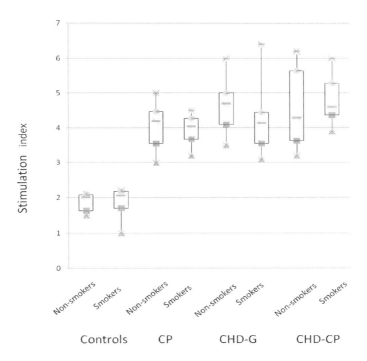

Figure 3. Boxplots showing median, interquartile range, minimum and maximum stimulation index of Human HSP60-induced lymphoproliferative responses in non-smokers and smokers (n=6 for each group). CP and CHD with or without CP responded significantly to HSP60 (ANOVA p<0.001)

CRP

The median (interquartile range) of serum CRP levels in the 4 groups was 0.64 (0.18-1.86) mg/L in the control group, 1.27 (1.01-2.83) mg/L in the CP group, 2.15 (1.03-2.94) in the CHD-G group and 2.0 (1.31-3.78) in the CHD-CP group (figure 4). There was a statistically significant difference amongst the groups by ANOVA (p=0.002). Post-ANOVA analysis revealed significant differences between the control group compared to the CP group (p=0.007) and the control group compared with the CHD-G group (p=0.001). However there was no significant difference between the CP compared with the CHD-CP group (p=0.383). It is tempting to interpret this to mean that CP influences CRP levels, however we do not have data on whether these responses may fluctuate with time, and what other innate or adaptive mechanisms determine the outcome; nor do we know how this impacts on CHD.

Serum CRP levels are not significantly associated with serum anti-human HSP60 IgG levels in the control group (r_s =0.115, p=0.583), in the CP group (r_s =-0.194, p=0.352) and in the CHD-G group (r_s =-0.099, p=0.637) (Table 3). However in the CHD-CP group there was an association between serum CRP levels and serum anti-human HSP60 IgG levels (r_s =0.417, p= 0.038) (Table 3).

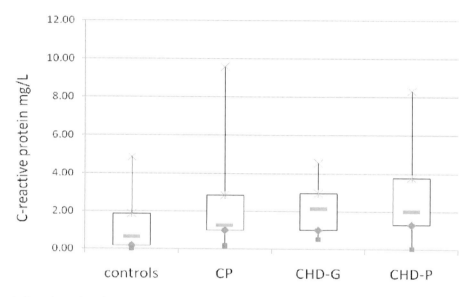

Figure 4. Boxplots showing median, interquartile range, minimum and maximum level of serum C-reactive protein amongst the 4 groups of patients

DISCUSSION

The results show that serum anti-human HSP60 IgG but not serum anti-microbial HSP65 IgG was elevated in patients with chronic periodontitis compared to the control group. No significant differences were noted in the level of serum anti-human HSP60 IgA and serum anti-microbial HSP65 IgA between the control group and patients with chronic periodontitis. These findings contrast with a study showing an elevation of serum anti-HSP65 IgG (Schett et al 1997a) and another study showing depression of serum anti-HSP65 IgA with no difference in serum anti-human HSP60 IgG and serum anti-microbial HSP 65 IgG in CP patients compared to the control group (Buhlin et al 2003). However these studies are difficult to compare directly as there are significant differences in demographical and clinical parameters. In one of these studies the patient group had a mean age of 37.5 ± 12.6 years range 26-65 years (Schett et al 1997); with this age range it is likely that more than one form of periodontitis was included. Our study included only patients with moderate-advanced chronic periodontitis or gingival health/mild gingivitis. The median age (interquartile range) of our patients with chronic periodontitis is 49 (43-53). Younger aged patients with advanced periodontitis may represent a different diagnostic category or a different spectrum of response from older patients suffering from chronic periodontitis (Ranney 2000), and may mount different immune responses (Gunsolley et al 1990).

The recruitment of patients who are undergoing treatment for chronic periodontitis (Buhlin et al 2003) is problematic and may yield conflicting results as treatment of CP has a modulating effect on humoral immune responses to HSP (Yamazaki et al 2004) and instrumentation may immunise patients with plaque antigens. To minimise the confounding effect of treatment in our results we recruited untreated cases.

Our findings are in agreement with studies where the mean ages of untreated chronic periodontitis were similar (Tabeta et al 2000, Lopatin et al 1999). These studies demonstrated a significant elevation in serum anti-human HSP 60 IgG compared to a control group (Tabeta et al 2000). Serum anti-microbial HSP65 IgG levels were either similar (Lopatin et al 1999) or elevated (Tabeta et al 2000) in chronic periodontitis patients compared to control patients.

It was important to match our patients for age, as clearly both CP and CHD occur with increasing frequency in older populations. In addition, the diagnosis of periodontal diseases is unfortunately age-dependent, so the distinction between early onset forms of periodontitis and chronic adult periodontitis becomes harder to establish when patients present at the age of 30-35. Until the behaviour of the disease can be determined it is difficult to be certain the correct diagnosis has been made without resorting to special tests and culture studies. We were therefore careful to match the age of patients to those presenting at the Coronary care unit, rather than those attending a Periodontal clinic where the patients tend to be three decades younger.

In this study whilst we demonstrated a statistically significant elevation in serum anti-human HSP60 IgG in the CHD-G group, there was no statistical difference in serum anti-microbial HSP65 IgG. A number of studies have demonstrated elevation in serum anti-microbial HSP65 IgG in patients with CHD (Ciervo et al 2002, Mahdi et al 2002, Prohászka et al 2001, Birnie et al 1998, Hoppichler et al 1996, Xu et al 1993) which was sustained over a number of years (Xu et al 1999) and predicted cardiovascular events (Veres et al 2002, Xu et al 1999). Most of these studies analysed subjects aged 60 years or over (Veres et al 2002, Ciervo et al 2002, Mahdi et al 2002, Xu et al 1999, Hoppichler et al 1996, Xu et al 1993) or did not include a healthy control group (Birnie et al 1998). Furthermore, the periodontal status of these patients was not determined. When a younger age group (less than 60 yrs old) was analysed for anti-HSP65 IgG, no significant difference was found compared with the control group (Xu et al 1993). In studies where the age group was comparable to our study, serum anti-HSP60 IgG was demonstrated to be elevated in the patient group compared to control (Bason et al 2003, Burian et al 2003, Prohászka et al 2001, Zhu et al 2001). Additionally, serum antibodies from these patients recognised human HSP60 peptide fragments (Bason et al 2003, Wysocki et al 2002). Older subjects have been shown to be more prone to chronic infections resulting in an increase in markers of inflammation including anti-microbial HSP65 (Kiechl et al 2001). The presence of anti-microbial HSP65 antibodies may reflect the cumulative effect of infections which increases with age. However this is still compatible with the hypothesis that cross-reactivity between microbial HSP65 and human HSP60 may lead to tissue damage in CP and CHD (Mayr et al 1999).

Serum anti-human HSP60 IgA when present with *Chlamydia pneumoniae* has been identified as a risk factor for future coronary events in patients who were initially healthy (Huittinen et al 2003, Huittinen et al 2002). Whilst we found there was no statistically significant difference in serum anti-human HSP60 IgA or serum anti-microbial HSP65 IgA between the control and the CHD-G group, it remains to be established whether antibody levels remain elevated or fluctuate in relation to intercurrent infections. It is clearly important to determine how innate, humoral and cellular immune responses change with time, infection, or coronary events in CP or CHD.

Cross reactivity between anti-microbial HSP65 antibodies and human HSP60 antibodies has been suggested to mediate macrophage lysis (Schett et al 1997b) and endothelial damage (Schett et al 1995). Serum anti-microbial HSP65 have been shown to recognise specific epitopes on human HSP60 in subjects with atherosclerosis (Perschinka et al 2003). In our study there was a moderate correlation between serum anti-human HSP60 IgG and serum anti-microbial HSP65 IgG in patients with CP and CHD-G, and therefore the possibility of cross-reactivity still exists. Shared epitopes within human HSP60 may help account for the association between CP and CHD and reveal a mechanistic link for tissue destruction. Once the epitopes recognised in CP and CHD have been mapped, the role of T and B cell epitopes in relation to inflammatory and anti-inflammatory responses can be elucidated.

Smoking is a risk factor for chronic periodontitis and CHD (Genco et al 2002). In addition smoking has been suggested to be a confounding variable in the association of CP with CHD (Hujoel et al 2000). Smoking is known to modulate immune response and in chronic periodontitis there is a direct correlation between serum cotinine levels and serum levels of intracellular adhesion molecule- a risk factor for CHD (Palmer et al 1999). Exposure of human monocytes and endothelial cells to freshly prepared filtrates of tobacco smoke induces expression of the inducible HSP70 (Vayssier-Taussat et al 2001). The role of smoking on the cellular and humoral immune responses to HSP in patients with chronic periodontitis and CHD has not been fully elucidated although, exposure to smoking reduces the release of TNF-α in human alveolar macrophages (Yamaguchi et al 1993) and PBMC (Ryder et al 2002). We found no difference between smokers and non-smokers in any of the subject groups suggesting that at least HSP-induced proliferation is not affected by smoking. It however remains to be determined how smoking affects HSP-induced T cell responses and inflammatory cytokine production in CHD and CP.

Serum CRP levels in patients with CP and CHD when compared to a healthy control group were significantly elevated. Previous studies have shown that serum CRP levels are elevated in CP (D'Aiuto et al 2004, Buhlin et al 2003, Ide et al 2003). Cross-sectional studies have shown that CRP levels are also raised in patients with angiographically recorded coronary heart disease (Garcia-Moll et al 2000, Rifai et al 1999) and in patients with symptoms of angina but normal coronary angiogram (Cosin-Sales et al 2003). In a prospective multiple risk factor intervention trial CRP was found to be an independent risk factor for coronary heart disease mortality in healthy but high risk individuals (Kuller et al 1996). Furthermore, CRP could be used to predict the risk of acute myocardial infarction and mortality of patients with angiographically recorded coronary heart disease (Bickel et al 2002, Zebrack et al 2002).

No significant correlation was shown between CRP and serum anti-HSP60 IgG levels in subjects, except in the CHD-CP group. This is in agreement with previous reports in the literature which do not demonstrate significant relationship between CRP and serum anti-human HSP60 levels (Veres et al 2002, Zhu et al 2001). These conflicting findings may simply reflect the complex nature of innate immunity and its diverse relationships to both inflammatory and anti-inflammatory mechanisms.

CONCLUSION

This study demonstrated that serum anti-human HSP 60 IgG but not serum anti-microbial HSP65 IgG is elevated in patients with CP with or without CHD indicating there are autoantibodies to human HSP60 in CP and CHD and together with our previous findings of autoimmune T cell response to human HSP provides further support for cross-reactivity in the pathogenesis of CP and CHD. Serum CRP levels were also significantly raised in the patient groups but there was no significant relationship between serum CRP levels with serum anti-human HSP60 IgG levels. If we are to determine successfuly whether the association between CP and CHD is real, HSP-induced inflammatory and anti-inflammatory mechanisms need to be further elucidated in relation to innate immunity.

REFERENCES

Amar, S., Gokce, N., Morgan, S., Loukideli, M., Van Dyke, T.E. & Vita, J.A. (2003) *Periodontal disease is associated with brachial artery endothelial dysfunction and systemic inflammation.* Arteriosclerosis, thrombosis, and vascular biology, 23, 1245-1249.

Ando, T., Kato, T., Ishihara, K., Ogiuchi, H. & Okuda, K. (1995) *Heat shock proteins in the human periodontal disease process.* Microbiology and immunology, 39, 321-327.

Badersten A., Nilveus R, Egelberg J. (1981) *Effect of nonsurgical periodontal therapy. I. Moderately advanced periodontitis.* Journal of clinical periodontology, 1, 57-72.

Bason, C., Corrocher, R., Lunardi, C., Puccetti, P., Olivieri, O., Girelli, D., Navone, R., Beri, R., Millo, E., Margonato, A., Martinelli, N. & Puccetti, A. (2003) *Interaction of antibodies against cytomegalovirus with heat-shock protein 60 in pathogenesis of atherosclerosis.* Lancet, 362, 1971-1977.

Beck J. Garcia R. Heiss G. Vokonas PS. Offenbacher S. (1996) *Periodontal disease and cardiovascular disease.* Journal of Periodontology. 67(10 Suppl):1123-37

Bickel, C., Rupprecht, H.J., Blankenberg, S., Espiniola-Klein, C., Schlitt, A., Rippin, G., Hafner, G., Treude, R., Othman, H., Hofmann, K.P. & Meyer, J. (2002) *Relation of markers of inflammation (C-reactive protein, fibrinogen, von Willebrand factor, and leukocyte count) and statin therapy to long-term mortality in patients with angiographically proven coronary artery disease.* The American journal of cardiology, 89, 901-908.

Birnie, D.H., Holme, E.R., McKay, I.C., Hood, S., McColl, K.E. & Hillis, W.S. (1998) *Association between antibodies to heat shock protein 65 and coronary atherosclerosis. Possible mechanism of action of Helicobacter pylori and other bacterial infections in increasing cardiovascular risk.* European heart journal, 19, 387-394.

Buhlin, K., Gustafsson, A., Pockley, A.G., Frostegard, J. & Klinge, B. (2003) *Risk factors for cardiovascular disease in patients with periodontitis.* European heart journal, 24, 2099-2107.

Burian, K., Kis, Z., Virok, D., Endresz, V., Prohaszka, Z., Duba, J., Berencsi, K., Boda, K., Horvath, L., Romics, L., Fust, G. & Gonczol, E. (2001*) Independent and joint effects of antibodies to human heat-shock protein 60 and Chlamydia pneumoniae infection in the development of coronary atherosclerosis.* Circulation, 103, 1503-1508.

Carroll, G.C. & Sebor, R.J. (1980) *Dental flossing and its relationship to transient bacteremia.* Journal of periodontology, 51, 691-692.

Ciervo, A., Visca, P., Petrucca, A., Biasucci, L.M., Maseri, A. & Cassone, A. (2002) *Antibodies to 60-kilodalton heat shock protein and outer membrane protein 2 of Chlamydia pneumoniae in patients with coronary heart disease.* Clinical and diagnostic laboratory immunology, 9, 66-74.

Cosin-Sales, J., Pizzi, C., Brown, S. & Kaski, J.C. (2003) *C-reactive protein, clinical presentation, and ischemic activity in patients with chest pain and normal coronary angiograms.* Journal of the American College of Cardiology, 41, 1468-1474.

Danesh, J., Collins, R. & Peto R. (1997) *Chronic infections and coronary heart disease: is there a link?* Lancet, 350, 430-436.

D'Aiuto, F., Parkar, M., Andreou, G., Suvan, J., Brett, P.M., Ready, D. & Tonetti, M.S. (2004) *Periodontitis and Systemic Inflammation: Control of the Local Infection is Associated with a Reduction in Serum Inflammatory Markers.* Journal of dental research, 83, 156-160.

DeStefano F. Anda RF. Kahn HS. Williamson DF. Russell CM. (1993) *Dental disease and risk of coronary heart disease and mortality.* BMJ. 306(6879):688-91

Desvarieux M. Demmer RT. Rundek T. Boden-Albala B. Jacobs DR Jr. Sacco RL. Papapanou PN. (2005) *Periodontal microbiota and carotid intima-media thickness: the Oral Infections and Vascular Disease Epidemiology Study (INVEST).* Circulation. 111(5):576-82

Direskeneli, H., Hasan, A., Shinnick, T., Mizushima, R., van der Zee, R., Fortune, F., Stanford, M.R. & Lehner, T. (1996) *Recognition of B-cell epitopes of the 65 kDa HSP in Behcet's disease.* Scandinavian journal of immunology, 43, 464-471.

Ellis RJ *Stress proteins as molecular chaperones.* (1995) In Stress proteins in medicine, eds. Willem V.E., Douglas B. Y & Mercel, D . 1st edition., pp. 1-26. Inc New york, Basel, Hong Kong.

Epstein SE. (2002) *The multiple mechanisms by which infection may contribute to atherosclerosis development and course.* Circulation Research. 90(1):2-4

Ford PJ. Gemmell E. Hamlet SM. Hasan A. Walker PJ. West MJ. Cullinan MP. Seymour GJ. (2005) *Cross-reactivity of GroEL antibodies with human heat shock protein 60 and quantification of pathogens in atherosclerosis.* Oral Microbiology & Immunology. 20(5):296-302

Ford PJ. Gemmell E. Timms P. Chan A. Preston FM. Seymour GJ. (2007) *Anti-P. gingivalis response correlates with atherosclerosis.* Journal of Dental Research. 86(1):35-40

Garcia-Moll, X., Zouridakis, E., Cole, D. & Kaski, J.C. (2000) *C-reactive protein in patients with chronic stable angina: differences in baseline serum concentration between women and men.* European heart journal, 21, 1598-1606.

Genco, R., Offenbacher, S. & Beck, J. (2002) *Periodontal disease and cardiovascular disease: epidemiology and possible mechanisms.* The Journal of the American Dental Association, 133 Suppl, 14S-22S.

Gunsolley, J.C., Tew, J.G., Gooss, C., Marshall, D.R., Burmeister, J.A. & Schenkein, H.A. (1990) *Serum antibodies to periodontal bacteria.* Journal of periodontology, 61, 412-419.

Haraszthy, V.I., Zambon, J.J., Trevisan, M., Zeid, M. & Genco, R.J. (2000) *Identification of periodontal pathogens in atheromatous plaques.* Journal of periodontology, 71, 1554-1560.

Hasan A, Sadoh D, Palmer R, Foo M, Marber M and Lehner T (2005) *The immune responses to human and microbial heat shock proteins in periodontal disease with and without coronary heart disease,* Clinical & Experimental Immunology, 142(3)585-594

Hoppichler, F., Lechleitner, M., Traweger, C., Schett, G., Dzien, A., Sturm, W. & Xu, Q. (1996) *Changes of serum antibodies to heat-shock protein 65 in coronary heart disease and acute myocardial infarction.* Atherosclerosis, 126, 333-338.

Hujoel, P.P., Drangsholt, M., Spiekerman, C. & Derouen, T.A. (2000) *Periodontal disease and coronary heart disease risk.* The journal of the American Medical Association, 284, 1406-1410.

Hujoel PP. Drangsholt M. Spiekerman C. Derouen TA.(2001) *Examining the link between coronary heart disease and the elimination of chronic dental infections.* Journal of the American Dental Association. 132(7):883-9

Huittinen T, Leinonen M, Tenkanen L, Manttari M, Virkkunen H, Pitkanen T, Wahlstrom E, Palosuo T, Manninen V& Saikku P. (2002). *Autoimmunity to human heat shock protein 60, Chlamydia pneumoniae infection, and inflammation in predicting coronary risk.* Arteriosclerosis, thrombosis, and vascular biology, 22, 431-437

Huittinen, T., Leinonen, M., Tenkanen, L., Virkkunen, H., Manttari, M., Palosuo, T., Manninen, V. & Saikku, P. (2003) *Synergistic effect of persistent Chlamydia pneumoniae infection, autoimmunity, and inflammation on coronary risk.* Circulation, 107, 2566-2570.

Ide, M., McPartlin, D., Coward, P.Y., Crook, M., Lumb, P. & Wilson, R.F. (2003) *Effect of treatment of chronic periodontitis on levels of serum markers of acute-phase inflammatory and vascular responses.* Journal of clinical periodontology, 30, 334-340.

Jindal S. Dudani AK. Singh B. Harley CB. Gupta RS. (1989) *Primary structure of a human mitochondrial protein homologous to the bacterial and plant chaperonins and to the 65-kilodalton mycobacterial antigen.* Molecular & Cellular Biology. 9(5):2279-83.

Kiechl, S., Egger, G., Mayr, M., Wiedermann, C.J., Bonora, E., Oberhollenzer, F., Muggeo, M., Xu, Q., Wick, G., Poewe, W. & Willeit, J. (2001*) Chronic infections and the risk of carotid atherosclerosis: prospective results from a large population study.* Circulation, 103, 1064-1070.

Kuller, L.H., Tracy, R.P., Shaten, J. & Meilahn, E.N. (1996) *Relation of C-reactive protein and coronary heart disease in the MRFIT nested case-control study. Multiple Risk Factor Intervention Trial.* American journal of epidemiology, 144, 537-547.

Kumar PS. Griffen AL. Barton JA. Paster BJ. Moeschberger ML. Leys EJ. (2003) *New bacterial species associated with chronic periodontitis.* Journal of Dental Research. 82(5):338-44,

Lang PN, Mombelli A & Attström R (1998) *Dental Plaque and Calculus*. In Clinical Periodontology and Implant Dentistry, eds. Lindhe, J., Karring, T. & Lang, N.P.. 3rd edition. p.102-137. Copenhagen: Munksgaard..

Listgarten MA. Loomer PM. (2003) *Microbial identification in the management of periodontal diseases. A systematic review*. Annals of Periodontology. 8(1):182-92

Lopatin, D.E., Shelburne, C.E., Van Poperin, N., Kowalski, C.J. & Bagramian, R.A. (1999) *Humoral immunity to stress proteins and periodontal disease*. Journal of periodontology, 70, 1185-1193.

Mahdi, O.S., Horne, B.D., Mullen, K., Muhlestein, J.B. & Byrne, G.I. (2002) *Serum immunoglobulin G antibodies to chlamydial heat shock protein 60 but not to human and bacterial homologs are associated with coronary artery disease*. Circulation, 106, 1659-1663.

Maron, R., Sukhova, G., Faria, A.M., Hoffmann, E., Mach, F., Libby, P. & Weiner, H.L. (2002) *Mucosal administration of heat shock protein-65 decreases atherosclerosis and inflammation in aortic arch of low-density lipoprotein receptor-deficient mice*. Circulation, 106, 1708-1715.

Mayr, M., Metzler, B., Kiechl, S., Willeit, J., Schett, G., Xu, Q. & Wick, G. (1999) *Endothelial cytotoxicity mediated by serum antibodies to heat shock proteins of Escherichia coli and Chlamydia pneumoniae: immune reactions to heat shock proteins as a possible link between infection and atherosclerosis*. Circulation, 99, 1560-1566.

Moore, W.E. & Moore, L.V. (1994) *The bacteria of periodontal diseases*. Periodontology 2000, 5, 66-77.

Palmer, R.M., Scott, D.A., Meekin, T.N., Poston, R.N., Odell, E.W. & Wilson, R.F. (1999) *Potential mechanisms of susceptibility to periodontitis in tobacco smokers*. Journal of periodontal research, 34, 363-369.

Perschinka, H., Mayr, M., Millonig, G., Mayerl, C., Van der Zee, R., Morrison, S.G., Morrison, R.P., Xu, Q. & Wick, G. (2003) *Cross-reactive B-cell epitopes of microbial and human heat shock protein 60/65 in atherosclerosis*. Arteriosclerosis, thrombosis, and vascular biology, 23, 1060-1065.

Pervin K. Childerstone A. Shinnick T. Mizushima Y. van der Zee R. Hasan A. Vaughan R. Lehner T. (1993) *T cell epitope expression of mycobacterial and homologous human 65-kilodalton heat shock protein peptides in short term cell lines from patients with Behcet's disease*. Journal of Immunology. 151(4):2273-82

Prohaszka, Z., Duba, J., Horvath, L., Csaszar, A., Karadi, I., Szebeni, A., Singh, M., Fekete, B., Romics, L. & Fust, G. (2001) *Comparative study on antibodies to human and bacterial 60 kDa heat shock proteins in a large cohort of patients with coronary heart disease and healthy subjects*. European journal of clinical investigation, 31, 285-292.

Pussinen, P.J., Jousilahti, P., Alfthan, G., Palosuo, T., Asikainen, S. & Salomaa, V. (2003) *Antibodies to periodontal pathogens are associated with coronary heart disease*. Arteriosclerosis, thrombosis, and vascular biology, 23, 1250-1254.

Ranney, R.R. (1993) Classification of periodontal diseases. Periodontology 2000 , 2, 13-25.

Rifai, N., Joubran, R., Yu, H., Asmi, M. & Jouma, M. (1999) *Inflammatory markers in men with angiographically documented coronary heart disease*. Clinical chemistry, 45, 1967-1973.

Ryder, M.I., Saghizadeh, M., Ding, Y., Nguyen, N. & Soskolne, A. (2002) *Effects of tobacco smoke on the secretion of interleukin-1beta, tumor necrosis factor-alpha, and transforming growth factor-beta from peripheral blood mononuclear cells.* Oral microbiology and immunology, 17, 331-336.

Saikku, P., Leinonen, M., Mattila, K., Ekman, M.R., Nieminen, M.S., Makela, P.H., Huttunen, J.K. & Valtonen, V. (1988) *Serological evidence of an association of a novel Chlamydia, TWAR, with chronic coronary heart disease and acute myocardial infarction.* Lancet, 2, 983-986.

Schett, G., Metzler, B., Kleindienst, R., Moschen, I., Hattmannsdorfer, R., Wolf, H., Ottenhoff, T., Xu, Q. & Wick, G. (1997a) *Salivary anti-hsp65 antibodies as a diagnostic marker for gingivitis and a possible link to atherosclerosis.* International archives of allergy and immunology, 114, 246-250.

Schett, G., Metzler, B., Mayr, M., Amberger, A., Niederwieser, D., Gupta, R.S., Mizzen, L., Xu, Q. & Wick, G. (1997b) *Macrophage-lysis mediated by autoantibodies to heat shock protein 65/60.* Atherosclerosis, 128, 27-38.

Schett, G., Metzler, B., Kleindienst, R., Amberger, A., Recheis, H., Xu, Q. & Wick, G. (1999) *Myocardial injury leads to a release of heat shock protein (hsp) 60 and a suppression of the anti-hsp65 immune response.* Cardiovascular research, 42, 685-695.

Silver, J.G., Martin, A.W. & McBride, B.C. (1977) *Experimental transient bacteraemias in human subjects with varying degrees of plaque accumulation and gingival inflammation.* Journal of Clinical Periodontology, 4, 92-99.

Tabeta, K., Yamazaki, K., Hotokezaka, H., Yoshie, H. & Hara, K. (2000) *Elevated humoral immune response to heat shock protein 60 (hsp60) family in periodontitis patients.* Clinical and experimental immunology, 120, 285-293.

Thole JE, Hindersson P, de Bruyn J, Cremers F, van der Zee J, de Cock H, Tommassen J, van Eden W, van Embden JD. (1988) *Antigenic relatedness of a strongly immunogenic 65 kDA mycobacterial protein antigen with a similarly sized ubiquitous bacterial common antigen.* : Microbial pathogenesis 4(1):71-83

Vayssier-Taussat, M., Camilli, T., Aron, Y., Meplan, C., Hainaut, P., Polla, B.S. & Weksler, B. (2001) *Effects of tobacco smoke and benzo[a]pyrene on human endothelial cell and monocyte stress responses.* American journal of physiology. Heart and circulatory physiology, 280, H1293-H1300.

Veres, A., Fust, G., Smieja, M., McQueen, M., Horvath, A., Yi, Q., Biro, A., Pogue, J., Romics, L., Karadi, I., Singh, M., Gnarpe, J., Prohaszka, Z. & Yusuf, S. (2002) *Relationship of anti-60 kDa heat shock protein and anti-cholesterol antibodies to cardiovascular events.* Circulation, 106, 2775-2780.

Wysocki, J., Karawajczyk, B., Gorski, J., Korzeniowski, A., Mackiewicz, Z., Kupryszewski, G. & Glosnicka, R. (2002) *Human heat shock protein 60 (409-424) fragment is recognized by serum antibodies of patients with acute coronary syndromes.* Cardiovascular pathology, 11, 238-243.

Xu, Q., Willeit, J., Marosi, M., Kleindienst, R., Oberhollenzer, F., Kiechl, S., Stulnig, T., Luef, G. & Wick, G. (1993) *Association of serum antibodies to heat-shock protein 65 with carotid atherosclerosis.* Lancet, 341, 255-259.

Xu, Q., Kiechl, S., Mayr, M., Metzler, B., Egger, G., Oberhollenzer, F., Willeit, J. & Wick, G. (1999) *Association of serum antibodies to heat-shock protein 65 with carotid atherosclerosis : clinical significance determined in a follow-up study.* Circulation, 100 , 1169-1174.

Yamaguchi, E., Itoh, A., Furuya, K., Miyamoto, H., Abe, S. & Kawakami, Y. (1993) *Release of tumor necrosis factor-alpha from human alveolar macrophages is decreased in smokers*. Chest, 103, 479-483.

Yamazaki, K., Ueki-Maruayama, K., Honda, T., Nakajima, T. & Seymour, G.J. (2004) *Effect of periodontal treatment on the serum antibody levels to heat shock proteins*. Clinical Experimental Immunology, 135, 478-482.

Zebrack, J.S., Anderson, J.L., Maycock, C.A., Horne, B.D., Bair, T.L. & Muhlestein, J.B. (2002) *Usefulness of high-sensitivity C-reactive protein in predicting long-term risk*. The American journal of cardiology, 89, 145-149.

Zhu, J., Quyyumi, A.A., Rott, D., Csako, G., Wu, H., Halcox, J. & Epstein, S.E. (2001) *Antibodies to human heat-shock protein 60 are associated with the presence and severity of coronary artery disease: evidence for an autoimmune component of atherogenesis*. Circulation, 103, 1071-1075.

In: Periodontitis Symptoms, Treatment and Prevention   ISBN: 978-1-61668-836-3
Editor: Rosemarie E. Walchuck, pp. 239-253   ©2010 Nova Science Publishers, Inc.

Chapter 11

CHRONIC PERIODONTITIS AND THE RISK OF ORAL CANCER

Mine Tezal[1, 2] and Maureen A. Sullivan[1, 2]
State University of New York at Buffalo, Buffalo, NY, USA[1]
Roswell Park Cancer Institute, Buffalo, NY, USA[2]

ABSTRACT

Morbidity and mortality from oral cancer are high and this has not improved in decades in spite of extensive research. A significant portion of research is concentrated on chemoprevention. However, advances in this field have not translated into a visible change in mortality and morbidity. In addition, existing chemoprevention strategies have two important obstacles: toxicity and reversal of the effects after cessation of treatment. Chronic infection and inflammation have been linked to carcinogenesis in a few organs. For oral cancer, substantial evidence has accumulated for the role of *human papillomavirus* (HPV). However, the development of an effective preventive vaccine strategy for oral cancer is still years away and the target population is largely unexplored. Therefore, safe and practical additional approaches are necessary to change the status quo of oral cancer. Periodontitis is a chronic oral infection caused by inflammatory reactions in response to gram negative anaerobic bacteria in the endogenous dental plaque. It leads to irreversible destruction of tissues around teeth clinically detectable as periodontal pockets and alveolar bone loss. Periodontal pockets have been suggested as reservoirs of HPV. Chronic proliferation and ulceration of the pocket epithelium may help HPV's initial infection and persistence. Our preliminary results from existing data at Roswell Park Cancer Institute suggest a robust independent association between the history of periodontitis and incident oral cancer. Our next step is to test the synergy between periodontitis and HPV for the risk of oral cancer. If this is true, it will translate to practical and safe prevention and treatment strategies. This chapter will review the evidence supporting the association between chronic periodontitis and oral cancer as well as HPV-periodontitis synergy.

INTRODUCTION

Oral cancer is a significant cause of morbidity and mortality and this has not changed for decades. It is estimated that 34,360 new cases of oral cancer and 7,550 deaths will occur in 2007 [1]. The incidence is open to debate because of the well-known field cancerization phenomenon in the head and neck region. Those with primary cancer of the oral cavity and pharynx are also at high risk for developing cancer of the esophagus, larynx, lung, and stomach. Oral cancer is notorious for its high rates of second primary cancers, recurrence, and distant metastases [2-4]. It often leaves the patients with disfiguration and loss of vital functions such as swallowing and breathing. Consequent psychological and social impairments are also very debilitating. The treatment is aggressive and often increases the morbidity without improving the survival significantly [5].

Even though oral cancer is largely preventable, the majority of funded research has been on treatment and diagnosis. However, advances in these fields have not translated into a visible change in grim oral cancer statistics. Primary prevention strategies against risk factors, mostly tobacco, alcohol and diet, are limited and have not been very effective. Most of the existing prevention strategies are secondary and tertiary. Preventive surgical resection, radiotherapy, photodynamic therapy and topical cytotoxic therapies had limited success [6, 7]. Chemoprevention, including retinoids, selenium, vitamin E, interferon- α (IFN-α), cyclo-oxygenase-2 (COX-2) and epidermal growth factor receptor (EGFR) tyrosine kinase inhibitors, have two important obstacles: toxicity and reversal of the effects after cessation of treatment [8-10]. Chronic infections with viruses, especially certain human papillomavirus strains (HPV 16 and 18) are another target for prevention. The vaccine targeting HPV types 6, 11, 16 and 18 became recently available for cervical cancer. However, the vaccine is prophylactic and is not effective for those who were previously exposed to the virus. It is expensive and requires 3 injections over a 6 month-period. Since the longest trial was 5 years, we don't know the length of immunity from the vaccine nor its long-term safety. Even though the vaccine is effective against infection, its effectiveness to prevent invasive cancer is not known [11-12]. Information concerning the role of viruses in oral cancer is fragmented and the development of an effective vaccine strategy may still be years away. The target population who would derive the most benefit from the vaccine is largely unexplored. Therefore, safe and practical additional approaches are necessary to change the status quo of oral cancer.

Although most studies assessing the infectious etiology of cancer are focused on viruses, the evidence on bacterial infections is also convincing [13-14]. Associations with *Helicobacter pylori* infection with gastric cancer and primary B-cell gastric lymphoma [15], *Chlamydia pneumonia* infection with lung cancer [16], *Salmonella typhi* infection with gallbladder cancer [17] and *Streptococcus bovis* infection with colon cancer [18] are a few examples. Recently, there are also a growing number of basic science studies identifying key molecular mechanisms [19-24].

Opposing effects of acute vs. chronic infection on cancer have been described. While chronic infection usually promotes cancer development, acute infection was shown to counteract cancer development. For example, a few studies showed that subjects who contracted *Salmonella typhi* but did not become carriers were not at higher risk for hepatobiliary carcinoma but only those who became chronic carriers were at high risk [25-

27]. The process of acute infection is self-limiting. Pro-inflammatory cytokines give way to anti-inflammatory cytokines as healing progresses. In chronic infection, on the other hand, active tissue destruction and repair proceed simultaneously. Angiogenesis and fibrosis are the chief components of this process and chronic inflammatory cells and mediators persist in the environment [28, 29]. Therefore, chronicity of the infection/inflammation appears to be the key factor for carcinogenesis.

CHRONIC PERIODONTITIS

Periodontitis is a chronic oral infection caused by inflammatory reactions in response to microorganisms in the endogenous dental plaque (Figure 1). The average prevalence of periodontitis in the general population is 30%; about 12% is a severe form [30-33].

The dental plaque is a biofilm. It is critical to understand the characteristics of the biofilm to effectively control periodontitis as well as its systemic sequela. Biofilms are sessile community of various types of bacteria embedded in a polymeric matrix irreversibly attached to a surface. The majority of bacteria in the body exist in biofilms. A main characteristic of biofilms is quorum sensing which is communication and group behavior of bacteria residing in the biofilm. The bacteria in the biofilm differ profoundly from their free floating counterparts and are resistant to antimicrobials as well to host defense [34]. Mechanical removal of the biofilm, by brushing and flossing, is required. In the presence of periodontitis, however, biofilm in the periodontal pockets is inaccessible to personal oral hygiene practices and professional treatment is needed. It is important to note that biofilm properties of the dental plaque contribute to the persistence of periodontitis in the absence of treatment. Treatment of chronic periodontitis is safe and is based on mechanical removal of the biofilm. Chemotherapy alone is not effective [30].

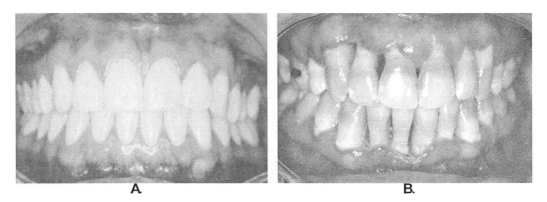

Figure 1. Comparison of healthy periodontium (A) with periodontitis (B).

Periodontitis results in a chronic release of inflammatory chemokines, cytokines, prostaglandins, growth factors and enzymes in saliva and to a lower degree in blood, all of which are also associated with carcinogenesis. The extent and severity of periodontitis are associated with the level of these inflammatory markers. The ensuing chronic inflammation is what leads to local pathologic anatomic changes, namely, periodontal pocket formation and alveolar bone loss [30]. As the disease progresses, epithelial attachment at the bottom of the periodontal pocket migrates apically along the root surface and the pocket depth increases. The pocket epithelium is characterized by continuous proliferation, formation of rete-ridges and ulcerations. In the connective tissue, there is increased angiogenesis, chronic inflammatory infiltrate, fibrosis and tissue loss (figure 2). Furthermore, periodontal pathogens and inflammatory mediators travel with saliva and blood from the affected tissues to distant sites and adversely affect systemic health. Multiple studies have shown that oral pathogens and cytokines are aspirated to lungs by saliva and are transported to arterial plaques by blood [31-38]. Most importantly, treatment of periodontal infections significantly prevents systemic adverse events [39-43]. We anticipate that the same mechanisms may play a part in the field cancerization of oral cancer.

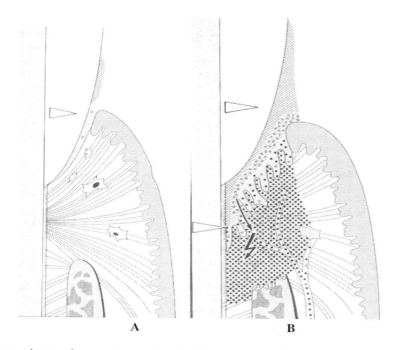

Figure 2. Tissue changes from periodontal health (A) to chronic periodontitis (B).

Poor oral hygiene (dental biofilm) is the cause of periodontitis but only small percentage of subjects with poor oral hygiene develops periodontitis [30]. A link between poor oral hygiene and the risk of oral cancer has also been suggested for a long time [44-54]. However, a definite association has not been established due to limited methodology of existing studies. We anticipate that among subjects with poor oral hygiene, those who develop periodontitis are at higher risk for oral cancer.

We are currently conducting an NIH funded study to test the hypothesis that chronic periodontitis is associated with increased risk of head and neck cancers using existing data at Roswell Park Cancer Institute (RPCI), Buffalo, NY. We have analyzed a subset of this population with a case-control study design. These preliminary analyses were restricted to subjects newly diagnosed with primary squamous cell carcinoma of tongue between June 15, 1999 and November 17, 2005. The control group consisted of subjects admitted during the same time period but not diagnosed with cancer. Children (age <21), edentulous, and those with prior history of cancer, cancer therapy and oral dysplasia were excluded. A total of 94 cases and 153 controls met the inclusion criteria. Histological diagnoses of cancer cases were available electronically from RPCI Tumor Registry. Cumulative history of periodontitis was measured by alveolar bone loss (ABL) from panoramic radiographs using an operator-interactive program on digitized radiographic images [55-58]. Accuracy and reliability of this technique have been established [59, 60]. ABL was measured in millimeter (mm) on mesial and distal sites of all teeth. One trained and calibrated examiner, blind to cancer status, performed all ABL measurements. Number of missing teeth, fillings, cavities and endodontic (root canal) treatments were also diagnosed from the radiographs. The independent effect of ABL on oral cancer was estimated from multiple logistic regression analysis by odds ratio (OR) and 95% confidence interval (CI). Each millimeter of alveolar bone loss was associated with 4.47 fold increase in the risk of tongue cancer (OR=4.47, 95% CI=2.80-7.15) after adjusting the effects of age at diagnosis, gender, race/ethnicity, smoking status, alcohol use and number of teeth. The remaining oral variables cavities, fillings, crowns and endodontic treatments were not significantly associated with the risk of tongue cancer (Table 1).

Table 1. Adjusted Odds Ratios for the Risk of Tongue Cancer (N=247)

	OR*	95% CI[#]	p
Mean ABL (per mm)	4.47	2.80 - 7.15	<0.001
At least 1 Site with ABL ≥4 mm (per site)	9.67	4.01 - 22.82	<0.001
Missing Teeth (per tooth)	1.02	0.98 - 1.05	0.357
Decayed Teeth (per tooth)	0.95	0.83 - 1.09	0.493
Filled Teeth (per tooth)	1.04	0.97 - 1.11	0.253
Crowns (per tooth)	0.91	0.83 - 1.01	0.080
Endodontic Treatments (per tooth)	0.89	0.74 - 1.06	0.197

*Odds ratios adjusted for age at diagnosis, gender, race, alcohol use, smoking status and number of teeth; [#] 95% Confidence intervals.

In summary, this study, analyzing existing patient records at a local comprehensive cancer center, confirmed our suspicions that the history of periodontitis may in fact be associated with oral cancer independent of smoking. However, the study had the classical shortcomings of secondary data analyses: Data on confounding variables was limited. In addition, the diagnosis of periodontitis was based on radiographs. Radiographic assessment of periodontal disease is not sensitive, does not reflect present disease status nor differentiate gingivitis from periodontitis. The encouraging results of this preliminary study provide the basis for further studies with quantitative clinical measures and comprehensive assessment of confounding.

BIOLOGICAL MECHANISM

The question of how infections can influence cancer has interested scientists for over one and a half centuries, but only now are the general principles and the real complexity of this subject emerging. Chronic infections, such as periodontitis, can play a direct or indirect role in carcinogenesis:

1) Direct Toxic Effect of Microorganisms

Microorganisms and their products such as endotoxins (LPS), enzymes (proteases, collagenases, fibrinolysin and phospholipase A) and metabolic by-products (H_2S, NH_3 and fatty acids) are toxic to surrounding cells and may directly induce mutations in tumor suppressor genes and protooncogenes or alter signaling pathways that affect cell proliferation and/or survival of epithelial cells [27]. *Porphyromonas gingivalis* is a major periodontal pathogen that is capable of invading epithelial cells. In a recent study, *P.gingivalis* induced a transient increase in keratynocyte DNA fragmentation; however, after prolonged incubation, *P. gingivalis* blocked apoptosis in keratynocytes [61]. Another example of direct bacterial stimuli is the association between *Helicobacter pylori* and primary B-cell gastric lymphoma, where chronic infection causes persistent B-cell activation culminating in chromosomal rearrangements that ultimately cause cancer [15]. Numerous other studies support the evidence that commensal bacteria can directly affect various stages of cell cycle in carcinogenesis [62-64].

2) Indirect Effect through Inflammation

Chronic infection may stimulate carcinogenesis through an indirect mechanism involving activation of surrounding host cells (neutrophils, macrophages, monocytes, lymphocytes, fibroblasts and epithelial cells) to generate:

*   Reactive oxygen species (hydrogen peroxide and oxy radicals), reactive nitrogen species (nitric oxides), reactive lipids and metabolites (malondialdehyhe, 4-hydroxy-2-nonenal) and matrix metalloproteases (MMPs) which can act as endogenous mutagens and can induce DNA damage in epithelial cells [28].
*   Cytokines, chemokines, growth factors and other signals which provide an environment for cell survival, proliferation, migration, angiogenesis and inhibition of apoptosis [65]. This environment:

    o   Help epithelial cells to accumulate mutations.
    o   Drive these mutant epithelial cells to proliferate, migrate and give them a growth advantage

Recently, a key molecular mechanism connecting inflammation and cancer was identified. It was shown that a pro-inflammatory gene is involved in cancer development and that inactivation of this gene could dramatically (80%) reduce tumor development [22]. A subsequent study showed that cancer metastasis was halted with inhibition of a pro-inflammatory protein, nuclear factor-kappa B (NF-κB) or an inflammatory mediator, tumor necrosis factor alpha (TNF-α) [23]. Another study showed how prostaglandin E_2 (PGE$_2$) promotes colorectal adenoma growth [24]. Numerous other studies have confirmed the associations of various players in inflammation to carcinogenesis in several organs [66-68] including the oral cavity [69-72].

3)   Biological Interactions of Periodontitis with Other Carcinogens

In addition to a plausible biological mechanism for an independent association, periodontitis may also biologically interact with other carcinogens such as tobacco, alcohol and certain viruses to increase the risk of oral cancer. For example, breaks in the mucosal barrier in the presence of periodontitis can lead to enhanced penetration of carcinogens [73]. An increased production of acetaldehyde (a known carcinogen) from ethanol was also shown in subjects with poor oral health [74, 75]. In addition, periodontal pockets may act as reservoirs for *human papillomavirus* (HPV), a suspected causal factor of oral cancer [76-78].

PERIODONTITIS-HPV SYNERGY

HPV is a DNA virus with a specific tropism for squamous epithelia. More than 120 different HPV types have been isolated to date. Low-risk HPVs, such as HPV-6 and HPV-11, induce benign hyperproliferations of the epithelium such as papillomas or warts which rarely progress to cancer. High-risk oncogenic types such as HPV-16 and HPV-18 are associated with squamous cell carcinoma (SCC). HPV-16 and HPV-18 are capable of transforming epithelial cells. This transforming potential is largely a result of the function of two viral oncoproteins, E6 and E7, which functionally inactivate two human tumor suppressor proteins, p53 and pRb, respectively. Expression of high-risk HPV E6 and E7 results in cellular proliferation, loss of cell cycle regulation, impaired cellular differentiation, increased frequency of mutations, and chromosomal instability [79]. HPV-16 and HPV-18 are a central cause of cervical cancer and are also being investigated for head and neck cancers [80-85].

The average prevalence of HPV DNA in normal mucosa is 10% [80]. In a review of 60 studies, the prevalence of HPV DNA in head and neck SCCs was 25.9%. This was 23.5% in oral, 35.6% in oropharyngeal, and 24.0% in laryngeal SCCs. HPV-16 accounted for a larger majority of HPV+ oropharyngeal SCCs (86.7%) compared with HPV+ oral (68.2%) and HPV+ laryngeal (69.2%) SCCs. Conversely, HPV-18 was rare in HPV+ oropharyngeal SCCs (2.8%) compared with HPV+ oral (34.1%) and HPV+ laryngeal (17.0%) SCCs. Aside from HPV-16 and HPV-18, other oncogenic HPV DNAs were rarely detected in HNCs [82]. Probability of HPV DNA being detected in the oral mucosa increases with increasing degree of dysplasia. Overall, HPV DNA is 2 to 3 times more likely to be detected in precancerous lesions and 4.7 times more likely to be detected in HNCs than in normal mucosa [80].

HPV infection is a necessary but not sufficient cause of cervical cancer. Although majority of the population is infected with HPV at least once in their lives, most HPV infections are cleared rapidly by the immune system and do not result in pathology [86, 87]. Persistence of HPV infection is the strongest risk factor in the development of cancer. Thus, the identification of factors that influence the persistence of HPV infection is critical to facilitate efforts to prevent carcinogenesis. Certain bacterial co-infections in the cervix were shown to act synergistically with HPV infection. For example, several studies have shown that concurrent infection with *Chlamydia trachomatis* is associated with HPV persistence and increased the risk of cervical cancer [88, 89]. Studies suggest that viruses and bacteria, mostly studied in isolation, may in fact cooperate synergistically and should probably be considered as a pathogenic consortium in future investigations [90-96]. In addition, elevated levels of inflammatory cytokines IL-6, IL-1, and TNF-α were shown to modulate HPV E6/E7 gene expression and proliferation in human epithelial cells [97-102].

The strictly epitheliotropic nature of HPV, with a specific anatomic site preference, limits its range of infectivity. HPV infects exclusively the basal cells of the epithelium. Naturally occurring HPV infection begins when the virus gains access to permissive basal cells through wounds or abrasions [79]. In the presence of periodontitis, the periodontal pocket epithelium is usually ulcerated facilitating the access of the virus. In addition, replication of virus is associated with proliferation of the basal and parabasal cells. The junctional epithelium, located at the bottom of the periodontal pocket, has a very high mitotic rate and consists of basal and parabasal cell layers. It shares properties similar to the squamous-columnar junction of the cervix uteri, where the majority of HPV-associated cancers arise [103]. Integrin $\alpha_6\beta_4$ and syndecan-1, candidate receptors for HPV, are expressed during wound-healing and are found in the pocket and junctional epithelium in the presence of periodontitis [79, 91].

It is not clear where latent HPV resides in the head and neck region. This is an important factor in the effectiveness of therapeutic methods. Latent state would require the presence of infected cells which fail to differentiate [79]. Theoretically, the junctional epithelium fully fits these criteria. It has only basal and suprabasal cell layers and does not differentiate. HPV types 6, 11 and 16 DNA is detected in gingival tissue, gingival cervicular fluid and subgingival plaque from periodontitis sites [104-107]. These observations suggest that periodontal pockets may serve as a reservoir of HPV in the oral mucosa. This could explain the development of gingival papillomas and condylomas frequently found in patients with AIDS and in patients with organ transplants receiving cyclosporin treatment [107]. In these patients, local reactivation of latent HPV infection could occur in gingival tissues.

In summary, chronic periodontitis may facilitate HPVs initial infection and persistence by: 1- providing anatomical predisposition, 2- stimulation of chronic inflammation, 3- causing epithelial damage, and 4- being a source of bacterial co-infections. Evidence of periodontitis-HPV synergy is important to understand the natural history of HPV infection and oral cancer. It has practical implications for intervention since there is no treatment for HPV infection but there is a safe treatment for periodontitis. If this synergy is real, it will provide us a clinical high-risk profile for HPV status as well as for oral cancer.

CONCLUSION

In spite of long years of research, the research of specific microbial etiology has not translated into effective intervention and prevention strategies for oral cancer. In most cases, the infectious agents are ubiquitous, but only a small fraction of infected individuals develop cancer. Our approach is to clinically identify those who are at high-risk of developing oral cancer among infected individuals. We hypothesize that chronic periodontitis increases the risk of oral cancer independently as well as by helping HPVs initial infection and persistence. If this hypothesis is true, it will shed light to the etiology of oral cancer and the results will translate into immediate and safe prevention and treatment strategies. Subjects with periodontitis may be targeted as a "high-risk" population, and survival from oral cancer may be improved by early diagnosis and treatment. Preventing or treating periodontitis may result in a decreased incidence, morbidity and mortality of oral cancer.

REFERENCES

[1]   Jemal A. Siegel R. Ward E. Murray T. Xu J. Thun MJ. *Cancer statistics,* 2007. CA Cancer J Clin. 2007;57(1):43-66.

[2]   Schwartz LH, Ozsahin M, Zhang GN, et al. *Synchronous and metachronous head and neck carcinomas.* Cancer 1994;74:1933-8.

[3]   Jones AS, Morar P, Phillips DE, et al. *Second primary tumors in patients with head and neck squamous cell carcinoma.* Cancer 1995;75:1343-53.

[4]   Adami HO, Hunter D, Trichopoulos D. *Oral and pharyngeal cancers.* In: Textbook of Cancer Epidemiology. Oxford University Press, Inc. New York, NY. 2000. p. 115-136.

[5]   Palme CE. Gullane PJ. Gilbert RW. *Current treatment options in squamous cell carcinoma of the oral cavity.* Surgical Oncology Clinics of North America. 13(1):47-70, 2004 Jan.

[6]   Lippman SM, Sudbø J, Hong WK. *Oral cancer prevention and the evolution of molecular-targeted drug development.* J Clin Oncol 2005;23:346-356.

[7]   Mignogna MD, Fedeleand S, Russo LL. *The World Cancer Report and the burden of oral cancer.* European Journal of Cancer Prevention 2004;13:139–142.

[8]   Khuri FR, Lee JJ, Lippman SM et al. *Randomized phase-II trial of low-dose isotretinoin for prevention of second primary tumors in stage I and II head and neck cancer patients.* J Natl Cancer Inst. 2006;98:441-50.

[9]   Kelloff GJ, Lippman SM, Dannenberg AJ. *Progress in Chemoprevention Drug Development: The Promise of Molecular Biomarkers for Prevention of Intraepithelial Neoplasia and Cancer. A Plan to Move Forward.* Clin Cancer Res. 2006;12(12):3661-3697.

[10]   ChoeMS, Zhang X, Shin HJ, Shin DM, ChenZG. *Interaction between epidermal growth factor receptor and cyclooxygenase 2-mediated pathways and its implications for the chemoprevention of head and neck cancer.* Mol Cancer Ther. 2005;4:1448-1455.

[11]   Muller M, Gissmann L. *A long way: History of the prophylactic papillomavirus vaccine.* Dis Markers. 2007;23(4):331-336

[12]   Raffle AE. *Challenges of implementing human papillomavirus (HPV) vaccination policy.* BMJ. 2007;335(7616):375-377.

[13]   Kuper H, Adami HO, Trichopoulos D: *Infections as a major preventable cause of human cancer.* J Intern Med 2000, 248:171-83.

[14]   Lax AJ and Thomas W. *How bacteria could cause cancer: one step at a time.* Trends Microbiol. 2002, 10:293-9.

[15]   Crowe SE:. *Helicobacter infection, chronic inflammation, and the development of malignancy.* Curr Opin Gastroenterol. 2005, 1:32-8.

[16]   Littman AJ, White E, Jackson LA, Thornquist MD, Gaydos CA, Goodman GE, Vaughan TL: *Chlamydia pneumoniae infection and risk of lung cancer.* Cancer Epidemiol Biomarkers Prev. 2004;3:1624-1630.

[17]   Vaishnavi C, Kochhar R, Singh G, Kumar S, Singh S, Singh K: *Epidemiology of typhoid carriers among blood donors and patients with biliary, gastrointestinal and other related diseases.* Microbiol Immunol. 2005; 49:107-112.

[18]   Gold JS, Bayar S, Salem RR: *Association of Streptococcus bovis bacteremia with colonic neoplasia and extracolonic malignancy.* Arch Surg. 2004, 139: 760-765.

[19] Huycke MM, Gaskins HR: *Commensal bacteria, redox stress, and colorectal cancer: mechanisms and models.* Exp Biol Med. 2004, 229:586-97.

[20] Lax AJ and Thomas W. *How bacteria could cause cancer: one step at a time.* Trends Microbiol. 2002, 10:293-9.

[21] Jordan RCK, Macabeo-Ong M, Shiboski CH, Dekker N, Ginzinger DG, Wong DTW, Schmidt BL. *Overexpression of matrix metalloproteinase-1 and -9 mRNA is associated with progression of oral dysplasia to cancer.* Clinical Cancer Research 2004;10:6460-6465.

[22] Greten FR, Eckmann L, Greten TF, Park JM, Li ZW, Egan LJ, Kagnoff MF, Karin M. *IKKβ links inflammation and tumorigenesis in a mouse model of colitis-Associated cancer.* Cell 2004; 118 (3):285-296.

[23] Luo JL, Maeda S, Hsu LC, Yagita H, Karin M. *Inhibition of NF-kappa B in cancer cells converts inflammation - induced tumor growth mediated by TNF alpha to TRAIL-mediated tumor regression.* Cancer Cell. 2004;6(3):297-305.

[24] Wang D, Wang H, Shi Q, Katkuri S, Walhi W, Desvergne B, Das SK, Dey SK, DuBois RN. *Prostaglandin E(2) promotes colorectal adenoma growth via transactivation of the nuclear peroxisome proliferator-activated receptor delta. [Journal Article]* Cancer Cell. 2004;6(3):285-95.

[25] Caygill CP, Hill MJ, Braddick M, Sharp JC: *Cancer mortality in chronic typhoid and paratyphoid carriers.* Lancet. 1994, 343:83-4.

[26] Lazcano-Ponce EC, Miquel JF, Munoz N, Herrero R, Ferrecio C, Wistuba II, Alonso de Ruiz P, Aristi UG, Nervi F: *Epidemiology and molecular pathology of gallbladder cancer.* CA Cancer J Clin. 2001, 51: 349-364.

[27] Mager DL, Haffajee AD, Devlin PM, Norris CM, Posner MR, Goodson JM: *The salivary microbiota as a diagnostic indicator of oral cancer: A descriptive, non-randomized study of cancer-free and oral squamous cell carcinoma subjects.* J Transl Med. 2005, 3:27.

[28] Philip M, Rowley DA, Schreiber H. *Inflammation as a tumor promoter in cancer induction.* Seminars in Cancer Biology. 2004;14:433-439.

[29] Balkwill F and Mantovani A. *Inflammation and cancer: back to Virchow?* Lancet. 2001:357;539-545.

[30] Loesche WJ, Grossman NS. *Periodontal disease as a specific, albeit chronic, infection: Diagnosis and treatment.* Clinical Microbiology Reviews. 2001;14(4):727-752.

[31] Armitage GC. *Periodontal diagnoses and classification of periodontal diseases.* Periodontology 2000. 2004;34:9-21.

[32] Champagne CME, Buchanan W, Reddy MS, Preisser JS, Beck JD, Offenbacher S. *Potential for gingival crevice fluid measures as predictors of risk for periodontal disease.* Periodontology 2000. 2003;31:167-180.

[33] Burt B. *Academy Report. Epidemiology of Periodontal Diseases.* J Periodontol 2005;76:1406-1419.

[34] Socransky SS, Haffajee AD. *Dental biofilms: Difficult therapeutic targets.* Periodontology 2000. 2002;28:12-55.

[35] Scannapieco FA, Wang B, Shiau HJ. *Oral bacteria and respiratory infection: Effects on respiratory pathogen adhesion and Epithelial Cell Proinflammatory Cytokine Production.* Annals of Periodontology. 2001;6(1):78-86.

[36] Scannapieco FA, Ho AW, DiTolla M, Chen C Dentino AR. *Exposure to the dental environment and respiratory illness in dental student populations.* J Can Dent Assoc. 2004;70:198-202.

[37] Scannapieco FA. *Pneumonia in Non-Ambulatory Patients: Role of oral bacteria and oral hygiene.* J Amer Dent Assoc. 2006;137(10 supplement):21S-25S.

[38] Scannapieco FA, Bush RM, Paju S. *Associations between periodontal disease and risk for nosocomial bacterial pneumonia and chronic obstructive pulmonary disease. A systematic review.* Annals Periodontol. 2003;8:54-69.

[39] Scannapieco FA. *Periodontal inflammation: From gingivitis to Systemic disease?* Compendium 2004;25(7);16-25.

[40] Timothy C. Nichols, Thomas H. Fischer, Efthymios N. Deliargyris, Albert S. Baldwin Jr. *Role of Nuclear Factor-Kappa B (NF-κB) in Inflammation, Periodontitis and Atherogenesis.* Annals of Periodontology. 2001 6:1, 20-29.

[41] Anthony M. Iacopino. *Periodontitis and Diabetes Interrelationships: Role of Inflammation.* Annals of Periodontology. 2001 6:1, 125-137.

[42] López, Isabel Da Silva, Joaquín Ipinza, Jorge Gutiérrez. *Periodontal Therapy Reduces the Rate of Preterm Low Birth Weight in Women With Pregnancy-Associated Gingivitis.* Journal of Periodontology. 2005, 76;11: 2144-2153.

[43] Jeffcoat MK, Hauth JC, Geurs NC, Reddy MS, Cliver SP, Hodgkins PM, *Goldenberg RL. Periodontal disease and preterm birth: Results of a pilot intervention study.* J Periodontol. 2003;74:8:1214-1218.

[44] Graham S, Dayal H, Rohrer T. *Dentition, diet, tobacco, and alcohol in the epidemiology of oral cancer.* J Natl Cancer Inst. 1977;59(6):1611-1618.

[45] Zheng T, Boyle P, Hu H, Duan J, Jiang P, Ma D. *Dentition, oral hygiene, and risk of oral cancer: A case-control study in Beijing, People's Republic of China.* Cancer Causes and Control. 1990;1(3):235-241.

[46] Marshall JR, Graham S, Haughey BP, Shedd D, O'Shea R, Brasure J. *Smoking, alcohol, dentition and diet in the epidemiology of oral cancer.* Oral Oncology, Eur J Cancer. 1992;28B(1):9-15.

[47] Velly AM, Franco EL, Schlecht N, Pintos J, Kowalski LP, Oliveira BV and Curado MP. *Relationship between dental factors and risk of upper aerodigestive tract cancer.* Oral Oncology. 1998;34:284-291.

[48] Moreno-Lopez LA, Esparza-Gomez GC, Gonzalez-Navarro A, Cerero-Lapiedra R, Gonzalez-Hernandez MJ, Dominguez-Rojas V. *Risk of oral cancer associated with tobacco smoking, alcohol consumption and oral hygiene: A case-control study in Madrid, Spain.* Oral Oncology. 2000;36:170-174.

[49] Homann N, Tillonen J, Rintamaki H, Salaspura M, Lindqvist C, Meurman JH. *Poor dental status increases acetaldehyde production from ethanol in saliva: a possible link to increased oral cancer risk among heavy drinkers.* Oral Oncology. 2001;37:153-158.

[50] Lissowska J, Pilarska A, Pilarski P, Samolczyk-Wanyura D, Piekarczyk J, Bardin-Mikollajczak A, Zatonski W, Herrero R, Munoz N, Franceschi S. *Smoking, alcohol, diet, dentition and sexual practices in the epidemiology of oral cancer in Poland.* Eur J Cancer Prev. 2003;12(1):25-33.

[51] Winn DM, Blot WJ, McLaughlin JK, Austin DF, Greenberg RS, Preston-Martin S. *Mouthwash use and oral conditions in the risk of oral and pharyngeal cancer.* Cancer Research. 1991;51:3044-3047.

[52] Talamini R, Vaccarella S, Barbone F, Tavani A, La Vecchia C, Herrero R. *Oral hygiene, dentition, sexual habits and risk of oral cancer*. British Journal of Cancer. 2000;83(9):1238-1242.

[53] Fernandez Garrote L, Herrero R, Ortiz Reyes RM, Vaccarella S, Lence Anta J, Ferbeye L. *Risk factors for cancer of the oral cavity and oropharynx in Cuba*. British Journal of Cancer. 2001;85(1):46-54.

[54] Balaram P, Sridhar H, Rajkumar T, Vaccarella S, Herrero R, Nandakumar A, Ravichandan K, Ramdas K, Sankaranarayanan R, Gajalakshmi V, Munoz N and Franceschi S. *Oral cancer in southern India: the influence of smoking, drinking, paan-chewing and oral hygiene*. Int. J. Cancer. 2002;98:440-445.

[55] Hausmann E, Allen K, Dunford R, Christersson L. *A reliable computerized method to determine the level of the radiographic alveolar crest*. J Periodont Res. 1989;24:368-369.

[56] Hausmann E, Allen K, Christersson L, Genco RJ. *Effect of X-ray Beam Vertical Angulation on Radiographic Alveolar Crest Level Measurement*. J Periodontal Res. 1989;24:8.

[57] Hausmann E, Allen K, Clerehugh V. *What alveolar crest level on a bite-wing radiograph represents bone loss?* J Periodontol .1991;62(9):570-2.

[58] Hausmann E, Allen K, Carpio L, Christersson LA, Clerehugh V. *Computerized methodology for detection of alveolar crestal bone loss from serial intraoral radiographs*. J Periodontol. 1992;63:657-662.

[59] Machtei EE, Christersson LA, Grossi SG, Dunford R, Zambon JJ, Genco RJ. *Clinical criteria for the definition of "established periodontitis"*. J Periodontol. 1992;63:207-215.

[60] Grossi SG, Genco RJ, Machtei EE, Ho AW, Koch, Dunford RG, Zambon JJ and Hausmann E. *Assessment of risk for periodontal disease (II), Risk indicators for alveolar bone loss*. J Periodontol. 1995;66;23-29.

[61] Nakhjiri SF, Park Y, Yilmaz O, Chung WO, Watanabe K, El-Sabaeny A, Park K, Lamont RJ. *Inhibition of epithelial cell apoptosis by Porphyromonas gingivalis*. FEMS Microbiology Letters. 2001:200:145-149.

[62] Lara-Tejero M, Galan JE: *A bacterial toxin that controls cell cycle progression as a deoxyribonuclease I-like protein*. Science. 2000;290:354-357.

[63] Baik S.C, Youn HS, Chung MH, Lee WK, Cho MJ, Ko GH, Park CK, Kasai H, Rhee KH: *Increased oxidative DNA damage in Helicobacter pylori infected human gastric mucosa*. Cancer Res. 1996;56:1279-1282.

[64] Sasaki M. Yamaura C. Ohara-Nemoto Y. Tajika S. Kodama Y. Ohya T. Harada R. Kimura S. *Streptococcus anginosus infection in oral cancer and its infection route*. Oral Diseases. 2005;11(3):151-6.

[65] Karin M. Lawrence T. Nizet V. *Innate immunity gone awry: linking microbial infections to chronic inflammation and cancer*. Cell. 2006;124(4):823-35.

[66] Sparmann A. Bar-Sagi D. *Ras-induced interleukin-8 expression plays a critical role in tumor growth and angiogenesis*. Cancer Cell. 2004;6(5):447-58.

[67] Dauer DJ. Ferraro B. Song L. Yu B. Mora L. Buettner R. Enkemann S. Jove R. Haura EB. *Stat3 regulates genes common to both wound healing and cancer*. Oncogene. 2005;24(21):3397-408.

[68] Cassatella MA. Huber V. Calzetti F. Margotto D. Tamassia N. Peri G. Mantovani A. Rivoltini L. Tecchio C. *Interferon-activated neutrophils store a TNF-related apoptosis-inducing ligand (TRAIL/Apo-2 ligand) intracellular pool that is readily mobilizable following exposure to proinflammatory mediators.* Journal of Leukocyte Biology. 2006;79(1):123-32.

[69] St John MA, Li Y, Zhou X, Denny P, Ho CM, Montemagno C, Shi W, Qi F, Wu B, Sinha U, Jordan R, Wolinsky L, Park NH, Liu H, Abemayor E, Wong DT. *Interleukin 6 and interleukin 8 as potential biomarkers for oral cavity and oropharyngeal squamous cell carcinoma.* Archives of Otolaryngology- Head & Neck Surgery. 2004;130(8):929-35.

[70] Vucicevic Boras V. Cikes N. Lukac J. Virag M. Cekic-Arambasin A. *Salivary and serum interleukin 6 and basic fibroblast growth factor levels in patients with oral squamous cell carcinoma.* Minerva Stomatologica. 2005;54(10):569-73 .

[71] Rhodus NL. Cheng B. Myers S. Miller L. Ho V. Ondrey F. *The feasibility of monitoring NF-kappaB associated cytokines: TNF-alpha, IL-1alpha, IL-6, and IL-8 in whole saliva for the malignant transformation of oral lichen planus.* Molecular Carcinogenesis. 2005;44(2):77-82.

[72] Rhodus NL, Ho V, Miller CS, Myers S, Ondrey F. *NF-kappa B dependent cytokine levels in saliva of patients with oral preneoplastic lesions and oral squamous cell carcinoma.* Cancer Detection & Prevention. 2005;29(1):42-5.

[73] Pollanen MT, Salonen JI, Uitto VJ. *Structure and function of the tooth–epithelial interface in health and disease.* Periodontology 2000. 2003;31:12–31.

[74] Homann N, Tillonen J, Rintamaki H, Salaspura M, Lindqvist C, Meurman JH. *Poor dental status 29. increases acetaldehyde production from ethanol in saliva: a possible link to increased oral cancer risk among heavy drinkers.* Oral Oncology. 2001;37:153-158.

[75] Visapaa JP, Gotte K, Benesova M, Li J, Homann N, Conradt C, Inoue H, Tisch M, Horrmann K, Vakevainen S, Salaspuro M, Seitz HK. *Increased cancer risk in heavy drinkers with the alcohol dehydrogenase 1C*1 allele, possibly due to salivary acetaldehyde.* Gut. 2004;53(6):871-6.

[76] Hormia M, Willberg J, Ruokonen H, Syrjanen S. *Marginal periodontium as a potential reservoir of human papillomavirus in oral mucosa.* J Periodontol. 2005;76(3):358-63.

[77] Saygun I, Kubar A, Ozdemir A, Slots J. *Periodontitis lesions are a source of salivary cytomegalovirus and Epstein-Barr virus.* J Periodontal Res. 2005;40(2):187-91.

[78] Pollanen MT, Salonen JI, Uitto VJ. *Structure and function of the tooth–epithelial interface in health and disease.* Periodontology 2000. 2003;31:12–31.

[79] Stubenrauch F, Laimins LA. *Human papillomavirus life cycle: Active and latent phases.* Semin Cancer Biol. 1999;9:379-386.

[80] Ragin CR, Modugno F, and Gollin SM. *The Epidemiology and Risk Factors of Head and Neck Cancer: a Focus on Human Papillomavirus.* J Dent Res. 2007;86(2):104-114.

[81] D'Souza G. Kreimer AR. Viscidi R. Pawlita M. Fakhry C. Koch WM. Westra WH. Gillison ML. Case-control *study of human papillomavirus and oropharyngeal cancer.* N Engl J Med. 2007;356(19):1944-1956.

[82] Miller CS, Johnstone B. *Human papillomavirus as a riskfactor for oral squamous cell carcinoma: A meta-analysis,1982-1997.* Oral Surg Oral Med Oral Radiol Endod. 2001;91:622-635.

[83] Puscas L. *The role of human papilloma virus infection in the etiology of oropharyngeal carcinoma* Curr Opin Otolaryngol HeadNeckSurg 13:212-216. 2005.

[84] Kreimer AR. Clifford GM. Boyle P. Franceschi S. *Human papillomavirus types in head and neck squamous cell carcinomas worldwide: a systematic review. [Review].* Cancer Epidemiology, Biomarkers & Prevention. 14(2):467-75, 2005 Feb.

[85] Gillison ML, Koch WM, Capone RB, Spafford M, Westra WH, LiWu, Zahurak ML, Daniel RW, Viglione MI,.Symer DE, Shah KV, Sidransky D. *Evidence for a causal association between human papilloma virus and a subset of head and neck cancers.* J Natl Cancer Inst. 2000;92:709–20.

[86] Giuliano AR, Sedjo RL, Roe DJ. *Clearance of oncogenic human papillomavirus (HPV) infection: effect of smoking (United States).* Cancer Cause Control. 2002;13:839-846.

[87] Molano M, vanden Brule A, *Plummer M. Determinants of clearance of human papillomavirus infections in Colombian women with normal cytology: a population-based, 5-year follow-up study.* Am J Epidemiol. 2003;158:486-494.

[88] Madeleine MM, Anttila T, Schwartz SM, Saikku P, Leinonen M, Carter JJ, Wurscher M, Johnson LG, Galloway DA, Daling JR. *Risk of cervical cancer associated with Chlamydia trachomatis antibodies by histology, HPV type and HPV cofactors.* Int J Cancer. 2007;120(3):650-655.

[89] Samoff E, Koumans EH, Markowitz LE, Sternberg M, Sawyer MK, Swan D, Papp JR, Black CM, Unger ER. *Association of Chlamydia trachomatis with persistence of high-risk types of human papillomavirus in a cohort of female adolescents.* Am J Epidemiol. 2005;162(7):668-675.

[90] Saygun I, Kubar A, Ozdemir A, Slots J. *Periodontitis lesions are a source of salivary cytomegalovirus and Epstein-Barr virus.* J Periodontal Res. 2005;40(2):187-91.

[91] Hormia M, Willberg J, Ruokonen H, Syrjanen S. *Marginal periodontium as a potential reservoir of human papillomavirus in oral mucosa.* J Periodontol. 2005;76(3):358-63.

[92] Kumar PS, Griffen AL, Barton JA, Paster BJ, Moeschberger ML, Leys EJ. *New bacterial species associated with chronic periodontitis.* J Dent Res. 2003;82(5):338-344.

[93] Slots, Kamma JJ, *Sugar C. The herpes virus-Porphyromonas gingivalis-periodontitis axis.* J Periodontal Res. 2003;38(3):318-23.

[94] Slots J. *Herpesviruses, the missing link between gingivitis and periodontitis?* Journal of the International Academy of Periodontology. 2004;6(4):113-9.

[95] Kamma JJ, Slots J. *Herpes viral-bacterial interactions in aggressive periodontitis.* Journal of Clinical Periodontology. 2003;30(5):420-6.

[96] Sugano N, Ikeda K, Oshikaa M, Idesawa M, Tanaka H, Sato S, Ito K. *Relationship between Porphyromonas gingivalis, Epstein-Barr virus infection and reactivation in periodontitis.* Journal of Oral Science. 2004;46(4):203-6.

[97] Woodworth CD, Simpson S. *Comparative lymphokine secretion by cultured normal human cervical keratinocytes, papillomavirus-immortalized, and carcinoma cell lines.* Am J Pathol. 1993;142:1544-1555.

[98] Woodworth CD, Notario V, Di Paolo JA. *Transforming growth factors beta 1 and 2 transcriptionally regulate human papillomavirus (HPV) type 16 early gene expression in HPV-immortalized human genital epithelial cells.* J Virol. 1990;64:4767-4775.

[99]   Woodworth CD, Lichti U, Simpson S, Evans CH, Di Paolo JA. *Leukoregulin and gamma-interferon inhibit human papillomavirus type 16 gene transcription in human papillomavirus-immortalized human cervical cells.* Cancer Res. 1992;52:456-463.

[100] Woodworth CD, Mc Mullin E, Iglesias M, Plowman GD. *Interleukin 1 alpha and tumor necrosis factor alpha stimulate autocrine amphiregulin expression and proliferation of human papillomavirus-immortalized and carcinoma-derived cervical epithelial cells.* Proc Natl Acad Sci USA. 1995;92:2840-2844.

[101] Iglesias M, Plowman GD, Woodworth CD. *Interleukin-6 and interleukin-6 soluble receptor regulate proliferation of normal, human papillomavirus-immortalized, and carcinoma-derived cervical cells in vitro.* Am J Pathol. 1995;146:944-952.

[102] Gaiotti D, Chung J, Iglesias M, Nees M, Baker PD, Evans CH. *Tumor necrosis factor-alpha promotes human papillomavirus (HPV) E6/E7 RNA expression and cyclin-dependent kinase activity in HPV-immortalized keratinocytes by aras-dependent pathway.* Mol Carcinog. 2000;27:97-109.

[103] Schroeder HE. *The junctional epithelium: Origin, structure and significance.* Acta Med Dent Helv. 1996;1:155-167.

[104] Madinier I, Doglio A, Cagnon L, Lefebvre JC, Monteil RA. Southern blot *detection of human papillomaviruses (HPVs) DNA sequences in gingival tissues.* J Periodontol. 1992;63:667-673.

[105] Parra B, Slots J. *Detection of human viruses in periodontal pockets using polymerase chain reaction.* Oral Microbiol Immunol. 1996;11:289-293.

[106] Saglam F, Onan U, Soydinc M, Yilmaz O, Kirac K, Sever MS. *Human papillomavirus in a patient with severe gingival overgrowth associated with cyclosporine therapy. A case report.* J Periodontol. 1996;67:528-531.

[107] Bustos DA, Grenon MS, Benitez M, de Boccardo G, PavanJV, Gendelman H. *Human papillomavirus infection in cyclosporin-induced gingival overgrowth in renal allograft recipients.* J Periodontol. 2001;72:741-744.

INDEX

B

D

K

kappa, 27, 79, 102, 172, 181, 244, 248, 251
kappa B, 27, 79, 102, 172, 181, 244, 248, 251
keratinocytes, 76, 78, 80, 84, 88, 89, 93, 95, 97, 98, 101, 182, 184, 192, 194, 195, 252, 253
keratosis, 102
kidney, 77, 101
killing, 92, 96
kinase, 79, 84, 88, 92, 192, 240, 253
kinase activity, 253
kinases, 76, 192, 194
kinetics, 84, 158
King, 221, 223
knee, 180

L

LAC, 149
lactose, 146, 149
lamellar, 78, 100
Langerhans cells, 77, 98
laryngeal, 245
larynx, 240
laser, 77, 78
lasers, 56
latency, 24
Latin America, 5
law, 120
LC, 68, 70, 248
LDL, 218, 223
leakage, 46, 128
lesions, 17, 18, 22, 30, 41, 45, 77, 88, 89, 93, 98, 109, 110, 112, 138, 169, 177, 179, 184, 186, 198, 200, 206, 207, 223, 245, 251, 252
leukemia, 89, 92, 112
leukocyte, 14, 27, 31, 112, 214, 219, 233
leukoplakia, 80, 88, 91, 99
lichen planus, 80, 88, 91, 99, 251
Lidocaine, ix, 141, 142, 145, 147, 152, 154, 163, 165
lifestyle, 3, 8, 37, 211
lifetime, 4
ligament, 4, 22, 31, 58, 62, 63, 113, 120, 123, 124, 127, 128
ligand, 12, 27, 172, 176, 181, 251
ligature-induced periodontitis, 7, 10, 12, 28
likelihood, vii, 1, 3, 21, 57, 109, 116, 135
limitations, 15, 88
line graph, 152, 159
linear, 39, 167, 174
lingual, 39, 43, 57, 63, 114, 125, 130, 131, 224
linkage, 212
links, 170, 180, 248

lipids, 11, 78, 244
lipopolysaccharide, 8, 32, 79, 92, 93, 102, 168, 176, 200, 210
lipopolysaccharides, 51, 169
liver, 199, 206, 249
local anesthetic, 48, 164
localization, 79, 98
location, 122, 126, 127, 134, 138, 212
locus, 116, 212, 214
London, 221, 225
long period, 130
longevity, 4, 119, 122
longitudinal studies, 3, 12, 13, 14, 16, 17, 137, 214
longitudinal study, 2, 10, 12, 17, 22, 24, 31, 33, 107
low-density, 99, 236
low-density lipoprotein, 99, 236
low-density lipoprotein receptor, 99, 236
LPS, 51, 79, 83, 210, 244
luciferase, 158
luciferin, 158
luminescence, 145, 164
lung, 85, 88, 91, 92, 95, 98, 178, 205, 240, 247
lung cancer, 183, 240, 247
lupus, 182
lymph node, 200, 205
lymphocyte, 91, 92
lymphocytes, 41, 77, 84, 85, 173, 177, 178, 244
lymphoma, 102, 240, 244
lysis, 223, 232, 237

M

machinery, 174
macrophage, 11, 83, 95, 168, 170, 223, 232
macrophage inflammatory protein, 83
macrophages, x, 15, 51, 52, 84, 95, 167, 168, 169, 176, 180, 244
maintenance, 3, 27, 37, 43, 46, 53, 57, 63, 64, 72, 114, 117, 124, 126, 134, 135, 137, 192, 193
Maintenance, 63, 68
major histocompatibility complex, 14
males, xi, 5, 17, 221
malignancy, 247
malignant, 251
malnutrition, 108, 109
Mammalian, 194
mammals, viii, 73, 75
management, 3, 10, 18, 47, 48, 51, 52, 53, 110, 127, 128, 136, 175, 180, 198, 236
mandible, 122
mandibular, 23, 26, 44, 122, 126, 127, 129, 132, 133, 138
manipulation, 177

N

O

U

V

W

X

Y

Z